Handbook
of the Physics
# of Radiation
Therapy

T0337404

Handbook of the Physics of Radiation Therapy

FAIZ M. KHAN, PhD

Professor Emeritus
Department of Therapeutic Radiology
University of Minnesota Medical School
Minneapolis, Minnesota

Contributors

John P. Gibbons, PhD
Medical Physics
Mary Bird Perkins Cancer Center
Baton Rouge, Louisiana

Hassaan Alkhatib, PhD
Radiation Oncology Department
Richland Memorial Hospital
Columbia, South Carolina

Dimitris N. Mihailidis, PhD
Medical Physics and Radiation Oncology
Charleston Radiation Therapy
Consultants and West Virginia University
Charleston, West Virginia

Wolters Kluwer | Lippincott Williams & Wilkins
Health

Philadelphia • Baltimore • New York • London
Buenos Aires • Hong Kong • Sydney • Tokyo

Senior Executive Editor: Jonathan W. Pine Jr.
Senior Product Manager: Emilie Moyer
Vendor Manager: Alicia Jackson
Senior Manufacturing Manager: Benjamin Rivera
Senior Marketing Manager: Angela Panetta
Creative Director: Doug Smock
Production Service: Aptara, Inc.

Library of Congress Cataloging-in-Publication Data
Khan's lectures : handbook of the physics of radiation therapy/Faiz M. Khan . . . [et al.].
    p. ; cm.
  Handbook of the physics of radiation therapy
  Abridged version of: The physics of radiation therapy/Faiz M. Khan. 4th ed. c2010.
  Includes bibliographical references and index.
  ISBN 978-1-60547-681-0 (alk. paper)
  1. Medical physics.   2. Radiotherapy.   I. Khan, Faiz M.   II. Khan, Faiz M. Physics of radiation therapy.   III. Title: Handbook of the physics of radiation therapy.
  [DNLM: 1. Health Physics–Examination Questions.   2. Health Physics–Handbooks.
  3. Radiometry–Examination Questions.   4. Radiometry–Handbooks.
  5. Radiotherapy–Examination Questions.   6. Radiotherapy–Handbooks.   WN 39]
  R895.K44 2012
  615.8'42–dc22   2011010654

Care has been taken to confirm the accuracy of the information presented and to describe generally accepted practices. However, the authors, editors, and publisher are not responsible for errors or omissions or for any consequences from application of the information in this book and make no warranty, expressed or implied, with respect to the currency, completeness, or accuracy of the contents of the publication. Application of the information in a particular situation remains the professional responsibility of the practitioner.

The authors, editors, and publisher have exerted every effort to ensure that drug selection and dosage set forth in this text are in accordance with current recommendations and practice at the time of publication. However, in view of ongoing research, changes in government regulations, and the constant flow of information relating to drug therapy and drug reactions, the reader is urged to check the package insert for each drug for any change in indications and dosage and for added warnings and precautions. This is particularly important when the recommended agent is a new or infrequently employed drug.

Some drugs and medical devices presented in the publication have Food and Drug Administration (FDA) clearance for limited use in restricted research settings. It is the responsibility of the health care provider to ascertain the FDA status of each drug or device planned for use in their clinical practice.

To purchase additional copies of this book, call our customer service department at (800) 638-3030 or fax orders to (301) 223-2320. International customers should call (301) 223-2300.

Visit Lippincott Williams & Wilkins on the Internet: at LWW.com. Lippincott Williams & Wilkins customer service representatives are available from 8:30 am to 6:00 pm, EST.

10 9 8 7 6

I dedicate this book to my students:
residents, graduate students, dosimetrists,
and radiation therapists,
from whom I learned how to teach

PREFACE

The objective of the Lectures is to provide a digest of the material contained in *The Physics of Radiation Therapy, Fourth Edition* ("the Textbook"). Key points of individual chapters are presented with a discussion that is condensed and often bulleted. For further details, the Textbook may be consulted. A problem set in the form of multiple choice questions is provided at the end of each chapter, with an answer key at the end of the book.

Like the Textbook, the lecture book is written for the radiotherapy team: radiation oncologists, medical physicists, dosimetrists, and therapists. The information presented is concise and to the point and may be used by those who need a quick review. As a companion book to the main Textbook, the *Khan's Lectures* will be most useful for those preparing for their board exams, whether for initial certification or renewal of certification. Teachers may use the material for their lecture presentations or writing exam questions for their classes.

As the author of *Khan's Lectures*, I was assisted by my former residents and contributors Drs. John Gibbons, Dimitris Mihailidis, and Hassaan Alkhatib. I greatly appreciate their providing editorial comments on the lectures and participation in writing the review questions.

I acknowledge Jonathan Pine, the Senior Executive Editor, Emilie Moyer, the Senior Product Manager, and other editorial staff of Lippincott Williams & Wilkins for their valuable contributions in making this publication possible.

Finally, I greatly appreciate my wife Kathy for her love and companionship she has given me for the last 45 years.

Faiz M. Khan

CONTENTS

CHAPTER 13: Treatment Planning III: Field Shaping, Skin Dose, and Field Separation

CHAPTER 14: Electron Beam Therapy

CHAPTER 15: Brachytherapy

CHAPTER 16: Radiation Protection

CHAPTER 17: Quality Assurance

CHAPTER 18: Total Body Irradiation

CHAPTER 19: Three-Dimensional Conformal Radiation Therapy

CHAPTER 20: Intensity-Modulated Radiation Therapy

CHAPTER 21: Stereotactic Radiation Therapy

CHAPTER 22: High-Dose-Rate Brachytherapy

CHAPTER 23: Prostate Implants

CHAPTER 24: Intravascular Brachytherapy

CHAPTER 25: Image-Guided Radiation Therapy

CHAPTER 26: Proton Beam Therapy

STRUCTURE OF MATTER

REFERENCE

Khan FM. *The Physics of Radiation Therapy*, 4th edition, 2009. Chapter 1 "Structure of Matter"

The Atom

TOPIC OUTLINE

The following topics will be discussed in this lecture:
- ➤ Atomic structure
- ➤ Specification of atoms
- ➤ Classification of atoms
- ➤ Nuclear stability
- ➤ Mass and energy equivalence
- ➤ Atomic energy levels
- ➤ Nuclear energy levels

ATOMIC STRUCTURE

Figure 1A.1 illustrates the structure of an atom.

An atom consists of a central nucleus packed with neutrons and protons and a surrounding cloud of electrons. The electrons revolve around the nucleus in various orbits. The radius of the atom as a whole is approximately 10^{-10} m. The radius of the nucleus is much smaller—on the order of 10^{-15} m. The subatomic particles are characterized by different masses and electrical charges.

- Protons have a unit positive charge.

- Neutrons have no charge.

- Electrons have a unit negative charge.

- A unit charge is equal to 1.60×10^{-19} coulombs.

- Number of protons in the nucleus equals the number of electrons revolving around the nucleus. So the atom is electrically neutral.

- If an electron is stripped from the atom by an ionizing event, the residual atom is called a positive ion (an atom with a net positive charge).

- If an extra electron is acquired by an atom, the atom is called a negative ion.

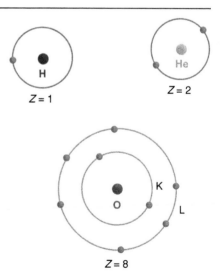

Figure 1A.1. Electron orbits for hydrogen, helium, and oxygen.

SPECIFICATION OF ATOMS

Each element is characterized by its basic constituent—the atom. An atom of an element is specified by

$$_Z^A X$$

where X is the chemical symbol for the element, A the mass number (the number of protons + neutrons in the nucleus), and Z the atomic number (the number of protons in the nucleus). The number of neutrons in the nucleus is given by $A - Z$.

CLASSIFICATION OF ATOMS

Atoms or elements are classified into isotopes, isotones, isobars, and isomers.

- *Isotopes*: Atoms that have the same number of protons but different number of neutrons (same Z but different A). EXAMPLE: $_6^{12}C$, $_6^{13}C$, $_6^{14}C$.

- *Isotones*: Atoms that have the same number of neutrons but different number of protons [same $(A - Z)$ but different A and Z]. EXAMPLE: $_{17}^{37}Cl$, $_{19}^{39}K$, $_{20}^{40}Ca$.

- *Isobars*: Atoms that have the same number of nucleons (protons + neutrons) but different number of protons and neutrons (same A, different Z). EXAMPLE: $_7^{17}N$, $_8^{17}O$, $_9^{17}F$.

- *Isomers*: Atoms that have the same number of protons and neutrons (same A and Z) but different nuclear energy states. EXAMPLE: $_{43}^{99m}Tc$ (m stands for metastable state) and $_{43}^{99}Tc$.

NUCLEAR STABILITY

Certain combinations of neutrons and protons result in stable (nonradioactive) nuclides. Stability depends on neutron-to-proton (n/p) ratio, but not linearly. Figure 1A.2 shows a plot of the ratio of neutrons to protons in stable nuclei.

From the figure we can see that:

- Stable nuclei in the low atomic number range ($Z \leq 20$) have an almost equal number of neutrons and protons.

- As Z increases more than 20, the neutron-to-proton ratio for stable nuclei becomes greater than 1.

- In general, if the nucleus is packed with more protons than neutrons, it tends to be unstable.

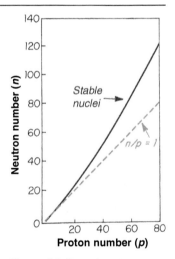

Figure 1A.2. A plot of neutrons versus protons in stable nuclei.

MASS AND ENERGY EQUIVALENCE

Masses of atoms and atomic particles are conveniently expressed in terms of atomic mass units (amu). An amu is defined as $1/12$ of the mass of a $_6^{12}C$ atom. Thus the $_6^{12}C$ atom is arbitrarily assigned a mass of 12 amu. In basic units of mass

$$1 \text{ amu} = 1.66 \times 10^{-27} \text{ kg}$$

The masses of subatomic particles in units of amu are as below:

- *Electron*: 0.000548

- *Proton*: 1.00727

- *Neutron*: 1.00866

Thus, neutron is slightly heavier than a proton, and electron is much lighter (~1/1,840 the mass of a proton).

Mass and energy are interconvertible. Einstein's famous equation, $E = mc^2$, where E is the energy, m the mass, and c the velocity of light, describes the relationship between matter and energy. Using this formula, one obtains

$$1 \text{ amu} = 931.5 \text{ MeV}$$

Because the rest mass of an electron is 0.000548 amu, its equivalent energy at rest (E_0) is

$$E_0 = 0.511 \text{ MeV}$$

MASS, VELOCITY, AND ENERGY OF A PARTICLE

- The mass of a particle depends on its velocity.
- If m is the mass of a particle moving with velocity v and m_0 is its mass at rest, then

$$m = \frac{m_0}{\sqrt{1 - v^2/c^2}}$$

- The kinetic energy (E_k) is given by

$$E_k = mc^2 - m_0c^2 = m_0c^2 \left[\frac{1}{\sqrt{1 - \dfrac{v^2}{c^2}}} - 1 \right]$$

DISTRIBUTION OF ORBITAL ELECTRONS

Electrons are restricted to discrete energy levels or shells. The innermost orbit or shell is the K shell. The next shells are L, M, N, and O.

- The maximum number of electrons that an orbit or shell can hold is given by $2\,n^2$, where n is the number of shell. EXAMPLE: The maximum number of electrons is 2 in the K shell, 8 in the L shell, 18 in the M shell, 32 in the N shell, and so on.
- A shell need not be completely filled before the electrons begin to fill the next shell.
- The maximum number of electrons that the outermost shell can hold is eight. Additional electrons begin to fill the next level to create a new outermost shell before more electrons are added to the lower shell. EXAMPLE: An atom of calcium has 20 electrons, with 2 in the K shell, 8 in the L shell, 8 in the M shell, and the remaining 2 in the N shell.
- Electrons in the outermost orbit are called the valence electrons. The chemical properties of an atom depend on the number of electrons in the outermost orbit.

ATOMIC ENERGY LEVELS

Electron orbits represent discrete energy states or energy levels. The energy in this case is the potential energy of the electrons. With opposite sign, it is also called the binding energy (Figure 1A.3).

The energy scale is arbitrarily set as zero at the position of the valence electrons when the atom is in the unexcited state (when all the valence electrons occupy the outermost orbit energy level). Below that position, the potential energy is given a negative sign and the binding energy is given a positive sign. Thus, the following can be noticed:

- The potential energy increases (becomes less negative) as we go from the lower to the higher energy orbits.
- Correspondingly, the binding energy decreases as we go from lower to higher energy orbits (reverse the energy sign in Figure 1A.3).
- The binding energy of electrons is the amount of energy required to remove an electron from its orbit. Electrons close to the nucleus have a higher

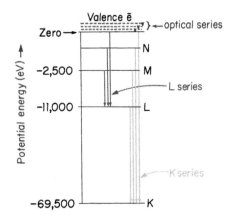

Figure 1A.3. A simplified energy-level diagram of the tungsten atom (not to scale). Only a few possible transitions are shown for illustration. Zero of the energy scale is arbitrarily set at the position of the valence electrons when the atom is in the unexcited state.

binding energy (are more tightly bound) compared to the outer orbit electrons. EXAMPLE: In a tungsten atom ($Z = 74$), the binding energies of K, L, and M shells are respectively 69.5, 11.0, and 2.5 keV.

- An electron can be ejected from its orbit if it receives energy greater than its binding energy. The vacancy thus created in the shell is filled by an outer shell electron, thereby creating another vacancy that is then filled by an outer orbit electron. These electronic transitions in which electrons cascade from outer to inner orbits give rise to characteristic x-rays (of energy equal to the energy difference between the shells involved).

- If an electron in the outermost orbit (a valence electron) is given energy of a few electron volts, it may be moved out to one of the optical orbits. But the electron cannot remain in any of the optical orbits for long and falls back to the outermost orbit of the atom (the unexcited state of the atom). In so doing energy is radiated as optical radiation.

NUCLEAR ENERGY LEVELS

The nucleus also has a shell structure. Nuclear particles (or nucleons) are arranged in shells that represent discrete energy states of the nucleus analogous to the atomic energy levels.

- A nucleus can be excited to a higher energy state if energy is imparted to it (e.g., by bombarding it with particles and having a particle overcome the nuclear barrier and penetrate it).

- When an excited nucleus returns to a lower energy state, it gives off energy equal to the energy difference of the two states.

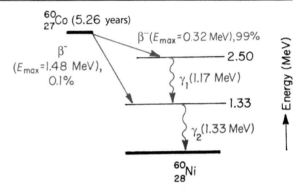

Figure 1A.4. Energy-level diagram for the decay of $^{60}_{27}$Co nucleus.

- The excess energy may be radiated in one or more steps. The nucleus may descend to intermediate states before it settles down to stable or ground state.

  Figure 1A.4 shows a decay scheme of a ^{60}Co nucleus that has been made radioactive in a reactor by bombarding stable ^{59}Co atoms with neutrons.

- The decay scheme shows that a ^{60}Co nucleus has two possible energy states to decay to before settling down to the stable or ground state. The predominant mode of decay is through two steps, giving rise to two γ-rays of 1.17 and 1.33 MeV.

1B

REFERENCE

Khan FM. *The Physics of Radiation Therapy*, 4th edition, 2009. Chapter 1 "Structure of Matter"

Forces of Nature and Fundamental Particles

 TOPIC OUTLINE

The following topics will be discussed in this lecture:
- ➤ Mass defect
- ➤ Forces of nature
- ➤ Nuclear potential barrier
- ➤ Fundamental particles
- ➤ Electromagnetic radiation

MASS DEFECT

Mass of an atom is less than the sum of the masses of its constituent particles. The reason for this is that when the nucleus is formed, a certain amount of mass is converted into energy that acts as a "glue" to keep the nuclear particles (nucleons) together. This mass difference is called the mass defect. The energy equivalence of the mass defect is called the binding energy of the nucleus. EXAMPLE: Mass of a deuterium ($_1^2$H) atom is 2.014102 amu. It is less than the sum of the masses of its individual constituent particles (ie, mass of 1 neutron + 1 proton + 1 electron = 2.016368 amu). The difference 0.002266 amu is the mass defect. When multiplied by 931 MeV/amu, it gives the nuclear binding energy of 2.11 MeV.

FORCES OF NATURE

At the very start of our universe, there was probably one force that governed it. The single force then broke down into four forces at the end of 10^{-10} seconds. Since then, the universe has managed itself with these four forces.

The four forces of nature today, in order of their strengths, are the following:

- *Strong nuclear force*: It is a short-range force that comes into play when the distance between particles becomes smaller than the nuclear diameter ($\sim 10^{-15}$ m).

- *Electromagnetic force*: It is called so because electricity and magnetism are fundamentally the same by nature. This force causes oppositely charged particles to attract each other and similarly charged particles to repel each other.

- *Weak nuclear force*: It is a weak nuclear force, as its name suggests. It comes into play in certain types of radioactive emissions such as β-particle decay.

- *Gravitational force*: It is the weakest of all the natural forces. It does not play any part at the nuclear or atomic level. However, gravity has played a huge part in the creation and evolution of our universe.

NUCLEAR POTENTIAL BARRIER

As a result of mass defect that provides the nuclear binding energy, a potential barrier exists against any nucleon to escape or enter the nucleus (Figure 1B.1).

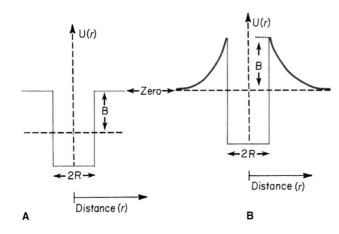

Figure 1B.1. Energy-level diagram of a particle in a nucleus. **A:** Particle with no charge. **B:** Particle with positive charge. $U(r)$ is the potential energy as a function of distance r from the center of the nucleus, B is the barrier height, and R the nuclear radius.

- A positively charged external particle, such as an α-particle approaching a nucleus, will experience repulsion because of the coulomb force of repulsion between the positively charged particle and the positively charged nucleus. However, if the particle is able to overcome the Coulomb force and get close enough to the nucleus so as to be within the range of the strong nuclear force, the repulsive forces would be overcome and the particle would be able to enter the nucleus.
- A particle with no charge such as a neutron has an easier time approaching a nucleus (no repulsive Coulomb force), but still experiences a nuclear barrier before it can enter the nucleus.
- Because particles have a dual nature, that is, they are particles of matter (have mass) but are also associated with waves (de Broglie waves), they can penetrate the nucleus with energies much lower than the height of the potential barrier.
- Particles within the nucleus are in continual motion but are constrained from escaping the nucleus by the nuclear barrier.
- In a stable nucleus, no particle attains enough energy to escape; however, in a radioactive or excited nucleus, a particle may attain enough energy (through random interactions with other nucleons) to escape the nucleus. The probability of this process occurring is pure chance. But in an aggregate of large number of excited nuclei such as in a chunk of a radioactive material, a certain percentage will disintegrate predictably in a given time (exponential radioactive decay).

FUNDAMENTAL PARTICLES

FUNDAMENTAL PARTICLES OF MATTER (FERMIONS)

Figure 1B.2 is a chart of fundamental particles according to the Standard Model. There are two kinds of fundamental particles of matter: quarks and leptons. There are six types of each of these, as listed below:

- *Quarks*: Up, down, charm, strange, top, and bottom;
- *Leptons*: Electron, electron neutrino, muon, muon neutrino, tau, and tau neutrino.
  - ➤ Besides the above 12 basic particles of matter, there are 12 corresponding basic particles of antimatter—with the same mass but opposite charge.
  - ➤ Quarks are the building blocks of heavier particles (hadrons) such as neutrons, protons, and mesons. EXAMPLE: It takes three quarks to make a proton (up, up, and down) and three quarks to make a neutron (up, down, and down).

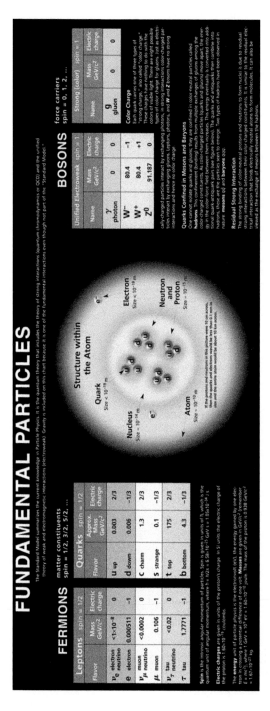

Figure 1B.2. A chart of fundamental particles and interactions. (Reproduced with permission from Contemporary Physics Education Project [CPEP], Lawrence Berkeley National Laboratory: Berkeley, CA. http://CPEPweb.org.)

➤ Quarks are held together by the messenger particles of strong nuclear force called gluons.

➤ The matter particles or fermions are characterized by mass, charge, and spin. They have non-integer spin (e.g., 1/2, 2/3, 3/2) and can travel at high speeds—but not quite the speed of light.

MESSENGER PARTICLES OF FORCE (BOSONS)

According to the quantum electrodynamic (QED) theory, messenger particles are the carriers of force in a force field. These particles are not material particles but quanta of the field like the photon. They are collectively called bosons. These are listed below:

• Photon (γ)   → Electromagnetic force

• Eight gluons   → Strong force

• W^+, W^-, Z^0 → Weak force

• Graviton (not yet discovered)   → Gravity

• Higgs particle (not yet discovered)   → Higgs field

➤ Bosons have no mass, have integer spin (e.g., 0, 1, 2), and travel at the speed of light (3×10^8 m/sec).

➤ Higgs field pervades the entire universe. Matter particles acquire their mass through interaction with the Higgs field.

ELECTROMAGNETIC RADIATION

WAVE MODEL

Electromagnetic radiation constitutes the mode of energy propagation for such phenomena as light, heat, radio waves, microwaves, ultraviolet rays, x-rays, and γ-rays.

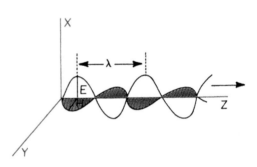

• These radiations are called "electromagnetic" because they consist of oscillating electric and magnetic fields that are perpendicular to each other and to the direction of energy propagation at any given instant of time (Figure 1B.3).

• The relationship between wavelength (λ), frequency (ν), and velocity (c) is given by

Figure 1B.3. Graph showing electromagnetic wave at a given instant of time. E and H are, respectively, the peak amplitudes of electric and magnetic fields. The two fields are perpendicular to each other.

$$c = \nu\lambda$$

• Velocity c is the speed of light (3×10^8 m/sec in vacuum)

• In the above equation, because c is constant, ν is inversely proportional to λ.

• The wave nature of electromagnetic radiation can be demonstrated by experiments involving phenomena such as interference and diffraction.

QUANTUM MODEL

Behavior of electromagnetic radiation such as photoelectric effect and Compton scattering can only be explained by considering their particle or quantum nature.

• The energy of a photon is given by

$$E = h\nu$$

Where E is energy, h the Planck's constant, and ν the frequency.

• If E is expressed in electron volts (eV) and λ in meters (m), then the above equation gives

$$E = \frac{1.24 \times 10^{-6}}{\lambda}$$

REVIEW QUESTIONS • Chapter 1

In multiple choice questions, more than one option may be correct.

✔ **TEST YOURSELF**

Review questions for this chapter are provided online.

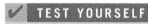

1. An atom is specified by ^A_ZX. What do the following stand for?

   a) X denotes chemical symbol for the element.
   b) A is the number of neutrons.
   c) Z is the number of protons.
   d) $(A + Z)$ is the number of nucleons.
   e) $(A - Z)$ is the number of neutrons.

2. Which of the following nuclide groups are classified correctly?

   a) $^{38}_{19}K$, $^{39}_{19}K$, $^{40}_{19}K$ are isobars.
   b) $^{99}_{43}Tc$, $^{99m}_{43}Tc$ are isomers.
   c) $^{40}_{20}Ca$, $^{40}_{19}K$, $^{40}_{18}Ar$ are isotopes.
   d) $^{41}_{20}Ca$, $^{40}_{19}K$, $^{39}_{18}Ar$ are isotones.

3. In general, nuclear stability depends on neutron-to-proton (n/p) ratio. A nucleus tends to be:

   a) Stable if n/p ≥ 1 and < 1.5
   b) Stable if n/p = 1 and Z ≤ 20
   c) Unstable if n/p < 1

4. Which of the following quantities is(are) correctly represented mathematically? [N_A is the Avogadro's number; A_W is the atomic weight; Z is the atomic number]

   a) Number of atoms/g $= \dfrac{N_A}{A_W}$

   b) Grams per atom $= \dfrac{A_W}{N_A}$

   c) Number of electrons/g $= \dfrac{N_A \cdot Z}{A_W}$

5. A $^{12}_6C$ atom has:

   a) 12 neutrons
   b) 6 protons
   c) A mass of 12 amu
   d) A mass equivalent to 931 MeV energy

6. What is the mass defect of the $^{12}_6C$ atom? [Masses of proton, neutron, and electron are 1.00727, 1.00866, and 0.00055 amu, respectively.]

   a) 0.09888 amu
   b) 0.08871 amu
   c) 0.8871 amu
   d) 6.0000 amu

7. An electron with a *kinetic* energy of 10 MeV has a *total* energy of:

   a) 10 MeV
   b) 10.051 MeV
   c) 10.151 MeV
   d) 10.511 MeV
   e) 10.931 MeV

8. What is the approximate velocity of an electron with a kinetic energy of 11 MeV?

   a) 0.250 c
   b) 0.500 c

   c) 0.750 c
   d) 0.999 c
   e) 1.250 c

9. Kinetic energy, in MeV, of a proton that travels with 96% of the speed of light is:
   a) 24
   b) 241
   c) 2,412
   d) 24,123

10. In a tungsten atom, what is the kinetic energy of an L-shell electron ejected by a photon that was created during the M–K shell transition of the atom? (Binding energies of K, L and M shell are 69.5, 11.0, and 2.5 keV, respectively).
    a) 56.0 keV
    b) 61.0 keV
    c) 67.5 keV

11. A tungsten K-shell electron is ejected and an L-shell electron fills the vacancy. What is the energy of the emitted characteristic x-ray?
    a) 11 keV
    b) 58.5 keV
    c) 69 keV
    d) 8.5 keV

12. Which of the following interactions is(are) matched correctly with the fundamental force involved?
    a) β-Decay of ^{60}Co → Weak force
    b) Coulomb scattering of electrons → Electromagnetic force
    c) Mutual attraction of nucleons → Strong force
    d) Bremsstrahlung → Strong force
    e) Rotation period of the moon → Gravitational force

13. A ^{60}Co source decays with the emission of:
    a) α-Particles
    b) β-Particles
    c) γ-Rays
    d) Neutrons

14. Blue light has a wavelength of 400 nm in vacuum. What is the frequency in hertz of its photon?
    a) 3.0×10^{12}
    b) 5.6×10^{13}
    c) 7.5×10^{14}
    d) 4.1×10^{15}

15. The blue light has a wavelength of 400 nm in vacuum. What is the energy of its photon?
    a) 0.031 eV
    b) 3.1 eV
    c) .333 eV
    d) 3.33 eV

16. What is the wavelength of a 6 MeV photon?
    a) 2.1 m
    b) 2.1 nm
    c) 0.21×10^{-3} nm
    d) 2.1 μm

2

NUCLEAR TRANSFORMATIONS

REFERENCE

Khan FM. *The Physics of Radiation Therapy*, 4th edition, 2009. Chapter 2 "Nuclear Transformations"

Radioactivity

 TOPIC OUTLINE

The following topics will be discussed in this lecture:
➤ Radioactivity
➤ Radioactive decay equation
➤ Radioactive series
➤ Radioactive equilibrium
➤ Modes of radioactive decay

RADIOACTIVITY

- Radioactivity was first discovered in 1896 by Antoine Henri Becquerel (1852–1908).

- Radioactivity is a process in which a nucleus with excess energy (excited nucleus) emits radiation to get rid of its excess energy. This can occur in one or more than one step.

- Figure 2A.1 shows a radium source, which is a naturally occurring radioactive material, emitting three types of radiation: α, β, and γ. Emitted radiation can be separated by applying a magnetic field. Because α-particles are positively charged and β-particles are negatively charged, they bend in different directions under the influence of the magnetic field. The γ-radiations, however, are unaffected.

DECAY CONSTANT (λ)

- Radioactive decay or disintegration is a statistical phenomenon in which a certain proportion of atoms (actually nuclei) in a radioactive material predictably disintegrate in a given interval of time. The process of emission is random—it is not possible to know when a particular atom will disintegrate.

- The number of atoms disintegrating per unit time (dN/dt) is proportional to the number of radioactive atoms (N) present at any given time. Mathematically

$$\frac{\mathrm{d}N}{\mathrm{d}t} \propto N$$

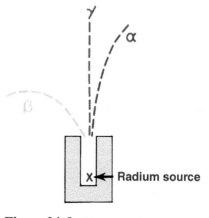

Figure 2A.1. Diagrammatic representation of the separation of three types of radiation emitted by radium under the influence of magnetic field (applied perpendicular to the plane of the paper).

- The above proportionality can be changed to an equation by inserting a constant λ, called the disintegration constant. The minus sign indicates that the rate of disintegration decreases with time

$$\frac{dN}{dt} = -\lambda N$$

- The solution of the above differential equation gives the following exponential equation

$$N = N_0 e^{-\lambda t}$$

where N_0 is the initial number of radioactive atoms and N the number present at time t.

ACTIVITY

- The rate of disintegration, dN/dt, is also called activity. Thus, if A_0 is the initial activity, the activity A after time t is given by the exponential equation

$$A = A_0 e^{-\lambda t}$$

- The unit of activity is curie (Ci).

$$1\,\text{Ci} = 3.7 \times 10^{10} \text{ disintegrations/sec}$$

- The SI (Système International) unit of activity is the becquerel (Bq), which is defined as 1 disintegration/sec or 1 dps.

$$1\,\text{Bq} = 1\,\text{dps} = 2.7 \times 10^{-11}\,\text{Ci}$$

HALF-LIFE AND MEAN LIFE

Figure 2A.2 shows exponential decay of a radioactive material.

- The term half-life ($T_{1/2}$) is defined as the time required for activity or atoms to decay to half the initial value. It can be shown that half-life is given by

$$T_{1/2} = \ln 2/\lambda = 0.693/\lambda$$

- The mean or average life (T_a) is the average lifetime for the decay of radioactive atoms. It can be shown that

$$T_a = 1/\lambda = 1.44\,T_{1/2}$$

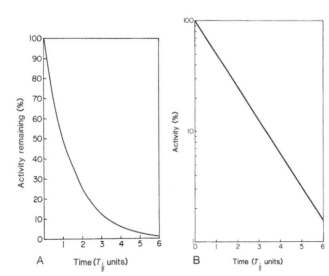

Figure 2A.2. A general decay curve. Activity as a percentage of initial activity plotted against time in units of half-life. **A:** Plot on linear graph. **B:** Plot on semilogarithmic graph.

Atomic number

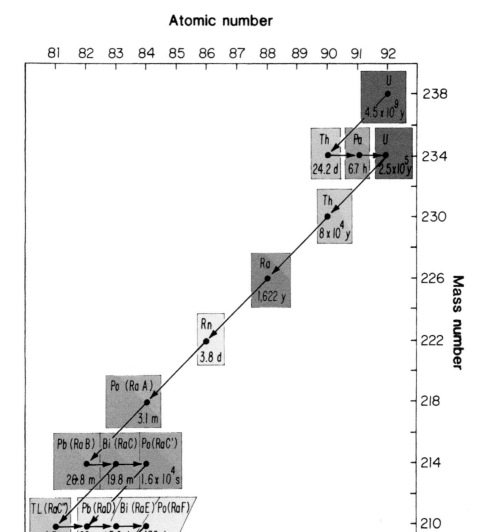

Figure 2A.3. The uranium series. (Data from U.S. Department of Health, Education, and Welfare. *Radiological Health Handbook*, Revised edition. Washington, DC: U.S. Government Printing Office; 1970.)

RADIOACTIVE SERIES

- All naturally occurring radioactive elements have been grouped into three series: the uranium, the actinium, and the thorium.

- The uranium series (Fig. 2A.3) originates with ^{238}U, the actinium series with ^{235}U, and the thorium series with ^{232}Th.

- All the series terminate at the stable isotopes of lead with mass numbers 206, 207, 208. EXAMPLE: Radium occurs in the uranium series and gives rise to many daughter products before settling down to stable lead.

RADIOACTIVE EQUILIBRIUM

- If the half-life of the parent radionuclide is longer than that of the daughter, then after a certain time, a condition of radioactive equilibrium is achieved.

- When in equilibrium, the ratio of the daughter activity to the parent activity is constant. Also, the apparent decay rate of the daughter is then governed by the half-life or disintegration rate of the parent.

- There are two kinds of radioactive equilibriums, depending on the half-lives of the parent and daughter nuclides: *secular equilibrium* and *transient equilibrium.*

- If the half-life of the parent is *much longer* than the half-life of the daughter, it will give rise to a secular equilibrium. EXAMPLE: ^{226}Ra ($T_{1/2} = 1,622$ years) decaying into ^{222}Rn ($T_{1/2} = 3.8$ days) gives rise to a secular equilibrium after an initial buildup of the daughter (see Figure 2A.4).

- At secular equilibrium and thereafter, the activity A_1 of the parent is equal to the activity A_2 of the daughter

$$A_2 = A_1$$

- If the half-life of the parent is *not much longer* than the half-life of the daughter, it gives rise to a transient equilibrium. EXAMPLE: Decay of ^{99}Mo ($T_{1/2} = 67$ hours) to ^{99m}Tc ($T_{1/2} = 6$ hours) (see Figure 2A.5).

- After the transient equilibrium has been achieved, the ratio of activity A_2 of the daughter to the activity A_1 of the parent is constant and is approximately given by

$$\frac{A_2}{A_1} = \frac{T_1}{T_1 - T_2}$$

where T_1 and T_2 are the half-lives of the parent and daughter, respectively.

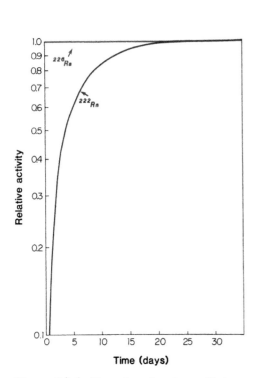

Figure 2A.4. Illustration of secular equilibrium by the decay of ^{226}Ra to ^{222}Rn.

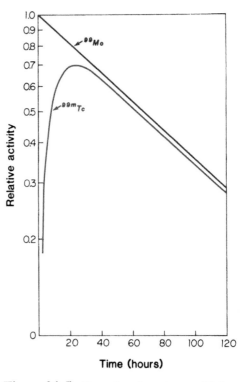

Figure 2A.5. Illustration of transient equilibrium by the decay of ^{99}Mo to ^{99m}Tc. It has been assumed that only 88% of the ^{99}Mo atoms decay to ^{99m}Tc.

MODES OF RADIOACTIVE DECAY

Radioactive nuclides (or radionuclides) decay because of excess energy. There are many different possible modes of nuclear decay but some of the common ones involve the following:

- α-Particle decay
- β-Particle decay
- Electron capture
- Internal conversion
- γ-Emission
- Isomeric transition

α-PARTICLE DECAY

This process occurs in radioactive nuclides with very high atomic number ($Z > 82$). It appears that as the number of protons in the nucleus increases beyond 82, the Coulomb forces of repulsion between the protons become large enough to overcome the nuclear forces that bind the nucleons together. EXAMPLE:

$$^{226}_{88}\text{Ra} \xrightarrow[1,622 \text{ years}]{T_{1/2}} {}^{222}_{86}\text{Rn} + {}^{4}_{2}\text{He} + 4.87 \text{ MeV}$$

The momentum of the α-particle ($^{4}_{2}$He nucleus) is equal to the recoil momentum of the radon nucleus. Because the radon nucleus is much heavier than the α-particle, the energy released in the above disintegration appears almost entirely as kinetic energy of the α-particle (4.78 MeV). The radon nucleus recoils with a negligibly small amount of kinetic energy (0.09 MeV).

β-PARTICLE DECAY

This process is characterized by the emission of a positive or negative electron as a result of nuclear decay. Neither of these particles exists as such in the nucleus but is created at the instant of decay. EXAMPLE:

$$^{1}_{0}\text{n} \rightarrow {}^{1}_{1}\text{p} + {}^{0}_{-1}\beta + \tilde{\nu} \ (\beta^- \text{ decay})$$

$$^{1}_{1}\text{p} \rightarrow {}^{1}_{0}\text{n} + {}^{0}_{+1}\beta + \nu \ (\beta^+ \text{ decay})$$

where, $^{1}_{0}$n, $^{1}_{1}$p, $\tilde{\nu}$, and ν stand for neutron, proton, antineutrino, and neutrino, respectively. The last two particles, namely, antineutrino and neutrino, are identical particles but with opposite spins. They carry no charge and practically no mass.

- The emission of a β-particle is always accompanied by a neutrino and the available energy (the energy of disintegration) is shared between the emitted particles (including γ-rays if emitted by the daughter nucleus).

- The β-particles are emitted with a spectrum of energies—all energies are possible, ranging from zero to the maximum energy characteristic of the β-transition.

- The Figure 2A.6 shows the distribution of energy among the β-particles of ^{32}P. The overall transition is

$$^{32}_{15}\text{P} \xrightarrow[14.3 \text{ days}]{T_{1/2}} {}^{32}_{16}\text{S} + {}^{0}_{-1}\beta + \tilde{\nu} + 1.7 \text{ MeV}$$

- The maximum β-particle energy (E_{max}) is characteristic of the particular nuclide (the end point of the β-ray energy spectrum). The average energy is approximately $E_{max}/3$.

- An example of positron-emitting β-decay is the decay of $^{22}_{11}$Na

$$^{22}_{11}\text{Na} \xrightarrow[2.60 \text{ years}]{T_{1/2}} {}^{22}_{10}\text{Ne} + {}^{0}_{+1}\beta + \nu + 1.82 \text{ MeV}$$

The released energy, 1.82 MeV, is the sum of the maximum kinetic energy of the positron, 0.545 MeV, and the energy of the γ-ray, 1.275 MeV, emitted by the daughter nucleus.

- The negatron (β^{-1})-emitting radionuclides tend to have a high neutron-to-proton (n/p) ratio, while positron (β^{+1})-emitting radionuclides have a low n/p ratio.

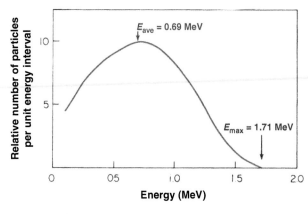

Figure 2A.6. β-Ray energy spectrum from ^{32}P.

- In the $β^{-1}$ *decay*, the mass number A remains the same but the atomic number increases from Z to $Z + 1$. The daughter atom must acquire another orbital electron to regain charge neutrality. Thus, the loss of electron in the decay process is balanced by the acquisition of orbital electron.

- In the $β^{+1}$ *decay*, the mass number A remains the same but the atomic number is decreased from Z to $Z - 1$. The daughter atom must release one of its orbital electrons to regain charge neutrality. So the loss of two electrons (the emitted positron and the released orbital electron) must be accounted for in the decay scheme.

- Because of the above-stated reason, the energy released for $β^{+1}$ decay is reduced by 1.022 MeV (energy equivalent of two electron masses).

- In the positron decay, at least 1.022 MeV must be available for the process to be energetically possible.

ELECTRON CAPTURE

The electron capture is a phenomenon in which one of the orbital electrons is captured by the nucleus, thus transforming a proton in the nucleus into a neutron

$$^1_1p + ^0_{-1}e → ^1_0n + ν$$

- Electron capture is an alternative process to the positron decay—the unstable nuclei with neutron deficiency may increase their n/p ratio to gain stability by electron capture.

- The resulting nucleus is still in the excited state and releases its excess energy almost instantaneously by the emission of a γ-ray photon.

- The electron capture involves mostly the K-shell electrons—the process is then referred to as *K capture*.

- As a result of electron capture, a vacancy is created in the involved shell, which is then filled by an outer orbit electron. This electronic transition can give rise to *characteristic x-rays* (also called *fluorescent x-rays*). Alternatively, this transition can cause the ejection of another electron, called the *Auger electron*.

- The kinetic energy of the Auger electron corresponds to the difference between the initial electronic transition energy and the binding energy of the electron shell from which the Auger electron is ejected.

- The relative emission of characteristic or fluorescent radiations to the number of vacancies is called the *fluorescent yield*.

- Fluorescent yield is favored for larger Z nuclides ($Z > 30$). Auger electrons tend to be produced by lower Z nuclides ($Z < 30$).

INTERNAL CONVERSION

A nucleus still left in the excited state after a nuclear transformation may get rid of its excess energy by the emission of γ-ray or by a process called internal conversion (Fig. 2A.7).

Internal Conversion

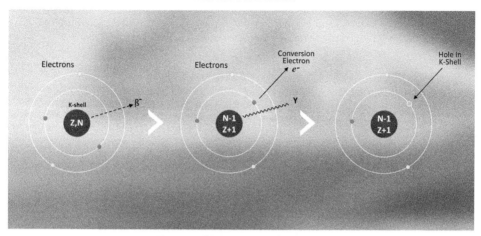

Energy of Conversion Electron
from K-Shell E = E_γ -E_K

Figure 2A.7. Schematic illustration of internal conversion. The nucleus (*left*) undergoes decay and creates a daughter nucleus (*right*), which is still in the excited state and decays by γ-emission. The γ-ray could be absorbed by the atom, ejecting a K-shell electron of energy ($E_\gamma - E_K$).

- In the internal conversion process, the excess nuclear energy is transferred to one of the orbital electrons, which is then ejected from the atom (analogous to internal photoelectric effect in which γ-ray photon escaping from the nucleus interacts with an orbital electron of the same atom).

- The kinetic energy of the internal conversion electron is equal to the energy released by the nucleus minus the binding energy of the electron shell from which the electron is ejected.

- As in the case of electron capture (discussed above), the ejection of orbital electron by internal conversion will create a vacancy in the involved shell, resulting in the production of characteristic x-ray or Auger electron (Fig. 2A.8).

Auger Electrons

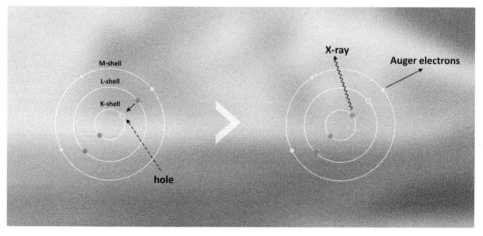

Energy of x-ray = E_K-E_L
Energy of Auger electron = $(E_K$ - $E_L)$ - E_M

Figure 2A.8. Schematic illustration of Auger electron emission. The steps involved in the process are the following: ejection of an orbital electron (e.g., by internal conversion) → creation of a hole in the shell (e.g., K shell) → filling of the hole by an electron from an outer shell (e.g., L shell) → emission of characteristic x-ray of energy ($E_K - E_L$) or → ejection of Auger electron (e.g., from the M shell) with energy ($[E_K - E_L] - E_M$).

γ-EMISSION

- In most radioactive transitions, the daughter nucleus is left in the excited state and loses the excess energy immediately in the form of γ-ray or by internal conversion.
- No radioactive nuclide, however, decays solely by γ-emission.

ISOMERIC TRANSITION

- In the case of some nuclides, the excited nuclear state following the emission of an α- or a β-particle persists with a finite half-life. In that case the nucleus is said to exist in the *metastable state* before decaying into the *ground state* with emission of a γ-ray or internal conversion.
- The transition from the metastable state to the ground is called the *isomeric transition*. The metastable nucleus is an isomer of the final product nucleus.
- Isomeric nuclei have the same atomic and mass number but differ in their states of energy. Isomeric transition does not involve change in the protons or neutrons.
- An isomeric transition results in either the γ-ray emission or internal conversion.
- An example of isomeric transition is ^{99m}Tc, which is produced by β-decay of ^{99}Mo, exists in its metastable state and decays into the ground state of ^{99}Tc with a half-life of 6 hours and the emission of 140 keV γ-ray.

REFERENCE

Khan FM. *The Physics of Radiation Therapy,* 4th edition, 2009. Chapter 2 "Nuclear Transformations"

LECTURE

2B

Nuclear Reactions

 TOPIC OUTLINE

The following topics will be discussed in this lecture:
➤ Nuclear reaction cross section
➤ Nuclear reaction energy
➤ Types of nuclear reaction
➤ Activation of nuclides
➤ Nuclear fission
➤ Nuclear fusion

NUCLEAR REACTION CROSS SECTION

Nuclear *cross section* is the probability of interaction between a bombarding particle and a target nucleus.

- Nuclear cross section, σ, is expressed as the area of cross section offered by the target nucleus to the bombarding particle for a nuclear reaction. The unit of σ is meter square per atom or barns per atom.
- 1 barn is equal to 10^{-28} m^2 (approximately the size of geometric cross section of atomic nucleus).

  [As the story goes, the term "barn" was coined when an early investigator exclaimed that a cross section that large would present a target "as big as a barn" for nuclear bombardment.]
- The rate of nuclear reaction of a particular type is given by

$$\frac{\Delta N}{\Delta t} = \Phi \sigma \rho_A$$

  where ΔN is the number of activations produced per unit volume in time Δt, Φ the particle flux density (number of particles incident on the target per unit area per unit time), σ the cross section for the reaction, and ρ_A the density of atoms in the target.

NUCLEAR REACTION ENERGY

A general reaction may be represented as

$$a + X \rightarrow Y + b + Q \quad \text{or} \quad X(a,b)Y + Q$$

where a is the bombarding particle, X the target nucleus, Y the resultant nucleus, b the emitted particle, and Q the energy released or absorbed during the nuclear reaction. $X(a,b)Y$ is a simplified notation for the reaction. The reaction energy Q is given by the difference in masses, converted to energy

$$Q = [(M_a + M_X) - (M_Y + M_b)]c^2$$

- If Q is positive, the reaction is exoergic. EXAMPLE: Fission reactions
- If Q is negative, the reaction is endoergic. EXAMPLE: Reactions requiring kinetic energy of the bombarding particle as threshold energy for the reaction.

TYPES OF NUCLEAR REACTIONS

- *(α,p) reaction:* EXAMPLE: $^{14}N(\alpha,p)^{17}O$
- *(α,n) reaction:* EXAMPLE: $^{9}Be(\alpha,n)^{12}C$
- *Proton bombardment:* EXAMPLE: $^{12}C(p,\gamma)^{13}N$
- *Deuteron bombardment:* EXAMPLE: $^{9}Be(d,n)^{10}B$
- *Neutron bombardment:* EXAMPLE: $^{59}Co(n,\gamma)^{60}Co$
- *Photodisintegration:* EXAMPLE: $^{63}Cu(\gamma,n)^{62}Cu$
- *Fission:* EXAMPLE: $^{235}U + n \rightarrow {}^{141}Ba + {}^{92}Kr + 3n + Q$
- *Fusion:* EXAMPLE: $^{2}H + {}^{3}H \rightarrow {}^{4}He + n + Q$

ACTIVATION OF NUCLIDES

- The product nucleus of certain nuclear reactions is radioactive. Radioactive materials can thus be produced by bombarding atoms or nuclides with particles.
- The yield of nuclear reaction depends on:
  - ➤ Bombarding particles: type, energy, flux density (Φ)
  - ➤ Cross section (σ) for the nuclear reaction
  - ➤ Target material: nature and density of target nuclei
- Activity of the activated isotope grows exponentially with time.
- Considering both the activation and decay of the activated material, the net growth curve achieves a saturation value after several half-lives. When that happens, the rate of activation equals the rate of decay.
- Examples of radioisotopes produced by activation are the following:
  - ➤ Radiation therapy sources (used for ^{60}Co teletherapy and brachytherapy), produced in nuclear reactors or with accelerators
  - ➤ Diagnostic imaging radioisotopes (used for positron emission tomography), produced with cyclotron accelerator or nuclear reactors
  - ➤ Nuclear medicine radioisotopes and tracers, produced with accelerators or in nuclear reactors

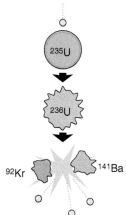

NUCLEAR FISSION

Nuclear fission is a process in which a heavy nucleus ($A > 200$) is made to split into two large fragments when sufficient excitation energy is provided. The most common way of adding the required excitation energy is by bombarding the target nuclei with neutrons. The nucleus, after absorbing the neutron, splits into two smaller nuclei as well as additional neutrons. EXAMPLE:

$$^{235}U + n \rightarrow {}^{141}Ba + {}^{92}Kr + 3n + Q$$

- Thermal neutrons (slow neutrons of average energy ~0.025 eV) are more effective in producing such reactions.

Figure 2B.1.
Illustration of nuclear fission process. (Image from Wikipedia Commons: http://en.wikipedia.org/wiki/File:Nuclear_fission.svg)

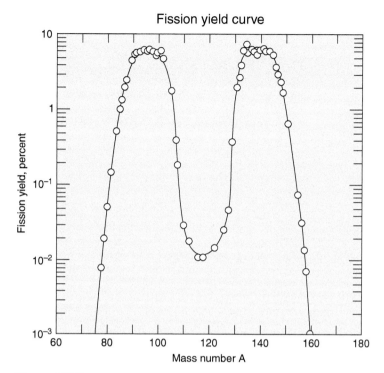

Figure 2B.2. Plot of nuclear fission yield (%) as a function of mass number of fission nuclei (fragments) produced. (From Professor Chung Chieh, with permission: http://www.science.uwaterloo.ca/~cchieh/cact/nuctek/ fissionyield.html)

- The product nuclei of a fission reaction are called fragments.
- There are many possible combinations of *A* and *Z* for the fission fragments.
  - ➤ The fission yield curve shows maximum yield at approximately *A* of 90 and 140.
  - ➤ The energy released in the above fission reaction (calculated by the mass difference between the original and the final particles) averages approximately 200 MeV per reaction.
  - ➤ The fission fragments carry most of the fission energy (~167 MeV).
  - ➤ In nuclear reactors, the fission process is made self-sustaining by chain reaction in which some of the fission neutrons are used to induce yet more fission.
  - ➤ Neutrons released during fission are fast neutrons. To induce a chain reaction, they have to be slowed down to thermal energies by collision with nuclei of low *Z* material (e.g., graphite, water, heavy water), called moderators.
  - ➤ The mass of the fissile material (e.g., ^{235}U) must exceed a certain critical mass to sustain a chain reaction.
  - ➤ In a nuclear reactor, the chain reactions are controlled and sustained in a steady state. In a nuclear bomb, on the other hand, the chain reaction is uncontrolled and occurs in a fraction of a second to cause explosion.

NUCLEAR FUSION

Nuclear fusion may be thought of as the reverse of nuclear fission; that is low mass nuclei are combined (fused together) to produce one nucleus. EXAMPLE:

$$^{2}_{1}\text{H} + ^{3}_{1}\text{H} \rightarrow ^{4}_{2}\text{He} + ^{1}_{0}\text{n} + Q$$

- Because the total mass of the product particles is less than the total mass of the reactants, energy *Q* of 17.6 MeV is released.

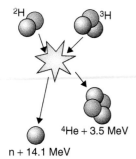

Figure 2B.3. Illustration of nuclear fusion process. Deuterium and tritium nuclei are made to fuse together, creating helium-4 and a neutron. Reaction energy of 17.6 MeV is released. (Image from Wikipedia Commons: http://en.wikipedia.org/wiki/File:Deuterium-tritium_fusion.svg)

- Fusion requires very high temperatures ($>10^{17}$ K) to bring the nuclei sufficiently close together so that the repulsive coulomb forces between nuclei are overcome and the short-range forces can initiate the fusion reaction.

- Fusion reactions are the source of our sun's energy.

REVIEW QUESTIONS • **Chapter 2**

In multiple choice questions, more than one option may be correct.

1. Cesium-137 source decays with a half-life of 30 years. It will decay by about 2% in how much time?

   a) 3 days
   b) 1 month
   c) 6 months
   d) 1 year
   e) 2 years

2. Activity of 1 g of radium is:

   a) 8.25 Ci
   b) 1.000 Ci
   c) 0.975 Ci
   d) 3.61×10^{10} Bq
   e) 3.7×10^{10} Bq

3. When will 10 mCi of ^{131}I (half-life = 8.05 days) and 4 mCi of ^{32}P (half-life = 14.3 days) have equal activities?

   a) 11.4 days
   b) 17.9 days
   c) 24.3 days
   d) 35.7 days

4. In the β-decay of ^{64}Cu, the maximum possible energy of β-particles is about 0.6 MeV. Which of the following statements is(are) true regarding the above decay?

   a) Maximum possible energy of neutrinos is 0.6 MeV.
   b) Average energy of beta particles is 0.2 MeV.
   c) Average energy of neutrinos is 0.4 MeV.

5. What percentage of the original activity of a radionuclide will remain after it decays for a time interval equal to its average life:

   a) 0
   b) 25
   c) 37
   d) 63

6. For a 100 mCi ^{137}Cs source how many total decays will have occurred when the source is completely decayed? [Half-life of cesium ~30 years]:

   a) 3.5×10^9
   b) 3.5×10^{10}
   c) 5.05×10^{10}
   d) 5.05×10^{18}

7. ^{13}N decays to ^{13}C via β$^+$ decay. If the total energy difference between the two atoms is 2.22 MeV, what is the maximum energy of the β-particle?

   a) 0.511 MeV
   b) 1.022 MeV
   c) 1.198 MeV
   d) 2.22 MeV

8. The K- and L-shell binding energies for iodine are approximately 33 and 5 keV, respectively. What is the energy of an Auger electron emitted from the L shell when another L shell electron fills a K-shell vacancy?

   a) 5 keV
   b) 23 keV

c) 28 keV

d) 33 keV

e) This process cannot take place

9. The activity of a certain radioisotope is 10% of its original activity after 197 days. What is its half-life?

a) 59.3 days

b) 74.2 days

c) 85.7 days

d) 197 days

10. A neutron beam of particle flux density of 10^{16} neutrons/m^2/sec strikes a uranium-235 target of density 3×10^{26} nuclei/m^3. If the cross section for fission is 500 barns, what is the rate of fission per unit volume of the target?

a) 1.5×10^{11} fission events/m^3

b) 1.5×10^{17} fission events/m^3

c) 1.5×10^{33} fission events/m^3

d) 1.5×10^{26} fission events/m^3

11. The decay of $^{66}_{27}$Co to $^{60}_{28}$Ni is an example of which decay process?

a) Nuclear fission

b) Electron Capture

c) Internal Conversion

d) β^- decay

e) β^+ decay

12. In β^+ decay:

a) Positrons are emitted with a kinetic energy equal to the nuclear transition energy.

b) Atomic mass of the daughter atom must be less than that of the parent atom by at least 1022 MeV in equivalent energy units.

c) Mass number is increased by 1.

d) Atomic number is decreased by 1.

13. Using the mean value of 200 MeV energy per fission, the fission rate (fissions/sec) to generate 1 W of power is:

a) 3.1×10^7

b) 3.1×10^{13}

c) 3.1×10^{10}

d) 3.1×10^3

3

PRODUCTION OF X-RAYS

REFERENCE

Khan FM. *The Physics of Radiation Therapy*, 4th edition, 2009. Chapter 3 "Production of X-rays"

X-Ray Tubes

 TOPIC OUTLINE

The following topics will be discussed in this lecture:
➤ Basic components of x-ray tube
➤ Focal spot
➤ Basic x-ray circuit
➤ X-ray tube voltage and generators

THE X-RAY TUBE

X-rays were discovered in 1985 by Wilhelm Conrad Roentgen (1845–1923). Later, in 1913, William D. Coolidge (1873–1975) developed the "hot cathode" x-ray tube that became the prototype for the modern x-ray tubes.

Figure 3A.1 is a schematic representation of a conventional x-ray tube. The basic components are the following:

- *Glass envelope*: It is a highly evacuated glass tube with a cathode (negative electrode) at one end and an anode (positive electrode) at the other, both hermetically sealed in the tube. A thin glass or beryllium window is provided in the tube envelope to allow the x-ray beam to emerge with as little attenuation as possible.

- *Cathode*: The cathode assembly in a modern x-ray tube (Coolidge tube) consists of a wire filament, a circuit to provide filament current, and a negatively charged focusing cup.

  ➤ The material of the cathode filament is tungsten, which is chosen because of its high melting point.

  ➤ The cathode filament, when heated by the filament current, emits electrons by a process known as *thermionic emission.*

  ➤ The function of the cathode cup is to direct the electrons toward the anode so that they strike the target in a well-defined area, the *focal spot.*

  ➤ Since the focal spot size depends on filament size, diagnostic tubes usually have two separate filaments to provide a "dual-focus", namely one small and one large focal spot.

- *Anode*: The anode is the tungsten target. Electrons emanating from the hot cathode filament are accelerated toward the anode by a high voltage applied between the cathode and the anode. These high-speed electrons bombard the target to produce x-rays.

  ➤ The choice of tungsten as target material is based on the criteria that the target must have high atomic number (Z) (to provide high efficiency of x-ray production) and high

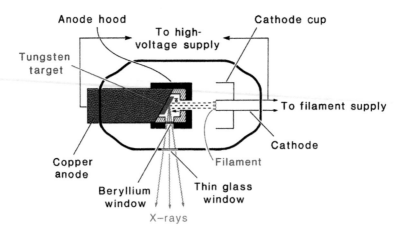

Figure 3A.1. Schematic diagram of a therapy x-ray tube with hooded anode.

melting point (to withstand intense heat produced in the target as a result of electronic bombardment). With $Z = 74$ and a melting point of 3,370°C, tungsten is the material of choice for the target.

➤ The heat generated in the target is conducted away to the outside of the tube by various methods, for example, target in contact with a thick copper anode, oil reservoir surrounding the tube (for cooling as well as electrical insulation), cooling water lines, air fan, and rotating anodes (for diagnostic x-ray tubes).

➤ Some stationary anodes are hooded by a copper and tungsten shield to prevent stray electrons from striking the walls or other nontarget components of the tube (copper to absorb stray electrons and tungsten to absorb x-rays produced as a result of stoppage of these electrons in the copper).

FOCAL SPOT

This is the area on the target from which the x-rays are emitted.

• The focal spot should be as small as possible for producing sharp radiographic images.

• However, smaller focal spots generate more heat per unit area of the target, thus limiting tube current and exposure.

• In therapy tubes, relatively larger focal spots are acceptable since the radiographic image quality is not the overriding concern.

• In the diagnostic as well as orthovoltage therapy tubes, the target is mounted on a steeply inclined surface of the anode. In the high-energy (megavoltage) x-ray machines (e.g., linear accelerators), transmission targets are used.

• For inclined targets, the apparent focal spot is much smaller than the real focal spot. This is known as the *line focus principle.* Referring to Figure 3A.2, if A is the side of the actual focal spot on a target sloped at an angle θ with respect to the perpendicular to the electron beam direction, the corresponding apparent (projected) side a is given by

$$a = A \sin \theta$$

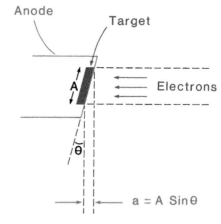

Figure 3A.2. Diagram illustrating the principle of line focus. The side A of the actual focal spot is reduced to side a of the apparent focal spot. The other dimension (perpendicular to the plane of the paper) of the focal spot remains unchanged.

Since the other side *B* of the actual focal spot is perpendicular to the electron beam direction, its apparent length remains the same as the original.

- The target angle θ in diagnostic tubes is quite small (6° to 17°) to produce apparent focal spot sizes ranging from 0.1 × 0.1 to 2 × 2 mm.

- In most orthovoltage therapy tubes, the target angle is larger (~30°) and the apparent focal spot ranges between 5 × 5 and 7 × 7 mm.

- Since the target is sloped and the x-rays are produced at various depths in the target, they suffer varying amounts of attenuation as they emerge from the target. There is greater attenuation of x-rays coming from greater depths than those from near the target surface. Consequently, the cross-sectional beam intensity decreases from the cathode to the anode direction. This intensity variation across the x-ray beam is called the *heel effect*.

- The heel effect is more pronounced in diagnostic tubes because the x-ray energy is low and target angles are steep.

- The heel effect, which adversely affects image quality, can be minimized by inserting compensating filters into the beam to improve cross-beam uniformity.

BASIC X-RAY CIRCUIT

A simplified diagram of a self-rectified x-ray unit is shown in Figure 3A.3. The circuit can be divided into two parts: the high-voltage circuit to provide accelerating potential for the electrons and the low-voltage circuit to supply heating current to the cathode filament.

- *Filament supply*: The voltage supply for electron emission usually consists of 10 V at about 6 A. This is accomplished by using a step-down transformer in the AC line voltage. The filament current can be adjusted by varying the voltage applied to the filament.

- *High-voltage supply*: High voltage to the x-ray tube (between cathode and anode) is supplied by the step-up transformer. The primary of this transformer is connected to an *autotransformer* and a *rheostat* to adjust the input voltage. This voltage is stepped up by the secondary of the transformer by a factor equal to the turn ratio of the transformer windings (no. of turns of secondary/no. of turns of primary).

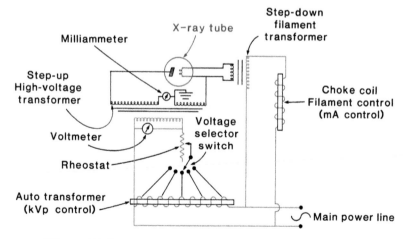

Figure 3A.3. Simplified circuit diagram of a self-rectified x-ray unit.

X-RAY TUBE VOLTAGE AND GENERATORS

Since the anode is positive with respect to the cathode only through half the voltage cycle, the tube current flows through only that half of the cycle. During the next half-cycle, the voltage reverses and the current cannot flow in the reverse direction. Thus, the tube current and the x-rays

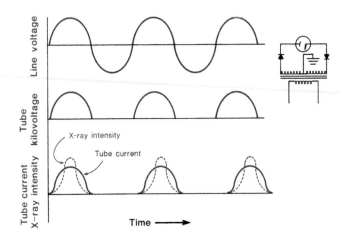

Figure 3A.4. Graphs illustrating the variation with time of the line voltage, the tube kilovoltage, the tube current, and the x-ray intensity for self- or half-wave rectification. The half-wave rectifier circuit is shown on the right. Rectifier indicates the direction of conventional current (opposite to the flow of electrons).

are generated only during the half-cycle when the anode is positive. A machine operating in this manner is called the *self-rectified* unit. The variation with time of the voltage, tube current, and x-ray intensity is illustrated in Figure 3A.4

- *Self-rectification*: The disadvantages of a self-rectified unit are the following: a) no x-ray production during the inverse voltage cycle and, therefore, low x-ray output of the machine; b) hot target (as a result of electron bombardment) emits electrons (by thermionic emission) that would flow from anode to cathode during the inverse voltage cycle, thereby destroying the film.

- *Half-wave rectification*: The problem of tube conduction during inverse voltage cycle can be solved by using voltage rectifiers placed in series in the high-voltage part of the circuit. This prevents the tube from conducting during the inverse voltage cycle. The x-ray output is still low because the x-rays are produced only during half the voltage cycle (when the anode is at positive potential relative to the cathode).

- *Full-wave rectification*: Rectifiers can be arranged so that the anode is positive and cathode is negative during both half-cycles of the voltage. This is shown in Figure 3A.5. With full-wave rectification, the effective tube current is higher (since the current flows during both half-cycles) and, as a result, the x-ray output is higher.

- *Three-phase power*: X-ray output can be further increased by applying three-phase power to the x-ray tube (Fig. 3A.6). The three-phase (3φ) power line is supplied through three separate

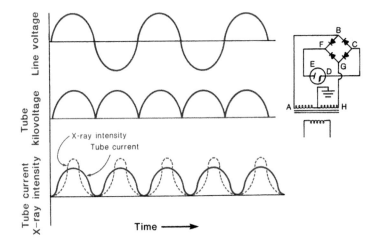

Figure 3A.5. Graphs illustrating the variation with time of the line voltage, the tube kilovoltage, the tube current, and the x-ray intensity for full-wave rectification. The rectifier circuit is shown on the right. The *arrow* on the rectifier diagram indicates the direction of conventional current flow (opposite to the flow of electronic current).

wires, requiring a step-up transformer with three separate windings and three separate iron cores. The voltage waveform in each wire is kept slightly out of phase with each other, so that the voltage across the tube is always near maximum.

➤ With the three-phase power and full-wave rectification, six voltage pulses are applied to the x-ray tube during each power cycle. This is known as a three-phase, six-pulse system. The voltage ripple, defined as $[(V_{max} - V_{min})/V_{max}] \times 100$, is 13% to 25% for this system.

➤ By creating a slight delay in phase between the three-phase rectified voltage waveforms applied to the anode and the cathode, a three-phase, twelve-pulse circuit is obtained. Such a system shows much less ripple (3% to 10%) in the voltage applied to the x-ray tube.

• *Constant potential*: The so-called constant potential x-ray generator (Fig. 3A.7) uses a three-phase line voltage coupled directly to the high-voltage transformer primary. The high voltage thus generated is smoothed and regulated by a circuit involving rectifiers, capacitors, and triode valves. The voltage supplied to the tube is nearly constant, with a ripple of less than 2%. Such a generator provides the highest x-ray output per milliampere second (mAs) exposure. However, it is a very large and expensive generator, used only for special applications.

• *High-frequency x-ray generators*: A much smaller and state-of-the-art generator that provides nearly a constant potential to the x-ray tube is the high-frequency x-ray generator.

This generator uses a single-phase line voltage, which is rectified and smoothed (using capacitors) and then fed to a chopper and inverter circuit. As a result, the smooth, direct current (DC) voltage is converted into a high-frequency (5 to 100 kHz) alternating current (AC) voltage. A step-up transformer converts this high-frequency low-voltage AC into a high-voltage AC, which is

Three-phase generators

A: Input Power

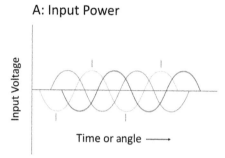

B: Tube voltage

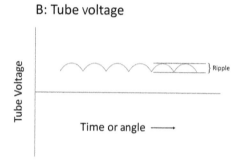

Figure 3A.6. Voltage waveforms in a three-phase x-ray generator.

Constant potential or high-frequency generator

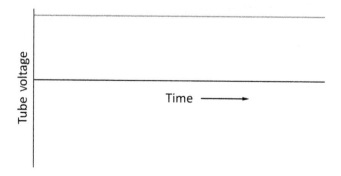

Figure 3A.7. Voltage waveforms in a high-frequency generator.

then rectified and smoothed to provide a nearly constant high-voltage potential (with a ripple of less than 2%) to the x-ray tube.

The principal advantages of a high-frequency generator are the following:

- Reduced weight and size
- Low-voltage ripple
- Greatest achievable efficiency of x-ray production
- Maximum x-ray output per mAs
- Shorter exposure times

REFERENCE

Khan FM. *The Physics of Radiation Therapy*, 4th edition, 2009. Chapter 3 "Production of X-rays"

Physics of X-Ray Production

 TOPIC OUTLINE

The following topics will be discussed in this lecture:
➤ Electron interactions with target
➤ Bremsstrahlung
➤ Angular distribution of x-rays
➤ Characteristic x-rays
➤ X-ray energy spectrum
➤ X-ray tube operating characteristics

ELECTRON INTERACTIONS WITH TARGET

Typical electron interactions with a target consist of the following:

• Ionization and excitation, with eventual generation of heat

• Ejection of orbital electrons, giving rise to characteristic x-rays and Auger electrons

• Occasional knock-on collisions to eject secondary electrons (called δ-rays) with enough kinetic energy to produce ionization tracks of their own

• Radiative collisions leading to bremsstrahlung

• Multiple Coulomb scattering with nuclei and orbital electrons without loss of energy

Further discussion of electron interactions in various media is presented in Chapter 14.

BREMSSTRAHLUNG

The process of bremsstrahlung (a German word meaning "break radiation") is a radiative collision (interaction) between a high-speed electron and a nucleus. The electron while passing near a nucleus may be deflected from its path by the action of Coulomb force of attraction. This sudden deflection causes the electron to accelerate momentarily and radiate a part or all of its kinetic energy as electromagnetic radiation or bremsstrahlung. The mechanism of bremsstrahlung production is illustrated in Figure 3B.1.

• Bremsstrahlung may result in partial or complete loss of electron energy.

• Events in which the electron loses all of its kinetic energy in one bremsstrahlung collision are rare. When it happens, the emitted photon has an energy $h\nu = E$, where E is the kinetic energy of the electron.

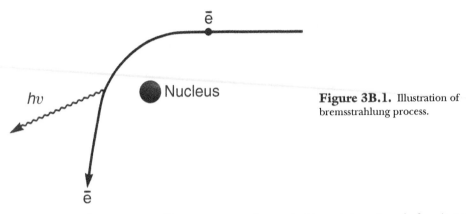

Figure 3B.1. Illustration of bremsstrahlung process.

- Because an electron may suffer one or more bremsstrahlung interactions before it comes to rest, the resulting photon may have any energy up to the initial energy of the electron.
- Bremsstrahlung photons in an x-ray beam show a continuous distribution of energies.

ANGULAR DISTRIBUTION OF X-RAYS

Angular distribution of bremsstrahlung x-rays around a transmission target is shown in Figure 3B.2.

- Direction of emission of bremsstrahlung photons depends on the energy of the incident electrons.
- At low electron energies (below 100 keV), x-rays are emitted more or less equally in all directions.
- As the kinetic energy of electrons increases, the direction of x-ray emission becomes increasingly forward.

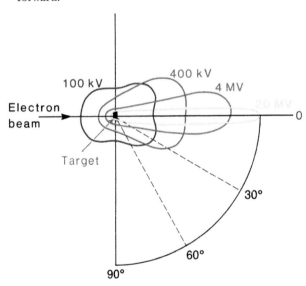

Figure 3B.2. Schematic illustration of spatial distribution of x-rays around a thin target.

EFFICIENCY OF X-RAY PRODUCTION

The term *efficiency* is defined as the ratio of output energy emitted as x-rays to the input energy deposited by electrons.

- Efficiency increases with the atomic number, Z, of the target material and the voltage, V, applied to the x-ray tube, as shown by the following equation:

$$\text{Efficiency} = 9 \times 10^{-10} \, ZV$$

EXAMPLE: Efficiency of x-ray production with tungsten target ($Z = 74$) bombarded by electrons accelerated through 100 kV is less than 1%. The rest of the input energy (~99%) appears as heat.

- Accuracy of the above equation is limited to a few megavolts.

CHARACTERISTIC X-RAYS

Electrons incident on a target may also produce characteristic x-rays (in addition to the bremsstrahlung). The mechanism of their production is illustrated in Figure 3B.3

An electron with kinetic energy E_0 may interact with the target atoms by ejecting an orbital electron, such as a K-, L-, or M-shell electron. The original electron will recede from the collision with energy $E_0 - \Delta E$, where ΔE is the energy given to the orbital electron.

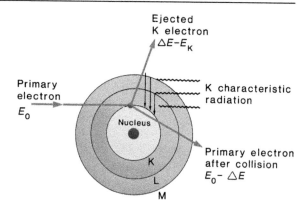

Figure 3B.3. Diagram to explain the production of characteristic radiation.

- Supposing that the ejected electron is the K-shell electron, its kinetic energy would be $\Delta E - E_K$, where E_K is the electron binding energy of the K shell. A vacancy thus created in the K shell will be filled by an outer orbit electron.

- Supposing that an electron from the L shell descends to fill the vacancy in the K shell, a photon may be emitted with energy $h\upsilon = E_K - E_L$, where E_L is the binding energy of the L-shell electron. Photons emitted in such transitions are called *characteristic x-rays* (characteristic of the atoms in the target and of the shells between which the transitions took place).

- Unlike bremsstrahlung x-rays, which are emitted with a spectrum of energies, the characteristic x-rays are emitted with discrete energies.

- The threshold energy that an incident electron must posses to eject an orbital electron is called the *critical absorption energy.*

- Characteristic x-rays contribute only a small fraction of the energy to the total spectrum of the x-ray beam, which is predominantly bremsstrahlung. They do not play an important role in therapeutic beams. However, they can be minimized by selective filtration using appropriate atomic number filters.

X-RAY ENERGY SPECTRUM

X-ray photons produced by an x-ray machine are heterogeneous in energy. The energy spectrum shows a continuous distribution of energies for the bremsstrahlung photons superimposed by characteristic radiation of discrete energies. A typical energy spectrum is shown in Figure 3B.4.

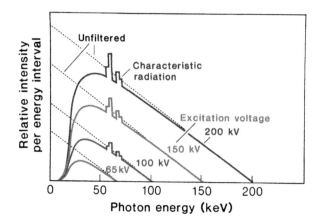

Figure 3B.4. Spectral distribution of x-rays calculated for a thick tungsten target using Equation 3.1. *Dotted curves* are for no filtration and *solid curves* are for a filtration of 1-mm aluminum. (Redrawn from Johns HE, Cunningham JR. *The Physics of Radiology*, 3rd edition. Springfield, IL: Charles C. Thomas; 1969, with permission.)

- If no filtration, inherent or added, of the beam is assumed, the calculated energy spectrum will be a straight line (shown as dotted lines in Figure 3B.4) and mathematically given by Kramer's equation

$$I_E = KZ(E_m - E)$$

where I_E is the intensity of photons with energy E, Z is the atomic number of the target, E_m is the maximum photon energy, and K is a constant.

- The maximum photon energy in the bremsstrahlung spectrum is equal to the energy of the incident electron. The maximum photon energy in keV is numerically equal to the applied peak voltage, kV_p.

- Added filtration enriches the beam with higher energy photons by absorbing the lower energy component of the spectrum. The transmitted beam is said to be *hardened.*

- The shape of the x-ray energy spectrum is the result of a) the alternating voltage applied to the tube, b) multiple bremsstrahlung interactions, and c) filtration.

- Even if the tube were to be energized with a constant potential, the x-ray beam would still be heterogeneous in energy because of the multiple bremsstrahlung processes that result in different energy photons.

- It is seen in Figure 3A.4 that the intensity of maximum energy photons is almost zero.

- The average energy of the x-ray beam, expressed in keV, is approximately equal (numerically) to $1/3$ kV_p. This is a rough approximation because it does not take into account the effect of filtration. The average energy does increase with an increase in filtration.

- Another parameter often used to measure x-ray beam quality is *half-value layer.* This topic is discussed in Chapter 7.

X-RAY TUBE OPERATING CHARACTERISTICS

Typical relationship between x-ray output, filament current, tube current, and tube voltage is shown in Figure 3B.5.

- Of all the parameters, x-ray output is most sensitive to the filament current. Therefore, constancy of filament current is critical to the constancy of x-ray output.

- There is a linear relationship between exposure rate and tube current.

- X-ray output increases more than linearly with increase in kilovoltage. It varies approximately as square of the kV_p.

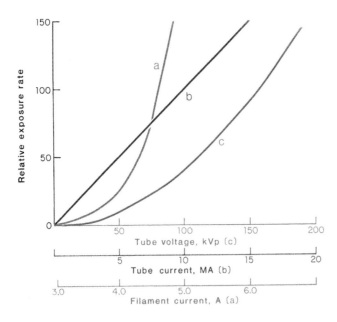

Figure 3B.5. Illustration of typical operating characteristics. Plots of relative exposure rate versus **a**, filament current at a given kVp; **b**, tube current at a given kVp; and **c**, tube voltage at a given tube current.

REVIEW QUESTIONS • Chapter 3

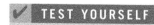

In multiple choice questions, more than one option may be correct.

Review questions for this chapter are provided online.

1. If the input line voltage is nominally 110 V, what is the peak voltage for a sinusoidal waveform?
   a) 110
   b) 155.6
   c) 220
   d) 233.4

2. What will be the peak voltage (kV_p) at the x-ray tube, if a line voltage of 220 V at 60 cycles/second is applied to the primary of the voltage transformer of 500:1 turn ratio?
   a) 77.8
   b) 110.0
   c) 155.6
   d) 220.0

3. Which factor(s) will impact the focal spot size of an x-ray tube?
   a) Anode angle
   b) Anode material
   c) kV_p
   d) mAs

4. In an x-ray tube, an electron beam deposits its energy in a 4 × 4 mm spot on the target angled at 30°. What is the projected focal spot length at the exit window?
   a) 1 mm
   b) 1.5 mm
   c) 2 mm
   d) 2.5 mm

5. A "heel effect" in an x-ray tube:
   a) Results from nonuniform intensity of electron beam incident on the target.
   b) Represents decreasing x-ray beam intensity from the cathode to the anode direction.
   c) Is caused by angled targets.
   d) Has adverse effect on image quality.

6. The average energy of the photon beam from an x-ray tube can be increased by:
   a) Increasing tube current
   b) Increasing tube voltage
   c) Increasing filament current
   d) Increasing filament voltage
   e) Increasing filtration

7. Rank the parameters that most affect x-ray tube output (largest to smallest):
   a) Tube voltage, tube current, filament current
   b) Tube current, filament current, tube voltage
   c) Filament current, tube voltage, tube current
   d) Tube voltage, tube current, filament current
   e) Filament currant, tube voltage, tube current

8. Which x-ray generator will require the highest mAs, given the same patient thickness and kV_p setting?
   a) Three phase
   b) High frequency
   c) Half-wave rectified
   d) Full-wave rectified

9. An x-ray beam generated by a constant potential will be:

   a) Monoenergetic
   b) Predominantly polyenergetic with a spectrum of photon energies
   c) Predominantly characteristic radiation of discrete energies
   d) Predominantly bremsstrahlung radiation

10. Efficiency of x-ray production increases with:

    a) Increasing electron energy
    b) Increasing atomic number
    c) Increasing mAs
    d) Increasing kV_p

11. What percentage of the 6 MeV electron energy is converted to x-rays on a tungsten ($Z = 74$) target?

    a) 33
    b) 40
    c) 66
    d) 100

12. The K-shell and L_{II}-shell binding energies for tungsten are 69.5 and 11.5 keV, respectively. What is the energy of a $K\alpha_1$ (L_{II}–K transition) characteristic x-ray shell from a 50-kV_p x-ray tube with a tungsten target:

    a) 69.5 keV
    b) 11.5 keV
    c) 58 keV
    d) 50 keV
    e) None

CLINICAL RADIATION GENERATORS

X-Ray and Electron Beams

 TOPIC OUTLINE

The following topics will be discussed in this lecture:
➤ Kilovoltage x-ray units
➤ Linear accelerator
➤ Microtron
➤ Cobalt teletherapy
➤ Penumbra

KILOVOLTAGE X-RAY UNITS

X-ray therapy in the kilovoltage range has been divided into following subcategories by the National Council on Radiation Protection and Measurements (NCRP Report 34, 1970):

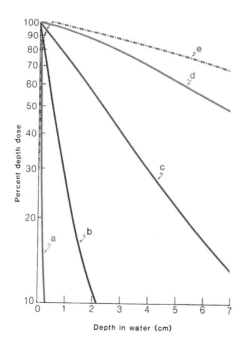

Figure 4A.1. Depth dose curves in water or soft tissues for various quality beams. **Line a:** Grenz rays, half-value layer (HVL) = 0.04 mm Al, field diameter 33 cm, source-to-surface distance (SSD) = 10 cm. **Line b:** Contact therapy, HVL = 1.5 mm Al, field diameter = 2.0 cm, SSD = 2 cm. **Line c:** Superficial therapy, HVL = 3.0 mm Al, field diameter = 3.6 cm, SSD = 20 cm. **Line d:** Orthovoltage, HVL = 2.0 mm Cu, field size = 10 × 10 cm, SSD = 50 cm. **Line e:** ^{60}Co γ-rays, field size = 10 × 10 cm, SSD = 80 cm. (Plotted from data in Cohen M, Jones DEA, Green D, eds. Central axis depth dose data for use in radiotherapy. *Br J Radiol.* 1978 [suppl 11]. The British Institute of Radiology, London, with permission.)

A. Grenz-ray Therapy: <20 kV$_p$

- Because of the very low depth of penetration (see Figure 4A.1) such radiations are no longer used in radiation therapy.

B. Contact (endocavitary) Therapy: 40–50 kV$_p$

- Treatments are delivered using endocavitary applicators at very short distances, for example, source-to-surface distance (SSD) of 2 cm or less.
- As seen in Figure 4A.1, this quality radiation is useful for tumors not deeper than 1 to 2 mm. The beam is rapidly absorbed and almost completely absorbed within 2 cm of soft tissue.
- Endocavitary therapy is still being used in the treatment of selected rectal cancers at some institutions. This method of treatment is also called the Papillon technique.

C. Superficial Therapy: 50–150 kV$_p$

- Aluminum filters of various thickness are used to obtain a beam quality in the range of 1 to 8 mm Al half-value layer (HVL). Treatments are delivered using applicators that provide an SSD in the range of 15 to 20 cm.
- As seen in Figure 4A.1, superficial therapy is useful for irradiating superficial tumors (e.g., skin cancers) confined to the depth of approximately 5 mm (~90% depth dose). Although such treatments can also be delivered by electron beams, the advantage of superficial therapy is in the design of shielding normal structures. A thin lead cutout (<1 mm thick) molded directly on the skin surface provides sufficient protection of the surrounding normal structures.

D. Orthovoltage or Deep Therapy: 150–500 kV$_p$

- Most orthovoltage equipment is operated at 200 to 300 kV$_p$ and 10 to 20 mA. The SSD is usually set at 50 cm.
- Beam quality is adjusted by using thin copper filters or combination of filters (e.g., Thoreaus filters) containing thin sheets of tin, copper, and aluminum (inserted in the beam in that order—with tin facing the source and aluminum facing the patient). With the use of these filters, a beam quality in the range of 1 to 4 mm Cu HVL can be obtained.
- As seen in Figure 4A.1, there are severe limitations in the use of orthovoltage beams (single or multidirectional fields) in treating lesions deeper than 2 to 3 cm. The biggest disadvantages are the lack of skin-sparing and excessive dose to bone.
- With the advent of cobalt teletherapy and linear accelerators, orthovoltage or deep therapy is now almost extinct.

E. Supervoltage Therapy: 500–1,000 kV$_p$

- Because conventional transformers are not suitable for producing potentials much greater than 300 kV$_p$, resonant transformers have been used for supervoltage therapy. Again, with the availability of ^{60}Co and linear accelerators, supervoltage therapy is no longer used.

F. Megavoltage Therapy: >1 MV

- X-ray beams of energy 1 MV or greater are known as megavoltage beams. γ-Ray beams of 1 MeV or greater (e.g., ^{60}Co) are also included in this category.
- Examples of clinical megavoltage machines include Van de Graaff generator, linear accelerator, betatron, microtron, and cobalt teletherapy. Of these, we will discuss only the linear accelerator, the microtron, and the cobalt teletherapy. The others, which are mostly of historic interest, are discussed in the Textbook.

LINEAR ACCELERATOR

Medical linear accelerators (linacs) are used for generating high-energy x-ray beams, mostly in the energy range of 4 to 25 MV, and electron beams in the range of 4 to 25 MeV. Current accelerators are also equipped with online imaging devices, which are discussed in Chapter 25 on image-guided radiotherapy.

- The linac is a device that uses high-frequency microwaves to accelerate charged particles such as electrons to high energies. Electrons are accelerated by the electric "E" field associated with the microwaves.

- The microwave frequency used in a radiotherapy linac is approximately 3,000 MHz (3 GHz).

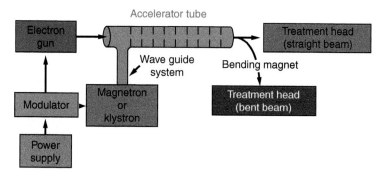

Figure 4A.2. A block diagram of typical medical linear accelerator.

BASIC COMPONENTS

Accelerator Structure

- The accelerator structure, in which the electrons are accelerated by microwaves, consists of a highly evacuated copper tube with its interior divided by copper discs or diaphragms of varying aperture and spacing.

- The accelerating structure can be of either a *traveling-wave* or a *stationary-wave* design.

- In the traveling-wave structure, the microwaves travel through the structure to its high-energy end, where they are absorbed by a terminating or "*dummy*" load to prevent backward reflection of the waves.

- In the standing wave structure, each end of the accelerator structure has a conducting surface. This provides maximum reflection of the microwaves at both ends of the structure. The combination of forward and reverse traveling waves gives rise to stationary waves.

- In some of the standing wave design, the microwave power is coupled into the structure by side coupling cavities. This provides the resonant coupling between the on-axis accelerating cavities and the side-coupled cavities.

- Because of the side-coupled resonant cavities, a standing-wave linac requires much shorter accelerator structure and is less bulky than a traveling-wave linac.

Circulator

- A standing-wave structure requires the installation of a circulator (or isolator) between the linac and the microwave source. This device prevents the microwave reflections from returning to the microwave power source (magnetron or klystron).

Modulator

- Modulator is a section of electronics where direct current (DC) voltage is converted into high-voltage flat-topped DC pulses of a few microseconds in duration. It contains the *pulse-forming network* and a high-voltage switch tube known as *hydrogen thyratron*.

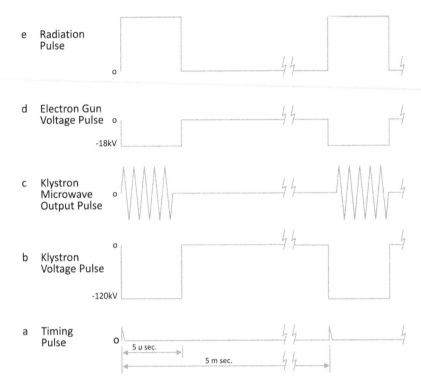

Figure 4A.3. Timing diagram for voltage, microwave, and radiation pulses. (From Karzmark CJ, Morton RJ. A Primer on Theory and Operation of Linear Accelerators in Radiation Therapy. Rockville, MD: U.S. Department of Health and Human Services, Bureau of Radiological Health; 1981, with permission.)

- High-voltage pulses from the modulator are delivered to the *magnetron* or *klystron* and simultaneously to the *electron gun.*
- Microwave pulses from the magnetron or klystron are injected into the accelerator structure through a *waveguide* system. At the proper instant, electrons from an electron gun are also injected into the accelerator structure.
- As illustrated in Figure 4A.3, the time duration of the klystron (or magnetron) voltage pulse, microwave pulse, electron gun voltage pulse, and radiation pulse is the same in each case (~5 μs). The interpulse duration is longer (~5 ms).

Wave Guide

- Waveguide is a rectangular copper tube to provide a path for microwaves to travel from the source (magnetron or klystron) to the accelerator structure. It is pressurized with Freon or sulfur hexafluoride gas to prevent electrical breakdown from E-field associated with the high-power microwaves.

Magnetron

- The magnetron is a device that produces microwaves. It functions as a high-power oscillator, generating microwave pulses of several microseconds duration and with a repetition rate of several hundred pulses per second.
- The frequency of microwaves within each pulse is about 3,000 MHz.
- Magnetron operation is illustrated in Figure 4A.4 and summarized below:

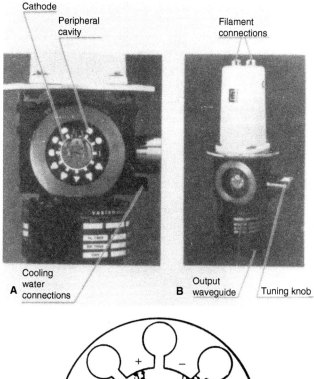

Cathode

Peripheral cavity

Filament connections

Cooling water connections

A

Output waveguide

Tuning knob

B

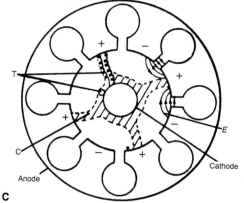

T

E

C

Anode

Cathode

C

Figure 4A.4. A,B: Cutaway magnetron pictures. **C:** Cross-sectional diagram showing principle of magnetron operation. (From Karzmark CJ, Morton RJ. *A Primer on Theory and Operation of Linear Accelerators in Radiation Therapy.* Rockville, MD: U.S. Department of Health and Human Services, Bureau of Radiological Health; 1981, with permission.)

- **Electrons emitted from cathode ➤ Electrons accelerated toward anode (with resonant cavities) by pulsed DC electric field ➤ Electrons made to move in complex spirals toward resonant cavities under simultaneous action of E-field and perpendicular static magnetic field ➤ Kinetic energy of spiraling electrons radiated in form of microwaves.**

Klystron

- Unlike magnetron, the klystron is not a generator of microwaves.
- Klystron is a microwave amplifier. It needs to be driven by a low-power microwave oscillator.
- Its operation is illustrated in Figure 4A.5 and summarized below:
- **Electrons emitted by hot cathode filament ➤ Electrons accelerated into buncher cavity by negative voltage pulse. Buncher cavity also energized by low power microwaves ➤ Microwaves in buncher cavity set up alternating E-field across cavity ➤ Electrons suffer velocity modulation—some speed up while others slow down, creating electron bunches ➤ Electron bunches then pass through field-free space in drift tube ➤ Electrons arriving at catcher cavity induce retarding E-field ➤ Electrons suffer deceleration ➤ Kinetic energy of electrons is converted into high-power microwaves.**

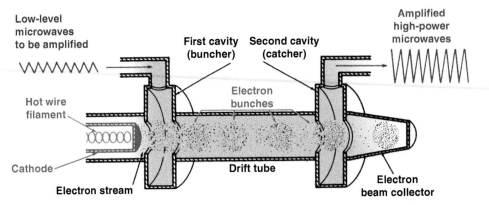

Figure 4A.5. Cross-sectional drawing of a two-cavity klystron. (From Karzmark CJ, Morton RJ. *A Primer on Theory and Operation of Linear Accelerators in Radiation Therapy*. Rockville, MD: U.S. Department of Health and Human Services, Bureau of Radiological Health, 1981, with permission.)

Electron Transport System

- Electron beam emerging from the exit window of the accelerator structure is a narrow pencil beam of about 2 to 3 mm diameter. In the low-energy linacs (up to 6 MV), the accelerator structure is short and the electrons are allowed to proceed straight on to strike a target to produce x-rays.

- In the higher-energy linacs, the accelerator structure is too long and, therefore, placed horizontally or at an upward angle with respect to the horizontal. The electrons are then bent through a suitable angle (usually about 90°–270°).

- The precision bending of the electron beam is accomplished by a *beam transport system* consisting of bending magnets, focusing coils, and other components.

Treatment Head

- Treatment head consists of a well-shielded shell of lead–tungsten alloy.

- It contains the following equipment:

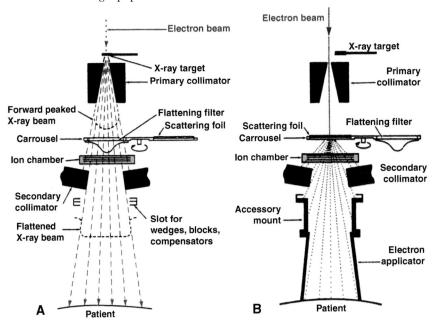

Figure 4A.6. Components of treatment head. **A:** X-ray therapy mode. **B:** Electron therapy mode. (From Karzmark CJ, Morton RJ. *A Primer on Theory and Operation of Linear Accelerators in Radiation Therapy*. Rockville, MD: U.S. Department of Health and Human Services, Bureau of Radiological Health; 1981, with permission.) (*continued*)

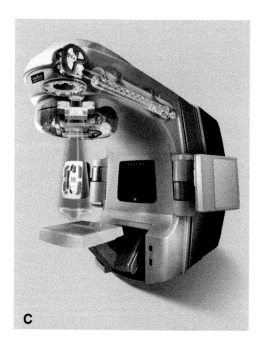

Figure 4A.6. (*continued*) **C:** A cut-away diagram of the linac (from Varian Medical Systems: www.varian.com, with permission).

> *Target*

• Transmission type tungsten target intercepts the electron beam to generate x-ray beam (bremsstrahlung).

• The focal spot is approximately 2 to 3 mm in diameter.

• The target moves out of the way when the accelerator is operated in the electron therapy mode.

> *Flattening Filter*

• Since the kinetic energy of electrons striking the target is in the megavoltage range, the x-ray beam intensity is peaked in the forward direction. To make the intensity uniform in cross section, a flattening filter is inserted in the beam.

• The flattening filter is usually made of a thick piece of lead and has a conical shape—thick in the middle and thin around the periphery—to provide differential attenuation.

> *Scattering Foil*

• In the electron mode of accelerator operation, both the target and the flattening filter move out of the way and a scattering foil is inserted to intercept the electron beam.

• The scattering foil is essentially a thin foil (<1 mm) of high atomic number material.

• The function of the scattering foil is to spread the pencil electron beam (by multiple Coulomb scattering) uniformly into a broad beam of electrons.

• An optimally designed scattering foil consists of a dual foil system—the first foil is uniform in thickness while the second foil is contoured (thicker in the middle). The combined effect of the two foils is to spread the beam more uniformly in cross section.

> *Beam Collimation and Monitoring*

• The first x-ray beam collimator is the *fixed primary collimator* that limits the beam to its maximum diameter.

• After passing through the flattening filter (in the case of x-ray beam) or the scattering foil (in the case of electron beam), the flat beam is incident on the *dose monitoring ion chambers*.

• Dose monitoring ion chambers (or simply monitor chambers) are usually transmission type, parallel-plate chambers. They monitor the treatment dose (when properly calibrated) as well as beam flatness.

• Dual monitor chambers assure redundancy and safety of dose delivery.

- After passing through the monitor chambers, the beam is collimated by a pair of continuously *movable x-ray collimators* (also called *x-ray jaws*) that provide a rectangular opening of 0×0 to 40×40 cm projected at the isocenter (100 cm from the target). They are made up of lead–tungsten alloy and are thick enough to have a primary beam transmission of approximately 1% or less.

- X-ray jaws are constrained to move along an arc so that the inside edge is always aligned with the radial line passing through the target.

- In addition to the x-ray jaws, modern accelerators are equipped with *multileaf collimators* to provide irregularly shaped field blocking and intensity modulation for intensity-modulated radiation therapy (IMRT).

- For electron beam therapy, additional beam collimation is provided by *electron applicators* that act as penumbra trimmers close to the patient surface.

MICROTRON

Microtron is an electron accelerator that combines the principles of both linear accelerator and cyclotron. Its operation is illustrated in Figure 4A.7.

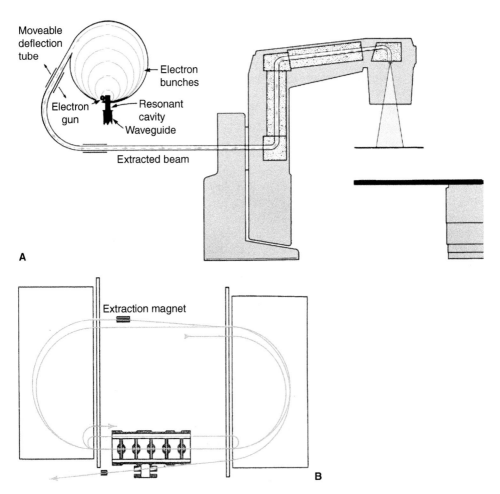

Figure 4A.7. A: Schematic diagram of a circular microtron unit. (Reprinted with permission from AB Scanditronix, Uppsala, Sweden.) **B:** Electron orbits and accelerating cavities in a racetrack microtron. (From Karzmark CJ, Nunan CS, Tanabe E. *Medical Electron Accelerators.* New York: McGraw-Hill; 1993, with permission.)

- **Electrons from electron gun injected into one or more microwave cavities ➤ Electrons accelerated by oscillating E-field associated with microwaves ➤ A magnetic field forces the electrons to move in a circular orbit and return to the cavity ➤ Electrons receive higher and higher energy by repeated passes through the cavity and describe orbits of increasing radius in the magnetic field ➤ Cavity voltage, frequency, and magnetic field are so adjusted so that electrons arrive each time in correct phase at the cavity ➤ Electrons extracted from orbit by a narrow deflection tube of steel that screens off magnetic field ➤ Electron beam is transported to the treatment head to produce x-rays or electron beams as in a linac.**

- Principal advantages of microtron over linear accelerator are easy energy selection, small energy spread, small size of machine, and ability to supply a beam to several treatment rooms.

- A racetrack microtron uses a standing wave linac structure (instead of a single cavity as in a circular microtron) to accelerate electrons. Such an accelerator is suited for higher energy beams (e.g., 50 MV).

COBALT TELETHERAPY

- The ^{60}Co source is produced by irradiating stable ^{59}Co material with neutrons in a reactor. The nuclear reaction can be represented by ^{59}Co$(n,\gamma)^{60}$Co.

- The ^{60}Co source decays to ^{60}Ni with the emission of β-particles and two photons per disintegration of energies 1.17 and 1.33 MeV. The decay scheme is presented in Figure 4A.8.

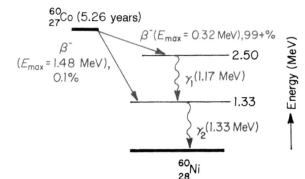

Figure 4A.8. Energy-level diagram for the decay of $^{60}_{27}$Co nucleus.

- β-Particles are absorbed in the source capsule and the useful beam consists of γ-rays of 1.17 and 1.33 MeV (average energy 1.25 MeV).

- The cobalt source used for teletherapy typically has an initial activity of 3,000 to 5,000 Ci but decays with a half-life of 5.26 years. Therefore, the source needs to be replaced about every 5 years so that the treatment times do not get to be unacceptably long.

- A typical cobalt teletherapy source consists of ^{60}Co disks encapsulated in a steel cylinder of diameter ranging from 1 to 2 cm. It is housed in a well-shielded shell, called the *sourcehead*.

- When the beam is tuned on, the source moves into position at the collimator opening with the circular end of the source capsule facing the patient. When the beam is turned off, the source moves back into its shielded position.

- Because of the relatively large source size (1–2 cm diameter), a ^{60}Co beam is associated with a much larger geometric penumbra than a linac x-ray beam that has a focal spot size of approximately 2 to 3 mm.

PENUMBRA

- The term *penumbra* means the region, at the edge of a radiation beam, over which the dose rate changes rapidly as a function of lateral distance.

- Dose gradation in the penumbra region is designated by the following three types of penumbra: transmission penumbra, geometric penumbra, and physical penumbra

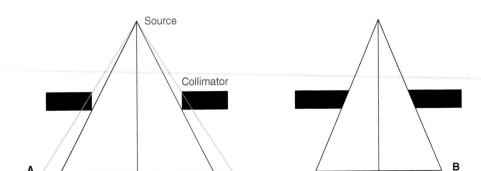

Figure 4A.9. Illustration of transmission penumbra: **A:** Nondivergent collimating block. **B**: Divergent collimating block.

➤ *Transmission penumbra* is the part of penumbra that is caused by photons transmitted through the edge of the collimating block.

➤ In diagram A of Figure 4A.9, transmission penumbra occurs due to the collimating blocks being straight (nondivergent). Transmission penumbra is removed by divergent collimating blocks as shown in diagram B.

➤ *Geometric penumbra* is caused by the source (or focal spot) having a finite size.

➤ The width of the geometric penumbra (P_d) at any depth (d) from the surface of a patient is given by

$$P_d = \frac{s(\text{SSD} + d - \text{SDD})}{\text{SDD}}$$

where SSD is the source-to-surface distance and SDD is the source to diaphragm distance, as shown in Figure 4A.10.

➤ The above equation shows that the width of the geometric penumbra increases with increase in source size s, SSD, and depth d. It decreases with increase in SDD.

➤ *Physical penumbra* is dose gradation zone caused by the combined effect of transmission penumbra, geometric penumbra, and lateral scatter of radiation (photon and electrons) within the patient. Dosimetrically, physical penumbra may be defined as the lateral distance between two specified isodose curves at a specified depth.

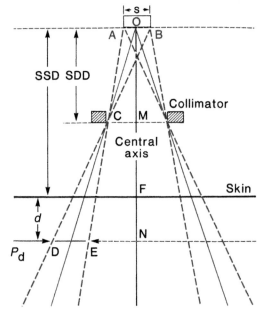

Figure 4A.10. Diagram for calculating geometric penumbra. SDD, source to diaphragm distance; SSD, source to surface distance.

REFERENCE
Khan FM. *The Physics of Radiation Therapy,* 4th edition, 2009. Chapter 4 "Clinical Radiation Generators"

Heavy Particle Accelerators

  TOPIC OUTLINE

The following topics will be discussed in this lecture:
➤ Heavy particle accelerators
➤ Neutron generators
➤ Protons and heavy ions
➤ Negative pions

HEAVY PARTICLE ACCELERATORS

Whereas x-rays and electrons are the main radiations used in radiotherapy, heavy particle beams offer special advantages with regard to dose localization and therapeutic gain (greater effect on tumor than on normal tissue).

- Heavy particles include neutrons, protons, deuterons, α-particles, negative pions, and heavy ions accelerated to high energies.

- Because of the enormous cost involved, only a few institutions have been able to acquire heavy particle beams for clinical use.

- Of all the heavy particle beams, protons have gained greater popularity in recent times. Proton beam therapy is discussed in Chapter 26.

➤ *Cyclotron*
- In radiation therapy, cyclotrons or synchrotrons are used to accelerate protons, deuterons, other heavy charged particles to high energies suitable for clinical use.

- High-energy protons and deuterons have also been used to generate neutron beams.

- The principle of cyclotron operation is illustrated in Figure 4B.1.

- The cyclotron consists essentially of a short metallic cylinder divided into two sections, usually referred to as *dees* (for their resemblance to letter D).

- The dees are highly evacuated and subjected to a constant strength magnetic field applied perpendicular to the plane of the dees.

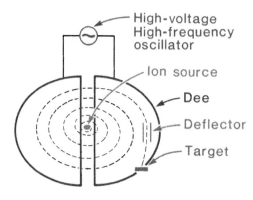

Figure 4B.1. Diagram illustrating the principle of operation of a cyclotron.

- A square wave of oscillating electric field is applied across the gap between the two dees.
- The cyclotron operation is outlined below:
- **Positively charged particles (e.g., protons or deuterons) injected at the center of the two dees ➤ Particles accelerated in the gap between dees by the electric field ➤ Particles travel in a circular orbit by the action of the magnetic field ➤ Polarity of the electric field switched at the exact time the beam enters the gap from the opposite direction ➤ Magnetic field confines beam in orbits of ever-increasing radii ➤ Beam extracted when the desired maximum energy is achieved.**

➤ *Synchrotron*

- As a particle reaches very high velocity (in the relativistic range), further acceleration causes the particle to gain in mass. This increases the transit time between the dees. As a result, the relativistic particles get out of step with the frequency of the alternating potential applied to the dees. This problem is solved in the synchrotron.
- In the synchrotron, the frequency of the accelerating potential is adjusted to compensate for the decrease in particle velocity.

NEUTRON GENERATORS

- Generators for high-energy neutron beams include: A) deuterium tritium (D-T) generators, B) cyclotrons, and C) linear accelerators
- The bombarding particles are either deuterons or protons and the target material is usually beryllium, except in the D-T generator in which tritium is used as the target.

A. D-T Generators

PRINCIPLE: A low-energy deuteron beam (100–300 keV) incident on a tritium target yields neutrons by the following reaction

$$_{1}^{2}H + _{1}^{3}H \rightarrow _{2}^{4}He + _{1}^{0}n + 17.6 \text{ MeV}$$

The disintegration energy of 17.6 MeV is shared between the helium nucleus (α-particle) and the neutron, with approximately 14 MeV given to the neutron.

- The neutrons thus produced are essentially monoenergetic and isotropic (same yield in all directions).
- The advantage of D-T generators over other neutron generators is that their size is small enough to allow isocentric mounting on a rotational gantry.
- The major problem is the lack of sufficient dose rate at the treatment distance. The highest dose rate that has been achieved so far is approximately 15 cGy/min at 1 m.

B. Cyclotron for Neutron Beams

PRINCIPLE: Deuterons accelerated to high energies (15–50 MeV) by a cyclotron bombard a low atomic number target such as beryllium to produce neutrons according to a *stripping* reaction

$$_{1}^{2}H + _{4}^{9}Be \rightarrow _{5}^{10}B + _{0}^{1}n$$

Neutrons are produced mostly in the forward direction with a spectrum of energies as shown in Figure 4B.2.

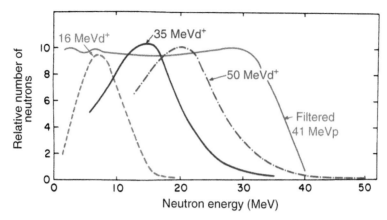

Figure 4B.2. Neutron spectra produced by deuterons on beryllium target. (From Raju MR. *Heavy Particle Radiotherapy.* New York: Academic Press, 1980. Data from Hall EJ, Roizin-Towle L, Attix FH. Radiobiological studies with cyclotron-produced neutrons currently used for radiotherapy. *Int J Radiol Oncol Biol Phys* 1975;1:33; and Graves RG, Smathers JB, Almond PR, et al. Neutron energy spectra of d[49]-Be and P[41]-Be neutron radiotherapy sources. *Med Phys* 1979;6:123, with permission.)

PROTONS AND HEAVY IONS

- Proton beams for therapeutic application range in energy from 150 to 250 MeV.

- The major advantage of high-energy protons and other heavy charged particles is the *Bragg peak.*

- As the heavy charged particle beam traverses the tissues, the dose deposited is approximately constant with depth until near the end of the range where the dose peaks out to a high value followed by a rapid falloff to zero. The region of high dose at the end of the particle range is called the Bragg peak (Figure 4B.3).

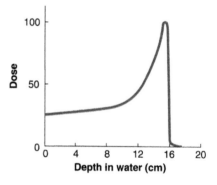

Figure 4B.3. Depth dose distribution characteristic of heavy charged particles, showing Bragg peak.

- The energy of heavy charged particles or stripped nuclei is often expressed in terms of kinetic energy per nucleon (*specific kinetic energy*) or MeV/u, where u is mass number of the nucleus.

- Particles with the same MeV/u have approximately the same velocity. EXAMPLE: 150 MeV protons, 300 MeV deuterons, and 600 MeV helium ions all have approximately the same velocity.

- For ions heavier than helium, the range for the same MeV/u is somewhat lower than that for protons.

- The range energy relationship for protons is plotted in Figure 4B.4.

- An approximate comparative range of heavy particles with the same initial velocity is given by

$$R_1/R_2 = (M_1/M_2)(Z_2/Z_1)^2$$

where R_1 and R_2 are particle ranges, M_1 and M_2 the masses, and Z_1 and Z_2 the charges of the two particles being compared.

- As can be deduced from the above equation, the range of heavy particles for the same initial velocity is dependent on A/Z^2, where A is the mass number and Z the nuclear charge.

- Because A/Z^2 decreases as the ions get heavier, the range of heavier ions is less than the range of lighter ones for the same MeV/u with the exception of protons.

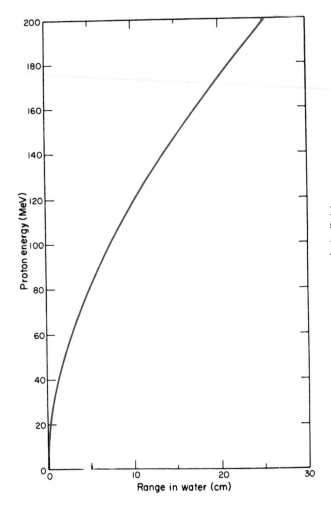

Figure 4B.4. Range energy relationship for protons. (From Raju MR. *Heavy Particle Radiotherapy.* New York: Academic Press, 1980, with permission.)

PIONS

- A pi meson (or pion) has a mass 273 times the mass of electron.
- A pion may have a positive, a negative, or a zero charge (neutral).
- The charged pions decay into mu mesons and neutrinos with a mean life of 2.54×10^{-8} seconds and the neutral pions decay into pairs of photons with a mean life of about 10^{-16} seconds.

$$\pi^+ \to \mu^+ + \nu$$
$$\pi^- \to \mu^- + \tilde{\nu}$$
$$\pi^0 \to h\nu_1 + h\nu_2$$

- Only negative pions have been used for radiation therapy.
- Negative pions of energy close to 100 MeV are of interest in radiation therapy, providing a range in water of approximately 24 cm.
- Beams of negative pions can be produced in a nuclear reaction as outlined below:
- **Protons of 400 to 800 MeV energy (produced in a cyclotron or a linear accelerator) ➤ Bombard a beryllium target ➤ Pions (positive, negative, and zero charge) produced with a spectrum of energies ➤ Negative pions of suitable energy extracted using bending magnets.**

- Negative pions, like other charged particles, deposit dose initially by ionization and excitation and exhibit Bragg peak as they slow down. But the Bragg peak is more pronounced because of the additional effect of nuclear disintegration produced by π^- capture.

- The phenomenon of π^- capture is also known as *star formation*. A negative pion is captured by a nucleus near the end of its range and results in the release of several other particles such as protons, neutrons, and α-particles.

- Although pion beams have attractive radiobiologic properties, they suffer from the problems of low dose rates, beam contamination, and high cost.

REVIEW QUESTIONS • Chapter 4

✔ TEST YOURSELF

Review questions for this chapter are provided online.

In multiple choice questions, more than one option may be correct.

1. In a medical linear accelerator:
   a) Magnetron is a generator of microwaves.
   b) Klystron is an amplifier of microwave power.
   c) Circulator protects the microwave power source from reflected microwaves.
   d) Bending magnets bend the x-ray beam through 90° to 270° depending on the gantry angle.

2. Which of the following is(are) true for medical electron linear accelerators?
   a) Electrons are accelerated toward an anode biased from 6 to 25 MeV.
   b) Microwave amplification occurs with either klystrons (for low-energy systems) or magnetrons (for high-energy systems).
   c) For the same maximum acceleration, side-coupled standing wave accelerator structures are shorter than traveling wave designs.
   d) High microwave frequencies of approximately 3 GHz are used within the accelerator structure.
   e) None of the above.

3. In a medical linear accelerator:
   a) Klystrons are more suited than magnetrons for higher energy (>10 MV) linacs.
   b) Magnetrons have a longer life span than klystrons.
   c) Modulator provides high-voltage direct current pulses to the magnetron or klystron and the electron gun, simultaneously.
   d) Accelerator structure contains Freon gas to conduct microwaves.

4. What is the approximate microwave pulse frequency in a medical linear accelerator?
   a) 100 MHz
   b) 300 MHz
   c) 1,000 MHz
   d) 3,000 MHz

5. Electron current in the x-ray mode versus electron mode in a linear accelerator is approximately:
   a) 10:1
   b) 100:1
   c) 1,000:1
   d) 1:1,000

6. Which of the following linac components require(s) to be cooled
   a) Klystron or magnetron
   b) Targets
   c) Wave guides
   d) Focusing coils
   e) Transformers

7. Geometric penumbra width increases with increase in
   a) Source (or focal spot) diameter
   b) Source–diaphragm distance
   c) Source–surface distance
   d) Depth in the patient
   e) All of the above

8. You are treating a patient to a depth of 5 cm with an 80 cm SSD Cobalt machine. Collimators are 35 cm from the source. If the source diameter is 2.1 cm, what is the geometric penumbra width?
   a) 1.1 cm
   b) 2.3 cm

c) 2.7 cm
d) 3.0 cm
e) 4.0 cm

9. Select an option from (a–d) in which the following components (1–5) are arranged in the *decreasing* order of their distance from the patient:

1. Monitor chamber
2. Target
3. Primary collimator
4. Jaws and secondary collimator
5. Flattening filter

a) 1, 2, 3, 4, 5
b) 1, 5, 2, 3, 4
c) 2, 3, 5, 1, 4
d) 2, 1, 5, 3, 4

10. Clinical proton generators consist of

a) Linacs
b) Microtrons
c) Synchrotrons
d) Betatrons
e) Cyclotrons

11. Which of the following is/are true for the production of high-energy neutrons for radio-therapy beams?

a) D-T generators produce neutrons with an energy spectra ranging from 0 to 14 MeV.
b) Deuterons accelerated by D-T generators always produce lower energy neutrons than cyclotron-accelerated deuterons incident on low Z materials.
c) Cyclotron produced neutrons are isotropic, whereas D-T generators produce forward-peaked neutron beams.
d) The peak energy of neutrons from D-T generators is proportional to the incident energy of the deuteron beam.
e) None of the above.

12. Which of the following nuclei has the largest range for the same initial velocity:

a) $^{4}_{2}\text{He}$
b) $^{1}_{1}\text{H}$
c) $^{2}_{1}\text{H}$
d) $^{12}_{6}\text{C}$
e) $^{20}_{10}\text{Ne}$

13. If the range of a 100 MeV proton in water is 7.6 cm, what would the range (in cm) of a deuteron with same initial velocity be?

a) 3.8
b) 7.6
c) 15.2
d) 30.4

14. High-energy deuterons bombarding on a beryllium target create neutrons by the process of:

a) Fission
b) Photodisintegration
c) Stripping
d) Deuteron capture

15. Bragg peak is exhibited by

a) Neutrons
b) Protons
c) Heavy charged particles
d) X- and γ-rays

INTERACTIONS OF IONIZING RADIATION

LECTURE

5A

REFERENCE

Khan FM. *The Physics of Radiation Therapy*, 4th edition, 2009. Chapter 5 "Interactions of Ionizing Radiation"

Photon Interactions

 TOPIC OUTLINE

The following topics will be discussed in this lecture:

➤ Ionizing radiation: definition
➤ Fluence: definition
➤ Photon beam attenuation
➤ Attenuation and absorption coefficients
➤ Photon interactions:
  • Coherent scattering
  • Photoelectric effect
  • Compton effect
  • Pair production
  • Photodisintegration
➤ Relative importance of different interactions

IONIZING RADIATION

• Ionization is the process by which a neutral atom acquires a positive or a negative charge. Stripping electron from an atom gives rise to an ion pair. The stripped electron quickly attaches itself to a neutral atom to create a negative ion and the atom from which the electron has been stripped becomes the positive ion.

• Charged particles of sufficient kinetic energy that produce ionization and excitation by collision with atoms are known as directly ionizing radiation. EXAMPLE:

  ➤ Electrons
  ➤ Protons
  ➤ α-Particles and heavier charged particles

• Uncharged particles of sufficient energy that liberate directly ionizing particles from atoms are known as indirectly ionizing radiation. EXAMPLE:

  ➤ Photons
  ➤ Neutrons

FLUENCE

- *Photon fluence* (Φ): It is the number of photons per unit area. Mathematically, it is the quotient dN by da, where dN is the number of photons that enter an imaginary sphere of cross-sectional area da.

$$\Phi = \frac{dN}{da}$$

- *Fluence rate or flux density* (ϕ): It is the fluence per unit time.
- *Energy fluence* (Ψ): The quotient of dE_{fl} by da, where dE_{fl} is the sum of the energies of all the photons that enter a sphere of cross-sectional area da.

$$\Psi = \frac{dE_{fl}}{da}$$

- *Energy fluence rate, energy flux density, or intensity* (ψ): It is the energy fluence per unit time.

PHOTON BEAM ATTENUATION

- A narrow monoenergetic beam of photons is attenuated exponentially by an absorber (Figure 5A.1):

$$I(x) = I_0 e^{-\mu x}$$

where $I(x)$ is the intensity transmitted by a thickness x, I_0 the intensity incident on the absorber, and μ the linear attenuation coefficient.

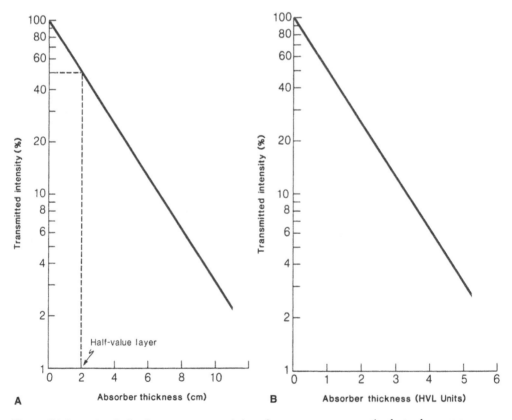

Figure 5A.1. A: Graph showing percent transmission of a narrow monoenergetic photon beam as a function of absorber thickness. For this quality beam and absorber material, half-value layer (HVL) = 2 cm and $\mu = 0.347$ cm^{-1}. **B:** Universal attenuation curve showing percent transmission of a narrow monoenergetic beam as a function of absorber thickness in units of HVL.

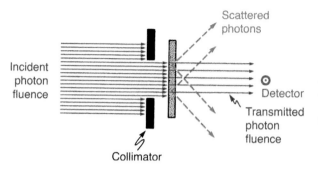

Figure 5A.2. Diagram to illustrate an experimental arrangement for studying narrow-beam attenuation through an absorber. Measurements are under "good geometry" (i.e., scattered photons are not measured).

- *Attenuation coefficient* (μ) characterizes a photon beam for its penetration power in a given medium. It depends on the beam energy and the material composition (density and atomic number) of the absorber or medium.

- Attenuation coefficient pertains to the primary beam. It is measured for a narrow beam and under "good geometry" conditions in which the scattered photons are excluded from measurement (Figure 5A.2).

- *Half-value layer* (HVL) is the thickness of an absorber required to attenuate the primary beam intensity to half its original value. It is measured for a narrow beam under "good geometry" conditions, as illustrated in Figure 5A.2.

- HVL layer and attenuation coefficient are related (analogous to half-life and disintegration constant in radioactivity) by the following relationship:

$$\text{HVL} = \frac{0.693}{\mu}$$

- For a typical x-ray beam, which has a spectrum of photon energies (bremsstrahlung), attenuation in a medium is not exactly exponential with a single value of μ. Similarly, a broad beam (containing scattered photons) will not follow exponential attenuation exactly.

- Practical megavoltage x-ray beams follow exponential attenuation in a medium only approximately in which an empirically determined "effective attenuation coefficient" may be assigned.

- *Energy transfer coefficient* (μ_{tr}) describes the fraction of photon energy transferred into kinetic energy of charged particles per unit thickness of absorber. This coefficient is related to μ as follows:

$$\mu_{tr} = \frac{\bar{E}_{tr}}{h\nu}\mu$$

where $\bar{E}_{tr}$ is the average energy transferred into kinetic energy of charged particles per interaction. The *mass energy transfer coefficient* is given by μ_{tr}/ρ, where ρ is the density of the medium. The mass energy transfer coefficient pertains to *kerma* which is the kinetic energy released per unit mass in the medium (see Chapter 8).

- *Energy absorption coefficient* is defined as the product of energy transfer coefficient and $(1 - g)$ where g is the fraction of the energy of secondary charged particles that is lost to bremsstrahlung in the material.

$$\mu_{en} = \mu_{tr}(1 - g)$$

As before, the mass energy absorption coefficient is given by μ_{en}/ρ. The mass energy absorption coefficient pertains to dose that is the energy absorbed per unit mass of the medium (see Chapter 8).

PHOTON INTERACTIONS

- There are five major types of interactions of photons with matter: coherent scattering, photoelectric effect, Compton effect, pair production, and photodisintegration.

COHERENT SCATTERING

- Coherent scattering interaction (also known as classical scattering or Rayleigh scattering) consists of a photon setting an orbital electron into oscillation. The oscillating electron reradiates energy at the same frequency as the incident photon (Figure 5A.3).

- No energy is absorbed in the medium from coherent scattering. The only effect is the scattering of photon at small angles.

- Coherent scattering is probable in high atomic materials and with photons of low energy.

Atom

PHOTOELECTRIC EFFECT

- The photoelectric effect is a phenomenon in which a photon is absorbed by an atom resulting in the ejection of an orbital electron.

Figure 5A.3. Diagram illustrating the process of coherent scattering. The scattered photon has the same wavelength as the incident photon. No energy is transferred.

- In the photoelectric process, the entire energy $h\nu$ of the photon is first absorbed by the atom and then transferred to an orbital electron. The kinetic energy of the ejected electron (called the photoelectron) is equal to $h\nu - E_B$, where E_B is the binding energy of the electron. Interactions of this type can take place with electrons in the K, L, M, or N shells.

- Ejection of a photoelectron may cause the emission of characteristic x-rays and Auger electrons (Figure 5A.4).

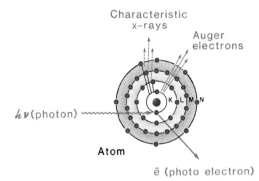

Figure 5A.4. Illustration of the photoelectric effect.

- Probability of photoelectric absorption depends on the photon energy as illustrated in Figure 5A.5, where the mass photoelectric attenuation coefficient (τ/ρ) is plotted as a function of photon energy.

- From the graph shown in Figure 5A.5, we get the following relationship between the mass photoelectric coefficient τ/ρ and photon energy E:

$$\tau/\rho \propto 1/E^3$$

- The data for various materials indicate that photoelectric attenuation depends strongly on the atomic number Z of the absorbing material. The following equation demonstrates approximate relationship:

$$\tau/\rho \propto Z^3$$

- Thus, the attenuation of photons in a medium depends inversely on E^3 and directly on Z^3.

- Attenuation by photoelectric effect is dramatically increased when the photon energy just equals the binding energy of a shell. This increased absorption is called the *absorption edge*.

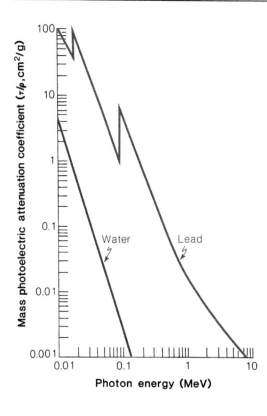

Figure 5A.5. Mass photoelectric attenuation coefficient (τ/ρ) plotted against photon energy. Curves for water ($Z_{\text{eff}} = 7.42$) and lead ($Z = 82$). (Data from Grodstein GW. *X-ray Attenuation Coefficients from 10 keV to 100 MeV.* Publication No. 583. Washington, DC: Bureau of Standards; 1957.)

COMPTON EFFECT

- The Compton interaction involves a collision between the photon and a "free" electron. The term *free* here means the binding energy of the electron is much smaller than the energy of the bombarding photon.

- In the Compton interaction, the electron receives some energy from the photon and is emitted at an angle θ. The photon, with reduced energy, is scattered at an angle ϕ (Figure 5A.6).

- In the Compton collision process, the energy and angle of scatter of the scattered photon and electron can be predicted by the application of the basic physics laws—*the laws of conservation of energy and momentum.*

- Compton interaction probability in water increases with photon energy from 10 to 150 keV. It then decreases with further increase in energy. However, it is the predominant mode of interaction in water for 30 keV to 24 MeV. That includes all photon beams used in radiation therapy.

- Compton probability is almost independent of Z. It depends on electron density (number of electrons per cm^3).

- Maximum energy of a photon scattered at 90° is 0.511 MeV, and at 180° it is 0.255 MeV.

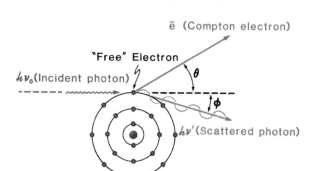

Figure 5A.6. Diagram illustrating the Compton effect.

PAIR PRODUCTION

- Pair production involves a high-energy photon interaction with the electromagnetic field of a nucleus. The entire energy of the photon is converted in creating a pair of electron (e^-) and positron (e^+) and providing them with kinetic energy (Figure 5A.7).
- The threshold energy for pair production is 1.02 MeV—just enough energy to create the electron–positron pair.
- Pair production probability increases slowly with photon energy beyond the 1.02 MeV threshold. It increases from approximately 6% at 4 MeV to 20% at 7 MeV (approximately, average energies of 12–21 MV x-ray beams, respectively).
- Pair production coefficient varies approximately as Z^2 per atom, Z per electron, and Z per gram.
- The reverse of the pair production process is *the electron–positron annihilation*, giving rise to two photons of each 0.511 MeV ejected in opposite direction (Figure 5A.8).

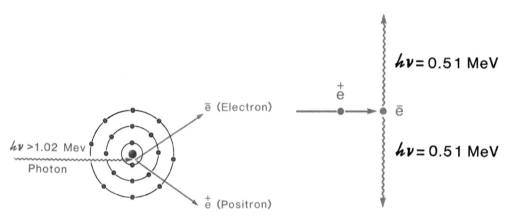

Figure 5A.7. Diagram illustrating the pair production process.

Figure 5A.8. Diagram illustrating the production of annihilation radiation.

PHOTODISINTEGRATION

- Photodisintegration involves a photon creating a nuclear reaction (described in section 2.8 F of the Textbook). In most cases it results in the emission of a neutron. The process is important only at high photon energies and is responsible for neutron contamination of therapy beams of energy greater than 10 MV.

RELATIVE IMPORTANCE OF PHOTON INTERACTIONS

- Table 5A.1 gives the relative importance of photoelectric, Compton, and pair production processes in water as a function of photon energy.
- Photon energy in column 1 of table 5A.1 is given in MeV. That means that the data presented here are for monoenergetic photons. For practical x-ray beams, one may apply these data (approximately) by assuming that the designated energy of an x-ray beam in MV is about three times its average energy (or energy of an equivalent monoenergetic beam) in MeV.
- The following approximate generalizations may be derived from the data in table 5A.1:
  - ➤ Photoelectric is predominant for beams of <75 kV.
  - ➤ Compton is predominant for beams of ~75 kV to 70 MV.
  - ➤ Pair production is predominant for beams of >70 MV.

TABLE 5A.1	Relative Importance of Photoelectric (τ), Compton (σ), and Pair Production (Π) Processes in Water		
	Relative Number of Interactions (%)		
Photon Energy (MeV)	τ	σ	Π
0.01	95	5	0
0.026	50	50	0
0.060	7	93	0
0.150	0	100	0
4.00	0	94	6
10.00	0	77	23
24.00	0	50	50
100.00	0	16	84

Data from Johns HE, Cunningham JR. *The Physics of Radiology*. 3rd edition. Springfield, IL: Charles C Thomas.

- In all clinically used megavoltage photon beams, the predominant interaction process in water or soft tissue is the Compton effect.

- Pair production threshold is at 1.02 MeV but its contribution is relatively small in clinical beams (~5% at 10 MV to ~20% at 25 MV).

REFERENCE

Khan FM. *The Physics of Radiation Therapy,* 4th edition, 2009. Chapter 5 "Interactions of Ionizing Radiation"

Particle Interactions

 TOPIC OUTLINE

The following topics will be discussed in this lecture:

➤ Charged particle interactions
  • Electrons
  • Protons
  • Heavy ions
➤ Stopping power
➤ Bragg peak
➤ Neutron interactions

CHARGED PARTICLE INTERACTIONS

• Charged particles may be classified as light or heavy, depending on their masses.

• Electrons and positrons are called "light" particles because of their very tiny mass (~1/1840 of mass of a proton).

• A charged particle is called "heavy" if its rest mass is large compared to the rest mass of an electron. EXAMPLE: Protons, mesons, α-particles, and atomic nuclei.

• All charged particles may undergo the following types of interactions in a medium to a varying degree, depending on their charge, mass, and velocity.

  1. **Inelastic collision with atomic electrons:** This process leads to ionization and excitation of the atoms. It is the most dominant process of energy loss for charged particles in low atomic number media (e.g., air, water, tissues).

     • In ionization, the energy transfer to an orbital electron exceeds its binding energy. The electron is stripped off the atom, thus creating an ion pair (the residual atom being a positive ion and another atom acquiring the stripped electron is the negative ion).

     • Secondary ionization is also possible if the stripped electron acquires sufficiently high kinetic energy to cause further ionization and excitation. The ejected electron is then called a secondary electron or δ-ray.

     • In excitation, the energy transfer to the orbital electron does not exceed its binding energy. The electron is raised to a higher energy level and may subsequently emit energy in the form of x-rays by returning to a lower energy state.

     • A certain amount of kinetic energy of the particle is lost at each ionization/excitation event, depending on the type and energy of the charged particle and the composition of the medium being ionized. EXAMPLE: Average energy loss per ion pair in dry air is approximately 34 eV for electrons and 35 eV for α-particles (ignoring small variation with particle energy).

- Both ionization and excitation can lead to breakage of molecular bonds. If the absorbing medium consists of body tissues, sufficient energy may be deposited within the cells, destroying their reproductive capacity. However, most of the absorbed energy is converted into heat, producing no biologic effect.

2. **Inelastic collision with nucleus:** This process can lead to bremsstrahlung (discussed in Chapter 3) in which a part of the kinetic energy of the particle is converted into x-rays. The process is more important for electrons than heavy charged particles.

3. **Elastic collision with nucleus:** The particle suffers Coulomb scattering with a nucleus without significant loss of energy.

    - Elastic collisions with nuclei are the main contributor of Coulomb scattering of charged particles.

    - Compared to the electron beams, the heavy charged particle beams have a smaller scattering angle and therefore sharper lateral distributions when traversing a dense medium.

4. **Elastic collision with atomic electrons:** The particle suffers Coulomb scattering with electrons without significant loss of energy.

5. **Nuclear reactions:** In addition to the Coulomb force interactions above, heavy charged particles can give rise to nuclear reactions (discussed in Chapter 2), thereby producing radionuclides. EXAMPLE: a proton beam passing through tissue can produce short-lived radioisotopes ^{11}C, ^{13}N, and ^{15}O, which are positron emitters.

STOPPING POWER

- The average rate of energy loss of a particle per unit path length in a medium is called the *stopping power*. The linear stopping power dE/dx is measured in units of MeV cm^{-1}.

- Related to the stopping power is the *linear energy transfer* (LET) of the particle. LET is the energy transferred to the medium (less that carried away by δ-rays) and is usually expressed as keV μm^{-1} in water. These basic parameters, namely stopping power and LET, are closely related to dose deposition in a medium and with the biologic effectiveness of radiation.

- The rate of energy loss of a charged particle due to ionization and excitation (collisional stopping power) is proportional to the electron density (electrons per unit volume) of the medium, the square of the particle charge, and inverse square of the particle velocity.

- As the particle continually loses energy in a medium, it slows down and the rate of energy loss per unit path length increases. As the particle velocity approaches zero near the end of its range, the rate of energy loss becomes maximum.

- The absorbed dose (energy absorbed per unit mass) follows the rate of energy loss in the medium. The sharp increase or peak in dose deposition at the end of the particle range is called the *Bragg peak* (Figure 5B.1).

- All heavy charged particles exhibit Bragg peak at the end of their range.

- Bragg peak is not observed for electron beams. Because electrons are very light particles, they suffer greater degree of scattering than heavy charged particles. Consequently, multiple changes in electron direction during the slowing down process smear out the Bragg peak.

- The rate of energy loss due to bremsstrahlung (radiative stopping power) increases with the increase in the kinetic energy of the particle and the atomic number of the medium. As stated earlier, the bremsstrahlung process is much more important with electrons than with heavy particles.

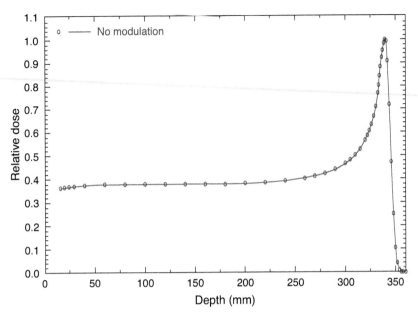

Figure 5B.1. Central axis depth dose distribution for an unmodulated 250 MeV proton beam, showing a narrow Bragg peak. (Data from synchrotron at Loma Linda University, CA. From Miller DW. A review of proton beam radiation therapy. *Med Phys.* 1995;22:1943–1954. Reproduced with permission.)

NEUTRON INTERACTIONS

- Neutron interactions in a medium may be classified into the following categories: a) elastic collisions with nuclei, b) inelastic collisions with nuclei, c) neutron capture

  ➤ *Elastic collisions with nuclei*: Elastic collision is a collision in which the total kinetic energy of the colliding bodies is the same before and after the collision.

    • Elastic collisions of neutrons with nuclei may be likened to billiard-ball collisions in which the kinetic energy of the neutron is redistributed after the collision between the neutron and the target nucleus.

    • The kinetic energy transferred to a stationary nucleus depends on the nuclear mass or its mass number.

    • Maximum transfer of kinetic energy will take place in a "head-on" collision along the original line of flight. By applying the principle of *conservation of energy and momentum,* the following relationship may be derived for a head-on collision:

$$E_\mathrm{f} = E_\mathrm{i}\left(\frac{M-m}{M+m}\right)^2$$

    where

    E_f = kinetic energy of final (scattered) neutron
    E_i = kinetic energy of incident neutron
    M = mass of targeted nucleus
    m = mass of neutron

    • The fraction of the original kinetic energy transferred, ΔE, to a nucleus of mass number A in a head on collision follows from the above equation:

$$\Delta E = \frac{4A}{(1+A)^2}$$

    where $\Delta E = (E_\mathrm{i} - E_\mathrm{f})/E_\mathrm{i}$

- From the above equation, we get a maximum value of 1.00 for a hydrogen nucleus that has $A = 1$. That means that all the kinetic energy of the neutron, in a "head-on" collision with a hydrogen nucleus, is transferred to the recoil proton.

- The energy transfer is less efficient for heavier nuclei.

- For the same reason, the most efficient absorbers of fast neutrons are the hydrogenous materials such as water, paraffin wax, polyethylene, and other plastics. Lead, which is a very efficient absorber for x-rays, is a poor shielding material against neutrons.

- Dose deposited in tissue from a high-energy neutron beam is predominantly contributed by recoil protons.

- Because of the higher hydrogen content, the dose absorbed in fat exposed to a neutron beam is approximately 20% higher than that in muscle.

➤ *Inelastic collisions with nuclei*: In this process, a neutron strikes a nucleus, is absorbed, and forms a compound nucleus. The compound nucleus is left in an excited state and de-excites with the emission of a neutron and a γ-ray photon. The reaction is denoted as (n, nγ). The general reaction is written as:

$$ {}^{A}_{Z}X + {}^{1}_{0}n \rightarrow {}^{A+1}_{Z}X^{*} \rightarrow {}^{A}_{Z}X + {}^{1}_{0}n + \gamma $$

Alternatively, the compound nucleus may de-excite by emitting a charged particle (a proton or an α-particle). The nuclear reactions are then denoted as (n, p) and (n, α).

- Inelastic collisions generally happen when high-energy neutrons interact with heavy nuclei.

- Nuclear disintegrations produced by neutrons in soft tissue result in the emission of heavy charged particles, neutrons, and γ-rays, thereby contributing approximately 30% of the tissue dose in patients treated with high-energy neutron beams.

➤ *Neutron capture (or radiative capture)*: This is the most common neutron capture reaction and is denoted as (n, γ). In this case the compound nucleus is raised to one of its excited states and then immediately returns to its normal state with the emission of a γ-ray photon. The emitted γ-ray is called the *capture γ-ray*. EXAMPLE:

$$ {}^{59}_{27}\text{Co} + {}^{1}_{0}n \rightarrow {}^{60}_{27}\text{Co} + \gamma $$

In the above neutron capture reaction, ^{60}Co nucleus is still in the excited state and decays (half-life = 5.26 years) into stable ^{60}Ni by the emission of β-particles and two γ-rays (energies of 1.17 and 1.33 MeV).

- The neutron capture probability is approximately inversely proportional to its velocity. The slower the neutron, the greater the time it spends in the vicinity of the target nucleus and, therefore, greater the probability of its capture.

- Thermal neutrons, which have an average energy of about 0.025 eV (in thermal equilibrium with their surroundings at a temperature of 20°C), have a higher probability of capture than the fast neutrons. At high energies (e.g., 10 MeV or greater), neutron capture has a low probability but it is not zero.

- **Fission:** Neutrons can induce a fission reaction in some heavy nuclei. For lighter elements (below lead), fission cross sections are negligible. Further discussion of fission is contained in Lecture 2B.

REVIEW QUESTIONS • Chapter 5

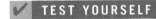

Review questions for this chapter are provided online.

In multiple choice questions, more than one option may be correct.

1. Photoelectric cross section varies with the photon energy E and atomic number Z of the absorber as:

   a) $1/E^3$
   b) $1/E$
   c) Z^3
   d) $1/Z$

2. In a Compton collision between a 10 MeV photon and an electron, the energy of the photon scattered at a right angle is approximately:

   a) 5 MeV
   b) 0.5 MeV
   c) 0.25 MeV
   d) 0.025 MeV

3. The threshold energy for a photon to interact by pair production is:

   a) 0.511 MeV
   b) 1.022 MeV
   c) 2.044 MeV
   d) 4.088 MeV

4. Which of the following photon energies are correctly matched with their most predominant interactions in soft tissue?

   a) 10 keV → Rayleigh scattering
   b) 150 keV → Photoelectric effect
   c) 1.25 MeV (cobalt-60 γ-rays) → Compton effect
   d) 10 MeV → Compton effect

5. A 14 MeV neutron collides "head-on" with a hydrogen nucleus. The kinetic energy of the recoil proton will be:

   a) 14 MeV
   b) 7 MeV
   c) 1.022 MeV
   d) 0.511 MeV

6. Compared to the electrons, protons:

   a) Scatter through smaller angles
   b) Generate more bremsstrahlung per unit path length
   c) Have greater LET
   d) Have a sharper lateral dose distribution at the field edges

7. What is the maximum energy a photon can have after Compton scattering at an angle of 30°?

   a) 512 keV
   b) 256 keV
   c) 3.8 MeV
   d) 4.3 MeV
   e) There is no maximum energy

8. Which of the following interaction processes is most likely for a 10 keV photon in water?

   a) Photoelectric effect
   b) Compton effect
   c) Pair production
   d) Rayleigh scattering
   e) None of the above

9. Which of the following statements are true:

    a) The energy threshold for a single photon pair production event is 511 keV.
    b) For a ^{60}Co beam, the mass attenuation coefficient in water is greater than in lead.
    c) For any given energy, the energy absorption coefficient, μ_{en}, is always less than the attenuation coefficient, μ.
    d) Photoelectric interaction can give rise to Auger electrons.
    e) None of the above.

10. The stopping power in MeV/cm due to ionization in water of an electron of energy E in the range of 2 MeV and above is S_E. What would the approximate stopping power of this particle be in aluminum if the energy was reduced to $E/2$?

    a) $0.09 \times S_E$
    b) $0.18 \times S_E$
    c) $1.3 \times S_E$
    d) $2.7 \times S_E$
    e) $5.4 \times S_E$

11. What percentage of its incident energy a 2 MeV neutron would transfer to a ^{11}B nucleus during a head-on collision?

    a) 8
    b) 15
    c) 31
    d) 100

12. The fraction of energy transferred in a head-on neutron collision with a lead nucleus ($A = 207$) would be:

    a) 0.01
    b) 0.02
    c) 0.1
    d) 0.2
    e) $\Delta E = 1$

13. A high-energy positron can undergo which of the following interactions as it traverses matter?

    a) Ionization and excitation
    b) Bremsstrahlung
    c) Coulomb scattering
    d) Compton scattering
    e) Annihilation

14. Attenuation of a photon beam by Compton effect in an absorber of thickness 1 g/cm^2:

    a) Depends on number of electrons/g
    b) Is greater in soft tissue than in bone
    c) Is greater in air than in water
    d) Is greater in hydrogen than in lead

15. Which statement (s) is (are) true about Compton effect?

    a) The electron may acquire any energy from 0 up to the energy of the incident photon.
    b) The wavelength of the scatter photon is less than that of the incident photon.
    c) The photon changes direction but does not lose energy.
    d) Maximum energy is imparted to the electron when the photon is scattered at 180°.

16. A 10 MeV photon interacts by pair production. What are the kinetic energies of the particles produced? [Assume available kinetic energy is shared equally between the particles.]

    a) 4.49 MeV
    b) 5.51 MeV
    c) 8.98 MeV
    d) Spectrum of energies equally shared between the particles

MEASUREMENT OF IONIZING RADIATION

LECTURE

6A

REFERENCE

Khan FM. *The Physics of Radiation Therapy*, 4th edition, 2009. Chapter 6 "Measurement of Ionizing Radiation"

Measurement of Exposure

 TOPIC OUTLINE

The following topics will be discussed in this lecture:
➤ Exposure: definition and units
➤ Electronic equilibrium
➤ Free-air ionization chamber
➤ Thimble chambers
➤ Exposure calibration of ion chambers
➤ Exposure measurement

EXPOSURE

- *Definition*: The International Commission on Radiation Units and Measurements (ICRU) defines exposure (X) as the quotient of dQ by dm where dQ is the absolute value of the total charge of the ions of one sign produced in air when all the electrons (negatrons and positrons) liberated by photons in air of mass dm are completely stopped in air.

$$X = \frac{dQ}{dm}$$

- *Units*: The SI unit for exposure is coulomb per kilogram (C/kg). The special unit is roentgen (R).

$$1R = 2.58 \times 10^{-4}\, C/kg\ air$$

- Note that the definition of exposure requires that "all the electrons (negatrons and positrons) liberated by photons in air of mass dm are completely stopped in air." In practical terms, that condition can only be met if an electronic equilibrium exists in the air volume from which the ions are collected.

- Also note that the term exposure applies only to x- and γ-radiations and is a measure of ionization in air only.

ELECTRONIC EQUILIBRIUM

The principle of electronic equilibrium is illustrated in Figure 6A.1. The ion collection volume is shown as shaded area enclosed by the collecting electrodes. According to the definition of exposure, the electrons produced in air by photons in the specified collection volume must spend all their energies in that volume by ionization and the total ionic charge of either sign should be measured. However, some electrons produced in the specified volume deposit their energy outside the region of ion collection and thus are not measured. Conversely, electrons produced outside the specified

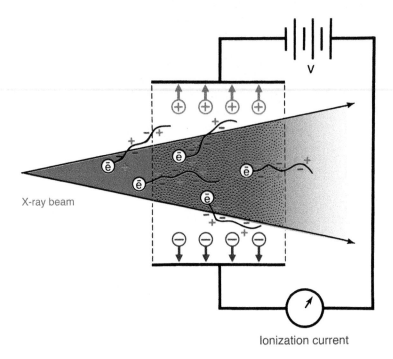

Figure 6A.1. Diagram illustrating electronic equilibrium in a free-air chamber.

volume may enter the ion-collecting region and produce ionization there. If the ionization loss is compensated by the ionization gained, a condition of *electronic equilibrium* exists. Under this condition, the definition of exposure is effectively satisfied. This is the principle of the *free-air ionization chamber.*

FREE-AIR IONIZATION CHAMBER

- *The free-air ionization chamber is an absolute ion chamber for measuring exposure.* It does not need calibration against another chamber or a standard. A free-air ionization chamber is represented schematically in Figure 6A.2.

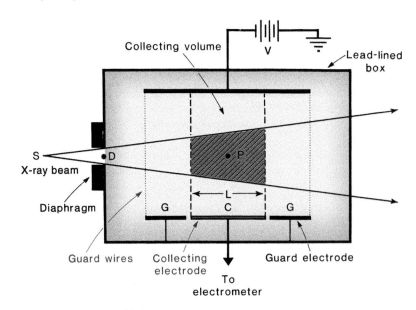

Figure 6A.2. A schematic diagram of a free-air chamber.

- There are limitations on the design of a free-air chamber for high-energy x-ray beams. Because the range of electrons librated by photons increases with photon energy, electronic equilibrium cannot be maintained in the collecting volume beyond a certain limit of photon energy. There is an upper limit on the photon energy above which the roentgen cannot be accurately measured. This limit occurs at approximately 3 MeV.

- Free-air ionization chambers are too delicate and bulky for routine use. Their main function is in the standardizing laboratories where they can be used to calibrate field instruments such as a thimble chamber for low-energy beams (e.g., superficial or orthovoltage x-rays).

THIMBLE CHAMBERS

- *Principle*: By compressing the volume of air required for electronic equilibrium, we can reduce its dimensions. In fact, the air volume required for electronic equilibrium can be substituted by a small air cavity with solid air-equivalent wall so that the electronic equilibrium is maintained in the air cavity. This is the principle of a thimble chamber, illustrated in Figure 6A.3.

- As before, it follows that the wall thickness of a thimble chamber must be equal to or greater than the maximum range of the electrons liberated in the thimble wall. If the wall is not thick enough, a close-fitting buildup cap is required to provide electronic equilibrium for the radiation in question.

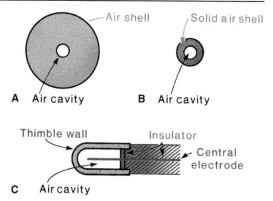

Figure 6A.3. Schematic diagram illustrating the nature of the thimble ionization chamber. **A:** Air shell with air cavity. **B:** Solid air shell with air cavity. **C:** The thimble chamber.

- *The thimble*: Figure 6.3C shows a typical thimble ionization chamber. The wall is shaped like a sewing thimble—hence the name. The inner surface of the thimble wall is coated by a special material to make it electrically conducting. This forms one electrode. The other electrode is a rod of low atomic number material such as graphite or aluminum held in the center of the thimble but electrically insulated from it. A suitable voltage is applied between the two electrodes to collect the ions produced in the air cavity.

  ➤ *Wall composition*: Ideally, the thimble wall (also called chamber wall) must be air-equivalent so that it interacts with photons the same way as air. That means it should have the same atomic number (Z) as air. However, exact Z equivalence of wall materials is neither possible nor necessary. Reason: The thimble chamber is a secondary ion chamber, that is, it must be calibrated against a standard chamber for the radiation beam in question. Thus, any small differences in Z are accounted for in its calibration factor.

  ➤ The most commonly used wall materials are made of graphite (carbon), Bakelite, or a plastic coated on the inside by a conducting layer of graphite or of a conducting mixture of Bakelite and graphite.

  ➤ *Sensitive volume (or cavity volume)*: The volume of air contained in the thimble cavity is the sensitive volume of the chamber. The thimble cavity usually contains air and communicates to the outside air through a tiny hole in the side of the chamber. During measurement with such a chamber, the temperature of air inside the cavity must be at equilibrium with the surrounding medium and the pressure of air must be the same as that of the surrounding atmosphere.

  ➤ Ionization produced in the air cavity is by electrons crossing the cavity, not by photon interactions with the cavity air. These electrons are ejected by photons as a result of their interactions with the chamber wall and the surrounding buildup cap or the medium in which the thimble might be embedded (e.g. chamber embedded in a water or plastic phantom).

CHAMBER CALIBRATION

- The ionization charge measured is contributed by the mass of air contained in the cavity. If Q is the ionization charge measured under equilibrium conditions and v the cavity volume (also called chamber volume), then the exposure X is given by: $X = Q/\rho_{air} v$, where ρ_{air} is the density of air. However, the volume of thimble chambers is not known with sufficient accuracy with this equation. Therefore, a thimble chamber must be calibrated against a standard instrument. *The thimble chamber is a secondary instrument.*

- In actual practice, the thimble chambers are calibrated against a free-air chamber for x-rays up to a few hundred kilovolts. For higher energies (up to ^{60}Co γ-rays), the thimble chambers are calibrated against a standard cavity chamber (e.g. spherical chambers with nearly air-equivalent walls and accurately known volume). In any case, the exposure calibration of a thimble chamber removes the need for knowing its cavity volume (see Chapter 8).

- When the calibration factor is applied to the chamber reading (corrected for changes in temperature and pressure of cavity air), it converts the value into true exposure in free air (without chamber). The exposure value thus obtained is free from the wall attenuation or the perturbing influence of the chamber.

CHAMBER CHARACTERISTICS

- *Chamber sensitivity*: It is defined as the ionization charge measured per roentgen. Sensitivity is directly proportional to the chamber-sensitive volume. EXAMPLE: The sensitivity of a Cutie Pie survey meter (volume ~600 mL) used for measuring low-level x-rays is approximately 1,000 times the sensitivity of a Farmer-type thimble chamber (volume ~0.6 mL) used for calibration of a treatment beam.

- *Stem leakage*: A chamber is known to have stem leakage if it records ionization produced anywhere other than its sensitive volume (extra-cameral ionization). The stem effect is caused by the measurement of a signal arising from ionization occurring in the chamber stem and the cable. Stem leakage depends on the chamber design, beam quality (modality and energy), and irradiation conditions (e.g. the extent of stem and cable exposed to radiation).

- *Bias voltage*: The voltage difference between the electrodes of an ion chamber is called the bias voltage.
  - ➤ As the bias voltage is increased from zero, the ionization current increases at first almost linearly and later more slowly. The curve finally approaches a *saturation* value for the given exposure rate (Figure 6A.4).
  - ➤ The initial increase of ionization current with voltage is caused by incomplete ion collection at low bias voltages. The negative and the positive ions tend to recombine unless they are quickly separated by the electric field. This recombination can be minimized by increasing the field strength (V/cm).
  - ➤ The chamber should be used in the saturation region so that small changes in the voltage do not result in changes in the ionic current.

- *Polarity effect*: If for a given exposure, the ionic charge collected by an ion chamber changes in magnitude as the polarity of the collecting voltage is reversed, the chamber is said to show a polarity effect.
  - ➤ With the chamber operating under saturation conditions, major causes of the polarity effects include the following:
    - High-energy electrons such as Compton electrons ejected by high-energy photons constitute a current (also called the *Compton current*) independent of gas (cavity air) ionization.

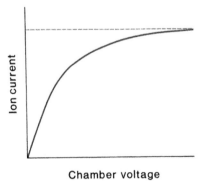

Figure 6A.4. Saturation curve for an ion chamber.

- Extracameral current collected outside the sensitive volume (e.g. stem, cable, and inadequately screened collector circuit points).

➤ The magnitude of polarity effect depends on chamber design, beam energy and modality, adequacy of bias voltage, and irradiation conditions.

➤ The errors caused by the polarity effect can be minimized but not eliminated by reversing the chamber polarity and taking the mean value of the collector current.

➤ Ideally, the difference between the ionization currents measured at positive and negative polarizing potential should be <0.5% for any radiation beam quality.

- *Efficiency of ion collection*: The ion collection efficiency is defined as the ratio of the number of ions collected to the number produced.

➤ Ideally, all the ions produced should be collected before they have a chance to recombine. That means the bias voltage on the chamber should be sufficiently high to minimize recombination losses, that is, bias voltage well within the saturation region (Figure 6A.4).

➤ Depending on the chamber design and the ionization intensity, a certain amount of ionization loss by recombination can be expected.

➤ At very high ionization intensity, such as is possible in the case of pulsed beams, significant loss of charge by recombination may occur even at bias voltages in the saturation region. Under these conditions, the *recombination losses* may have to be accepted and the correction has to be applied for these losses.

➤ One method (*the half-voltage method*) of determining ion recombination correction (P_{ion}) at the selected bias voltage V_1 is to measure ionization at another bias voltages V_2, so that $V_2 = V_1/2$. The ratio of the two readings (Q_1/Q_2) is related to P_{ion} (Figure 6A.5).

- *Temperature and pressure correction* ($P_{T,P}$): If the ion chamber is open to the atmosphere, its response is affected by temperature and pressure of the air in the chamber cavity.

➤ In the United States, the calibration laboratories [National Institute of Standards and Technology (NIST) and Accredited Dose Calibration Laboratories (ADCLs)] provide chamber calibration factors for reference environmental conditions of temperature $T_0 = 22°C$ and pressure $P_0 = 760$ mm Hg or 101.33 kilopascal (kP$_a$) (1 atm). The temperature and pressure correction, $P_{T,P}$, at different conditions is given by:

$$P_{T,P} = \left(\frac{760}{P} \right)\left(\frac{273.2 + T}{273.2 + 22.0} \right) \quad [\text{for } P \text{ in mm Hg}]$$

or

$$P_{T,P} = \left(\frac{101.33}{P} \right)\left(\frac{273.2 + T}{273.2 + 22.0} \right) \quad [\text{for } P \text{ in kP}_a]$$

Note: Temperatures in the above equations are converted to the absolute scale of temperature (in degrees Kelvin) by adding 273.2 to the Celsius temperatures.

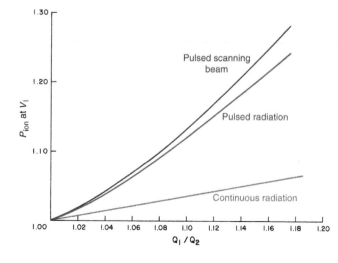

Figure 6A.5. Ion recombination correction factors (P_{ion}) for continuous radiation (^{60}Co, Van de Graaff), pulsed radiation (accelerator-produced x-rays and electron beams), and pulsed scanning beams. These data are applicable when $V_1 = 2V_2$. (From AAPM. A protocol for the determination of absorbed dose from high-energy photon and electron beams. *Med Phys.* 1983;10:741, with permission.)

EXPOSURE MEASUREMENT

The general equation for the measurements of exposure (X) in free air in units of roentgens (R) is the following:

$$X = M \cdot N_X \cdot P_{T,P} \cdot P_{ST} \cdot P_{ion}$$

where M is the chamber reading (coulombs) measured under equilibrium conditions and corrected for any polarity effect, N_X the chamber exposure calibration factor (R/coulomb) for the given quality beam, $P_{T,P}$ the temperature and pressure correction, P_{ST} the stem leakage correction, and P_{ion} the ion recombination correction.

➤ The quantity X is the exposure that would be expected in air at the point of measurement in the absence of the chamber. In other words, the correction for any perturbation produced in the beam by the chamber is inherent in the chamber calibration factor N_X.

➤ For low-energy beams such as superficial and orthovoltage x-rays, the thimble chambers are usually calibrated and used without a buildup cap. For higher energies such as ^{60}Co, a Lucite (acrylic) buildup cap is used unless the chamber wall is already thick enough to provide electronic equilibrium (e.g. Victoreen high-energy chambers).

➤ The above exposure measurements are made in free air with the chamber positioned in the beam in a configuration similar to the one used for its calibration (usually with its axis perpendicular to the beam axis). The use of the thimble chamber for the determination of absorbed dose in a phantom is discussed in Chapter 8.

REFERENCE
Khan FM. *The Physics of Radiation Therapy,* 4th edition, 2009. Chapter 6 "Measurement of Ionizing Radiation"

Chambers and Electrometers

 TOPIC OUTLINE

The following topics will be discussed in this lecture:
➤ Farmer-type chambers
➤ Thimble chambers for beam scanning
➤ Parallel-plate chambers
➤ Electrometers

FARMER-TYPE CHAMBERS

The original Farmer chamber was introduced by FT Farmer in 1955. A modified version of the original Farmer chamber by Aird and Farmer is shown in Figure 6B.1.

The *Farmer-type chambers* are constructed similar to the original Farmer chamber but vary mostly with respect to the composition of the wall material and the central electrode.

- Farmer-type chambers are the most commonly used ion chambers for the calibration of radiation therapy beams.

- Several Farmer-type chambers are commercially available. They are similar in overall design but differ significantly in materials and construction techniques. EXAMPLE: PTW, Capintec, NEL, Exradin, and others, each with several models and refinements.

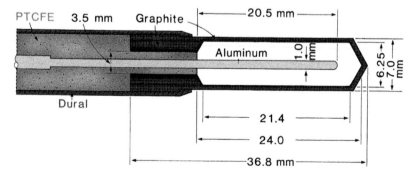

Figure 6B.1. Farmer graphite/aluminum chamber. Nominal air volume, 0.6 mL. PTCFE, polytrichlorofluorothylene. (Redrawn from Aird EGA, Farmer FT. The design of a thimble chamber for the Farmer dosimeter. *Phys Med Biol.* 1972;17:169, with permission.)

COMPONENTS AND CHARACTERISTICS

- *Chamber wall*: The thimble wall material may be graphite or plastic, such as PMMA (acrylic), nylon, AE (air-equivalent) plastic, and TE (tissue-equivalent) plastic.
  - ➤ In the case of a plastic thimble, the inner surface of the wall is made conducting with a thin coating of graphite.
  - ➤ The wall thickness of Farmer-type chambers varies between different makes and models. The approximate range is 0.04 to 0.09 g/cm^2.
- *Outer electrode*: The outer electrode is the thimble wall (if made of a conducting material) or the inner surface of the thimble wall coated with a conducting material.
- *Central electrode*: The central electrode consists of a thin aluminum rod of 1 mm diameter. It is the collector electrode, delivering the ionic current to a charge-measuring device, the electrometer.
- *Guard electrode*: A cylindrical conductor that wraps around the insulator surrounding the central electrode in the stem of the chamber. A second insulator wraps around the guard electrode, separating the guard from the outer electrode. The guard is kept at the same potential as the central electrode. Because there is no potential difference between the guard and the central electrode, any charge leakage does not get to the central electrode.
  - ➤ The function of the guard is to reduce the leakage of any extraneous charge to the collecting electrode.
- *Chamber (or cavity) volume*: Because the thimble is vented to the outside, the cavity volume determines the mass of air in the cavity and, therefore, the sensitivity (charge measured/unit exposure) of the chamber. Farmer-type chambers have a cylindrical cavity with a nominal volume of 0.6 mL. The cavity radius is approximately 0.3 cm.
- *Energy dependence*:
  - ➤ Energy dependence (change in response/unit exposure with beam energy) for an ion chamber, in general, depends on the composition and thickness of the wall material.
  - ➤ The energy response of the chamber designed by Aird and Farmer is shown in the form of a plot of calibration factor as a function of beam half-value layer (see Figure 6B.2). The response is almost constant from 0.3 mm Cu HVL upward and within 4% from 0.05 mm Cu upward.
- *Stem effect*: As discussed in the previous lecture, the stem effect arises out of irradiation of the stem and the radiation-induced signal in the cable, if exposed.
  - ➤ The stem effect originating in the stem is directly related to the length of the unguarded stem.
  - ➤ The stem effect (originating either in the stem or the cable) is a function of energy as well as type of beam (photon or particle).
  - ➤ The magnitude of stem effect in commonly used Farmer-type chambers, irradiated in a ^{60}Co beam, is in the range of 0.1% to 0.6%.

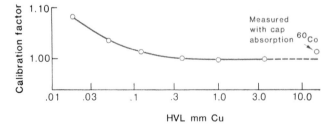

Figure 6B.2. Energy response of the chamber shown in Figure 6B.1. HVL, half-value layer. (Redrawn from Aird EGA, Farmer FT. The design of a thimble chamber for the Farmer dosimeter. *Phys Med Biol.* 1972;17:169.)

THIMBLE CHAMBERS FOR BEAM SCANNING

These chambers are used in beam data acquisition systems. A typical system consists of a water phantom equipped with two thimble chambers, one referred to as the probe A and the other monitor B. Whereas the probe is arranged to move in the tank of water to sample the dose rate at various points, the monitor is fixed at some point in the field to monitor the beam intensity with time. The ratio of the probe to the monitor response (A/B) is recorded as the probe is moved in the phantom.

- The desirable features of a scanning chamber are a good spatial resolution and a good signal-to-noise ratio.

- For good spatial resolution, the chamber should have a small sensitive volume, for example, cavity should have a small diameter and a small length. Too small a sensitive volume, however, runs counter to having a good signal-to-noise ratio. So a compromise needs to be achieved in which both features provide an acceptable accuracy of measuring relative depth dose distribution.

- The commonly used chambers (e.g., PTW, Capintec, Scanditronix-Wellhofer, and Exradin) for scanning have a range of cavity dimensions: sensitive volume, 0.1 to 0.3 mL; cavity diameter, 3.5 to 6 mm, and cavity length, 5.5 to 16 mm.

PARALLEL-PLATE CHAMBERS

Parallel-plate chambers have the two electrodes in the shape of flat plates parallel to each other. The air gap between the two electrodes constitutes the sensitive volume.

- There are two kinds of parallel-plate chambers: A) the *extrapolation chamber* with variable volume; B) the *plane-parallel chamber* with fixed volume.

A. Extrapolation Chamber

Figure 6B.3 shows a schematic diagram of an extrapolation chamber designed by Failla in 1937.

- In this chamber, the beam enters through a thin foil which is carbon coated to form the upper electrode. The lower or the collecting electrode is a small coin-shaped region surrounded by a guard ring and is connected to an electrometer.

- The electrode spacing can be varied accurately by micrometer screws. By measuring the ionization per unit volume as a function of electrode spacing, one can determine the surface dose by extrapolating the ionization curves to zero electrode spacing.

- Extrapolation chambers are not as practical as plane-parallel chambers with the fixed plate separation. However, they are the most accurate ion chambers for measuring surface dose or buildup of dose in a phantom.

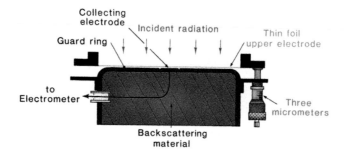

Figure 6B.3. Extrapolation ion chamber by Failla. (Redrawn from Boag JW. Ionization chambers. In: Attix FH, Roesch WC, eds. *Radiation Dosimetry.* Vol 2. New York: Academic Press; 1969:1, with permission.)

B. Plane-Parallel Chambers

Figure 6B.4 shows a Markus chamber, as an example.

- Plane-parallel chambers are similar to extrapolation chambers except that they have a fixed electrode spacing (~1–2 mm).

- A thin wall or window (e.g., foils of 0.01–0.03-mm-thick Mylar, polystyrene, or mica) allows measurements practically at the surface of a phantom without significant wall attenuation.

- By adding layers of phantom material on top of the chamber window, one can study the variation in dose as a function of depth at shallow depths where cylindrical chambers are unsuitable because of their larger cavity diameter.

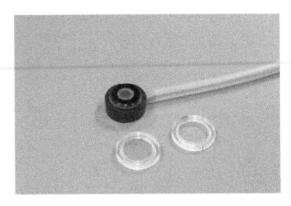

Figure 6B.4. Photograph of a 0.02 cm^3 Advanced Markus chamber (PTW Type 34045).

- Among the practical ion chambers, plane-parallel chambers are the dosimeters of choice for measuring dose at the surface of a phantom or in the buildup region where the dose increases rapidly with depth.

- The width of the guard ring should be sufficiently large to prevent electrons scattered by the side and back walls of the chamber from affecting the ionization in the ion-collecting volume of the cavity.

- The commonly used plane-parallel ion chambers (e.g., PTW Markus, Memorial, Capintec, Pitman) have a range of specifications with regard to sensitive volume, electrode spacing, entrance window thickness, width of guard ring, and so on, depending upon their usage and desired accuracy. EXAMPLE: The Advanced Markus chamber (PTW Type 34045) has a vented sensitive volume of 0.02 mL, electrode spacing of 1 mm, entrance window of 0.03 mm thick graphite-coated polyethylene membrane, guard ring of 2 mm width, and lower collector electrode of graphite-coated acrylic of diameter 5.4 mm. The chamber is waterproof when used with its protective acrylic cover of 0.87 mm thickness.

ELECTROMETERS

The electrometer is a charge-measuring device. Since the ionization current or charge to be measured by an ion chamber is very small, special electrometer circuits have been designed to measure it accurately. The most commonly used electrometers for ion chamber dosimetry are *negative-feedback operational amplifiers* (OP-AMP).

NEGATIVE-FEEDBACK OPERATIONAL AMPLIFIERS

Figure 6B.5 schematically shows three simplified circuits that are used to measure ionization in the integrate mode, rate mode, and direct-reading dosimeter mode. The OP-AMP is shown as a triangle with two input points. A negative feedback is provided by connecting a capacitor (Figure 6B.5A and 5C) or a resistor (Figure 6B.5B) between the negative input terminal (inverting terminal) and the output terminal. [The term negative feedback here means that some or all of the output is fed back into the inverting input terminal.]

- The operational amplifier has a very high open-loop gain (>10^4) and a very high input impedance (>10^{12} Ω).

- Because of these conditions, it can be shown that in a negative-feedback operational amplifier:

  ➤ Essentially no current flows into the amplifier. The current flows through the feedback circuit.

  ➤ The output voltage is dictated by the feedback element, independent of the open-loop gain.

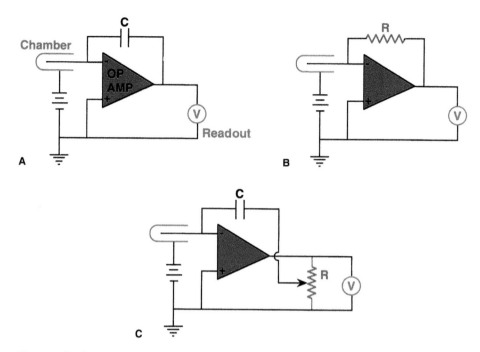

Figure 6B.5. Schematic diagrams of ion chambers connected to negative-feedback operational amplifiers. **A:** Integrate mode. **B:** Rate mode. **C:** Direct-exposure reading mode.

➤ The potential between the positive and negative inputs of the amplifier (called the error voltage) is maintained very low (<100 mV) and, consequently, the current through the amplifier (called the offset current) is very low.

➤ The gain of the circuit can be controlled precisely by the feedback element.

• *Integrate mode*: In this circuit, the ionization charge produced by the ion chamber is deposited on the capacitor C of the feedback element (see Figure 6B.5A). The voltage across C is measured by voltmeter *V*. The accumulated charge *Q* is given by

$$Q = CV$$

where *Q* is charge in coulombs, *C* capacitance in farads, and *V* voltage in volts.

➤ The response of an electrometer with such a feedback circuit is independent of the amplifier gain.

➤ The accuracy is totally dependent on the feedback element and the readout device (voltmeter).

➤ The very low offset current of the amplifier does not alter the transferred charge.

➤ The very high input impedance of the amplifier does not allow the charge to bleed away during short intervals.

• *Rate mode*: In this configuration (shown in Figure 6B.5B), the ionization current *I* from the ion chamber flows through the feedback resistor *R*. The output voltage *V* is given by

$$V = RI$$

where *V* is in volts, *R* in ohms, and *I* amperes.

➤ The output voltage is a measure of the input current.

➤ The very low offset current of the amplifier has a negligible effect on the input current *I*.

• *Direct-exposure reading mode*: If a variable fraction of the output voltage is fed back to the input as by a voltage divider (Figure 6B.5C), the electrometer can be converted into a direct-exposure reading (*R* or *R*/min) instrument for a given chamber and a given quality of radiation.

REVIEW QUESTIONS • Chapter 6

✔ **TEST YOURSELF**

Review questions for this chapter are provided online.

In multiple choice questions, more than one option may be correct.

1. A free air ionization chamber has a 10 mm diameter aperture, a plate separation of 90 mm, and a collection length of 70 mm. Neglecting divergence of the beam, what is the mass of air in the collection region, using $p_{air} = 1.293$ kg/m^3?

   a) 7 µg
   b) 10 µg
   c) 7 mg
   d) 8 mg
   e) 10 mg

2. An unsealed ion chamber is compared to a sealed ion chamber with all dimensions exactly twice the size. If the internal pressure is 3 atm, what should the sensitivity of the new chamber be relative to the unsealed one?

   a) 1/24
   b) 1/6
   c) The same
   d) 6
   e) 24

3. For small recombination corrections, P_{ion} for a pulsed ion beam is approximately given by the following equation:

$$P_{ion} = \left[\left(1 - \frac{V_H}{V_L}\right) \middle/ \left(\frac{M_H}{M_L} - \frac{V_H}{V_L}\right)\right]$$

   where M_H and M_L are the measured readings for bias voltages V_H and V_L respectively. If M_H is 1% higher than M_L when the bias voltage is doubled, what is the value of P_{ion}?

   a) 0.98
   b) 0.99
   c) 1.00
   d) 1.01
   e) 1.02

4. Calculate the temperature and pressure correction applied to a calibrated ion chamber reading for an environmental pressure of 745 mm Hg and a temperature of 25°C:

   a) 0.970
   b) 0.990
   c) 1.000
   d) 1.010
   e) 1.031

5. A monoenergetic photon beam of 25 keV energy interacts by photoelectric process with 3×10^4 atoms/mm^3 in dry air of density 1.205 kg/m^3. Assuming that the charged particle equilibrium exits and $W/e = 33.97$ J/C, what is the exposure X of this beam? [Assume a binding energy for dry air of 0.5 keV.]

   a) 40 C/kg
   b) 2.9×10^{-3} C/kg
   c) 1.8×10^{-6} R
   d) 53 C/kg
   e) 7.8×10^{-4} C/kg

6. What would be the approximate average pressure in mm Hg at a site with an elevation of 3,600 feet? [Assume pressure drop of about 1 inch Hg per 1,000 feet.]

   a) 668.6
   b) 724.0
   c) 754.6
   d) 756.4

7. If an ion chamber, which bears a calibration factor specified at 760 mm Hg and 22°C, is used to calibrate a linear accelerator located at the above site, what would be the temperature and pressure correction factor applied to the chamber reading if the pressure is equal to the average pressure and the temperature is 24°C?

   a) 1.012
   b) 1.022
   c) 1.057
   d) 1.145

8. If the pressure is erroneously measured to be 760 mm Hg in the above problem, what would be the percentage error in calibration?

   a) 0.05
   b) 0.10
   c) 4.9
   d) 13.7
   e) 14.5

9. In the above problem, the calibration error would cause:

   a) The patients to be underdosed significantly.
   b) The patients to be overdosed significantly.
   c) The patients to be underdosed but not significantly.
   d) The patients would be overdosed but not significantly.

10. A thimble chamber has a sensitive volume of 0.6×10^{-6} m^3. If the air density is 1.205 kg/m^3 and the exposure is 100 R, what is the charge collected? [Assume electronic equilibrium, air equivalence of wall, no wall attenuation, no stem effect, and no ion recombination.]

    a) 1.44×10^{-8} C
    b) 1.87×10^{-8} C
    c) 2.91×10^{-8} C
    d) 3.12×10^{-8} C

11. In the above problem, what is the chamber calibration factor in units of roentgens/coulomb, specified at 760 mm Hg and 22°C?

    a) 3.21×10^{9} R/C
    b) 3.43×10^{9} R/C
    c) 5.34×10^{9} R/C
    d) 5.79×10^{9} R/C

12. Chamber polarity effect:

    a) Is caused by positive ions being heavier than negative ions.
    b) Can be caused by Compton current independent of cavity air ionization.
    c) Is, in general, more severe for measurements in electron beams than photon beams.
    d) Can be corrected by taking the mean of readings at both polarities.

13. Ion collection efficiency is:

    a) Greater for positive ions than for negative ions.
    b) In general, less for pulsed radiation than for continuous radiation at the same dose rate (dose/minute).
    c) Always 100% at the saturation bias voltage.
    d) Dependent on the atmospheric temperature and pressure.

14. Negative-feedback operational amplifiers used in electrometers:

   a) Amplify ionic current by a factor of 1,000 or more.
   b) Have high open-loop gain ($>10^4$).
   c) Have high input impedance ($>10^{12}$ Ω).
   d) Allow the ionic current to flow unimpeded through the amplifier.

15. Regarding the guard electrode in an ion chamber:

   a) The guard electrode in a Farmer-type chamber prevents leakage from the high-voltage collector electrode.
   b) The guard ring in a plane-parallel chamber makes the chamber waterproof.
   c) The guard ring electrode better defines the ion-collecting volume.
   d) The guard electrode minimizes polarity effect.

QUALITY OF X-RAY BEAMS

LECTURE

7

REFERENCE
Khan FM. *The Physics of Radiation Therapy*, 4th edition, 2009. Chapter 7 "Quality of X-ray Beams"

Specification and Measurement of X-Ray Beam Quality

 TOPIC OUTLINE

The following topics will be discussed in this lecture:

➤ Parameters of x-ray beam quality
  • Half-value layer
  • Peak voltage
  • Mean energy
  • Effective energy
  • Energy spectrum
  • Depth dose distribution
➤ Measurement of energy spectrum
➤ Specification of clinical beam quality

PARAMETERS OF X-RAY BEAM QUALITY

The ideal way to describe the quality of an x-ray beam is to specify its spectral distribution, that is, energy fluence in each energy interval. However, spectral distributions are difficult to measure and, furthermore, such a complete specification of the beam quality is not necessary in most clinical situations. The following beam quality parameters are used depending on their practical use in clinical situations.

HALF-VALUE LAYER

Since the biologic effects of x-rays are not very sensitive to the quality of the beam, in radiotherapy one is interested primarily in the penetration of the beam into the patient rather than its detailed energy spectrum to specify its quality. Thus, a crude but simpler description of the beam quality is often used, namely the *half-value layer*.

• The term half-value layer (HVL) is defined as the thickness of an absorber of specified composition required to attenuate the intensity of the beam to half its original value.

• HVL of an x-ray beam depends on the energy spectrum, which is a function of primarily the peak voltage and the filtration (inherent and added).

• The HVL of a beam is related to the linear attenuation coefficient (μ) by the following equation:

$$\text{HVL} = \frac{0.693}{\mu}$$

- Like the attenuation coefficient, the HVL pertains to the primary beam (scattered photons are excluded).

- HVL is measured under narrow-beam or "good geometry" conditions to exclude scattered photons from the measurement. Good geometry can be achieved by using a narrow beam and a large distance between the absorber and the detector when measuring beam transmission.

- HVL for clinical x-ray beams is measured in different absorber materials such as aluminum, copper, or lead, depending on the beam energy. EXAMPLE:

  ➤ Diagnostic or superficial x-ray beams → HVL in mm Al

  ➤ Orthovoltage x-ray beams → HVL in mm Cu

  ➤ Megavoltage x-ray or γ-ray beams → HVL in mm Pb

- HVL of diagnostic or superficial therapy beams can be modified by adding aluminum filters of different thicknesses. For orthovoltage, the filters are usually made up of thin copper plates of thickness ranging from 0.25 to a few mm.

- HVL for orthovoltage beams can be optimized by special filters such as the *Thoreaus filters*. The optimization is intended to increase HVL with the least reduction in beam output. This may be achieved by the use of *combination filters* such as the Thoreaus filters.

- A Thoreaus filter consists of three filters: tin, copper, and aluminum. EXAMPLE: Thoreaus I filter has 0.2 mm Sn + 0.25 mm Cu + 1 mm Al.

- The principle of Thoreaus filters in optimizing HVL in an orthovoltage beam is illustrated in Figure 7.1.

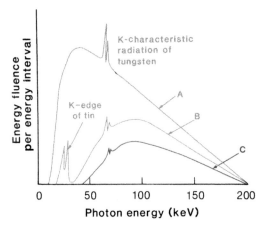

Figure 7.1. Schematic graph showing changes in spectral distribution of 200-kV$_p$ x-ray beam with various filters. Curve A is for Al, B for Sn + Al, and C for Sn + Cu + Al.

Figure 7.1 shows the following:

  ➤ Tin preferentially reduces K-characteristic radiation produced in the tungsten target;

  ➤ Copper preferentially filters out K-characteristic radiation from tin;

  ➤ Aluminum effectively absorbs K-characteristic radiation from copper.

- It is important that the combination filters be arranged in the proper order, with the highest atomic number material nearest to the x-ray target. Thus, a Thoreaus filter is inserted with tin facing the x-ray tube and the aluminum facing the patient, with the copper sandwiched between the tin and the aluminum plates.

PEAK VOLTAGE (kV$_p$ OR MV)

The maximum energy of an x-ray beam corresponds to the kinetic energy of electrons striking the target.

- In diagnostic or orthovoltage x-ray machines, the maximum photon energy in keV is numerically equal to the kV$_p$.

- In megavoltage beams, such as generated by linear accelerators, the maximum photon energy corresponds to the electron energy striking the target but is designated by MV, as if the beam were produced by applying that voltage across an x-ray tube.

➤ Peak voltage (kV$_p$) applied to an x-ray tube can be measured directly (e.g., voltage divider, sphere gap method) or indirectly (e.g., fluorescence, attenuation, or a penetrameter device such as an Adrian-Crooks cassette).

➤ Peak energy (MV) of a megavoltage x-ray beam can be measured by scintillation spectrometry or by photoactivation of appropriate foils (e.g., photoactivation ratio method). Most commonly used methods, however, are indirect such as comparing measured percentage depth dose distribution in water with published data.

MEAN ENERGY

The spectral distribution of an x-ray beam is characterized by the distribution of photon fluence (Φ) or energy fluence (Ψ) with respect to energy.

The mean energy ($\bar{E}$) based on photon fluence can be calculated as:

$$\bar{E} = \frac{\int_0^{E_{max}} \Phi_E \cdot E \cdot dE}{\int_0^{E_{max}} \Phi_E \cdot dE}$$

where $\Phi_E = \dfrac{d\Phi(E)}{dE}$.

Similarly, the mean energy based on energy fluence (Ψ_E) distribution is given by:

$$\bar{E} = \frac{\int_0^{E_{max}} \Psi_E \cdot E \cdot dE}{\int_0^{E_{max}} \Psi_E \cdot dE}$$

The above two expressions, however, lead to different values of $\bar{E}$ because $\Phi_E \neq \Psi_E$. Thus it is important to specify the type of distribution used in calculating the mean energy.

• The mean energy parameter is useful in dosimetry such as in the calculation of a detector response as a function of beam energy.

EFFECTIVE ENERGY

Because x-ray beams are heterogeneous in energy, it is convenient sometimes to express the quality of an x-ray beam in terms of effective energy.

• The *effective (or equivalent) energy* of an x-ray beam is the energy of photons in a monoenergetic beam that is attenuated at the same rate as the radiation in question.

• The effective energy may also be defined as the energy of a monoenergetic photon beam that has the same μ or HVL as the given beam.

• Figure 7.2 shows the relationship between effective energy and HLV for x-ray beams in the superficial and orthovoltage range.

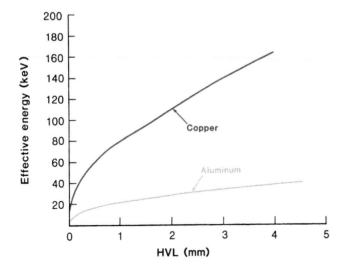

Figure 7.2. Plot of effective energy as a function of half-value layer (HVL). Data calculated from attenuation coefficients of monoenergetic photon beams.

- For a heavily filtered x-ray beam, the effective or average energy is approximately one third of the peak energy. EXAMPLE: A 6 MV x-ray beam from a linear accelerator has an average energy of approximately 2 MeV.

ENERGY SPECTRUM

Although the HVL is a practical parameter characterizing therapeutic beams, it is only approximate and cannot be used in systems that are sensitive to spectral distribution of photons. EXAMPLE:

- Radiation detectors that show a large variation in response to different photon energies (e.g., film, diodes), and even ion chambers, are more or less energy dependent. In such instances, spectral distribution is the relevant parameter of beam quality.
- In this and other investigative work (e.g., beam modeling), it is important to determine spectral distributions of photon beams.
- The energy spectrum of an x-ray beam may be calculated (e.g., Monte Carlo) or measured (e.g., scintillation spectrometry).
- The scintillation spectrometer consists of a crystal or phosphor, usually sodium iodide, attached to a photomultiplier tube (Figure 7.3).

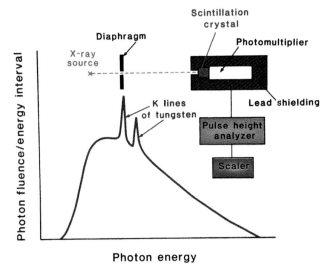

Figure 7.3. Energy spectrum of an x-ray beam determined by scintillation spectrometer (shown in the inset).

- The principle of spectrometry is as outlined below:
- **X-ray photons incident on phosphor crystal ➤ Ionization and excitation by ejected electrons produce phosphor scintillation (production of light photons in the optical or ultraviolet region) ➤ Scintillations detected by photocathode in the photomultiplier tube ➤ Ejection of low-energy photoelectrons ➤ Collection and multiplication of electrons (~ million times) by photomultiplier dynodes ➤ Generation of output pulses, each proportional to the original energy of individual x-ray photons entering the crystal ➤ Different size pulses sorted out by a multichannel analyzer ➤ Each channel accumulates pulses corresponding to a particular input photon energy ➤ Spectrum displayed in terms of photon fluence per unit energy interval as a function of photon energy (Figure 7.3).**

SPECIFICATION OF CLINICAL BEAM QUALITY

The quality of clinical photon beams is usually described by parameter(s) related to the penetrating ability of the beam, for example, HLV, kV_p, or MV, percentage depth dose at a specified depth in water or ratio of depth doses under reference conditions. The following are the recommended or most commonly used parameters for specifying quality of clinical photon beams:

- *Superficial and orthovoltage beams:* HVL and kV_p, in preference to HVL alone (recommended by ICRU Report 10b, 1964).

- *γ-Ray beams:* The energy of γ-rays or the nuclide of origin. EXAMPLE: The quality of a γ-ray beam emitted from a ^{60}Co source can be stated in terms of 1.17 and 1.33 MeV (average 1.25 MeV) or simply ^{60}Co beam.

- *Megavoltage x-ray beams:* MV (which is numerically equal to the maximum photon energy or the kinetic energy of electrons incident on the target). Because the x-ray beam is heterogeneous in energy (bremsstrahlung spectrum), its maximum energy is designated by MV (megavolts), as if the beam were generated by applying that voltage across an x-ray tube.

REVIEW QUESTIONS • Chapter 7

In multiple choice questions, more than one option may be correct.

The following table used in problems 1 to 3 describes the measured beam intensity as a function of aluminum filter thickness:

Filter Thickness [mm]	Reading/Unit Time [nC]
0	100
1.0	67.0
2.0	54.9
3.0	48.0
5.0	40.1
10.0	31.0
15.0	26.5
17.0	25.3
18.0	24.7
20.0	23.7

1. What is the first HVL for this beam?

   a) 1.7 mm Cu
   b) 2.0 mm Al
   c) 2.7 mm Al
   d) 0.5 mm Al
   e) 0.5 mm Cu

2. What is the attenuation coefficient μ for this beam in aluminum?

   a) 0.26 mm^{-1}
   b) 0.35 mm^{-1}
   c) 0.41 mm^{-1}
   d) 1.4 mm^{-1}
   e) 2.0 mm^{-1}

3. The homogeneity coefficient is defined as the first HVL divided by the second. What is the homogeneity coefficient for this beam?

   a) 0.15
   b) 0.18
   c) 1
   d) 5.6
   e) 6.5

4. Suppose there were three photon beams with the same peak energy; one from an x-ray machine without filtration, one from an x-ray machine with 2.0 mm Al filtration, and one monoenergetic. Which beam would have the largest HVL?

   a) Unfiltered x-ray beam
   b) Filtered x-ray beam
   c) Monoenergetic beam
   d) All three will have the same HVL
   e) Not enough information is given

5. The beam quality for megavoltage photon beams is sometimes specified in terms of their ionization ratio, or the ratio of the doses at depths of 20 to 10 cm for a fixed source–detector distance and meter setting. If a nominal 6 MV photon beam has an ionization ratio of 0.68, what is the approximate attenuation coefficient of this beam, neglecting scatter radiation?

   a) $0.029\ cm^{-1}$
   b) $0.039\ cm^{-1}$
   c) $0.049\ cm^{-1}$
   d) $0.059\ cm^{-1}$
   e) $0.069\ cm^{-1}$

6. HVL should be measured under "good geometry" conditions that require:

   a) A narrow beam with negligible scatter
   b) A broad beam with full scatter
   c) Detector positioned far away from the absorber to avoid scatter
   d) Chamber imbedded in a phantom at a sufficient depth to provide full buildup scatter

7. A Thoreaus filter for orthovoltage beams must be inserted with:

   a) Aluminum filter facing the patient
   b) Tin filter facing the patient
   c) Copper filter facing the patient
   d) Lead filter facing the x-ray tube

8. The following instrument(s) can be used to measure kV_p *directly* if the high tension leads of the x-ray tube are accessible:

   a) Penetrameter
   b) Voltage divider
   c) Sphere-gap apparatus
   d) Wisconsin test cassette

9. HLV measured for a 6 MV beam turned out to be 13.3 mm Pb. For this beam: [Hint: Consult Table A-7 in the Appendix of the Textbook.]

   a) The mass attenuation coefficient is $4.59 \times 10^{-3}\ m^2\,kg^{-1}$ in lead.
   b) The mass energy absorption coefficient in lead is the same as in water.
   c) The mass attenuation coefficient is greater than the mass energy absorption coefficient.
   d) The effective energy is approximately 2 MeV.

10. The peak photon energy in a megavoltage beam can be determined by:

   a) Measuring HLV layer in lead
   b) Comparing depth dose distribution with published data
   c) Measuring MV_p using a voltage divider
   d) Measuring photoactivation ratio

8

MEASUREMENT OF ABSORBED DOSE

REFERENCE

Khan FM. *The Physics of Radiation Therapy*, 4th edition, 2009. Chapter 8 "Measurement of Absorbed Dose"

Dosimetry Concepts

 TOPIC OUTLINE

The following topics will be discussed in this lecture:

➤ Absorbed dose: definition and units
➤ Relationships: kerma, exposure, and absorbed dose
➤ Bragg-Gray cavity theory
➤ Dose calibration protocols
➤ Exposure rate constant for radioactive sources

ABSORBED DOSE: DEFINITION AND UNITS

- The quantity *absorbed dose*, or simply *dose*, is defined as the energy absorbed per unit mass of any material. Mathematically, dose is the quotient $\dfrac{\mathrm{d}\bar{E}}{\mathrm{d}m}$, where $\mathrm{d}\bar{E}$ is the mean energy imparted by ionizing radiation to material of mass $\mathrm{d}m$.

- The old unit of dose is the *rad* (an acronym for radiation absorbed dose) and represents the absorption of 100 ergs of energy per gram of absorbing material.

$$1\,\mathrm{rad} = 100\,\mathrm{ergs/g} = 10^{-2}\,\mathrm{J/kg}$$

The *SI unit* for absorbed dose is the *gray* (Gy) and is defined as:

$$1\,\mathrm{Gy} = 1\,\mathrm{J/kg}$$

Thus, the relationship between gray, centigray (cGy), and rad is:

$$1\,\mathrm{Gy} = 100\,\mathrm{rad} = 100\,\mathrm{cGy}$$

or

$$1\,\mathrm{rad} = 10^{-2}\,\mathrm{Gy} = 1\,\mathrm{cGy}$$

RELATIONSHIPS: KERMA, EXPOSURE, AND ABSORBED DOSE

KERMA

The quantity kerma (K) is the kinetic energy released in the medium per unit mass. Mathematically, kerma is the quotient of $\mathrm{d}E_{\mathrm{tr}}$ by $\mathrm{d}m$, where $\mathrm{d}E_{\mathrm{tr}}$ is the sum of the initial kinetic energies of all the charged particles (electrons and positrons) liberated by uncharged particles (photons) in a material of mass $\mathrm{d}m$.

The unit for kerma is the same as for dose, that is, J/kg.

- Kerma can be divided into two parts: collision kerma, K^{col}, and radiative kerma, K^{rad}. Mathematically:

$$K = K^{col} + K^{rad}$$

where

$$K^{col} = \Psi\left(\frac{\bar{\mu}_{en}}{\rho}\right)$$

and

$$K^{rad} = \Psi\left(\frac{\bar{\mu}_{en}}{\rho}\right) \times \left(\frac{\bar{g}}{1 - \bar{g}}\right)$$

where Ψ is the photon energy fluence, $\frac{\bar{\mu}_{en}}{\rho}$ is the average mass energy absorption coefficient, and $\bar{g}$ is the average fraction of an electron energy lost to radiative (bremsstrahlung) processes.

EXPOSURE AND KERMA

Exposure is the ionization equivalent of the collision kerma in air. Mathematically:

$$X = (K^{col})_{air} \times \left(\frac{e}{\overline{W}}\right)$$

where $\overline{W}$ is the mean energy required to produce an ion pair in dry air and e the electronic charge. $\overline{W}$ is almost constant for all electron energies and has a value of 33.97 eV/ion pair. The energy absorbed per unit charge of ionization in dry air is $\frac{\overline{W}}{e} = 33.97$ J/C.

ABSORBED DOSE AND KERMA

The relationship between absorbed dose and kerma is illustrated in Figure 8A.1 for a megavoltage beam of photons as it enters a medium.

The absorbed dose in a medium from a photon beam is related to kerma by the following general relationship:

$$D = \beta \cdot K^{col}$$

where D is the absorbed dose and β the quotient of absorbed dose at a given point and the collision part of kerma at the same point.

- Whereas, kerma is maximum at the surface and decreases with depth, the dose initially builds up to a maximum value and then decreases at the same rate as kerma.
- $\beta < 1$ in the initial dose buildup region.
- $\beta = 1$ where dose and collision kerma are equal (electronic equilibrium).
- $\beta > 1$ where dose exceeds collision kerma (transient electronic equilibrium).

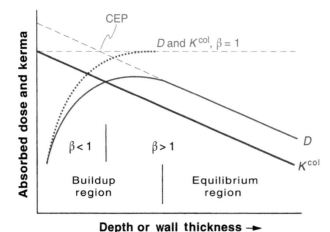

Figure 8A.1. Relationship between absorbed dose (D) and collision kerma (K^{col}) for a megavoltage photon beam. β is the ratio of absorbed dose to collision kerma. The point designated as CEP is the center of electron production (see text). (From Loevinger RA. Formalism for calculation of absorbed dose to a medium from photon and electron beams. *Med Phys.* 1981; 8:1, with permission.)

Absorbed Dose to Air

Under charged particle equilibrium (CPE), dose to air is given by:

$$D_{air} = (K^{col})_{air} = X \times \frac{\overline{W}}{e}$$

If exposure X is given in roentgens (R), the dose to air in centigrays (cGy) is given by:

$$D_{air}(cGy) = 0.876 \, X \, (R)$$

- The *roentgen-to-cGy conversion factor* for air is 0.876. In other words, 1 R = 0.876 cGy.

Absorbed Dose to Any Medium

Under CPE, the roentgen-to-cGy conversion factor for any medium (f_{med}) is given by:

$$f_{med} = 0.876 \frac{(\overline{\mu}_{en}/\rho)_{med}}{(\overline{\mu}_{en}/\rho)_{air}}$$

- f_{med} depends on composition of the medium and the photon beam energy. EXAMPLE: For 20 keV x-rays, cGy/R is 0.876 in air, 0.892 in water, and 4.07 in bone; for ^{60}Co γ-rays, cGy/R is 0.876 in air, 0.971 in water, and 0.96 in bone.

DOSE CALCULATION IN A MEDIUM FROM EXPOSURE

Exposure measured in *free air* can be converted into dose to any medium at the same point, provided CPE exists at the point of measurement. For example, dose in free space, $D_{f.s.}$ (dose to a small mass of tissue of equilibrium thickness located in free air), can be calculated from exposure X in free air by:

$$D_{f.s.} = X \cdot f_{tissue} \cdot A_{eq}$$

where A_{eq} is the transmission factor representing the ratio of the energy fluence at the center of the equilibrium mass of tissue to that in free air at the same point.

Similarly, an exposure measurement in any medium (e.g., exposure at the center of chamber cavity) can be converted to dose to the medium at the point of measurement (in the absence of the cavity) by:

$$D_{med} = X \cdot f_{med} \cdot A_m$$

where A_m is the transmission factor for the photon energy fluence at point P when the chamber cavity is replaced by the medium.

- The above two equations have been used in the past to calibrate low-energy beams (up to ^{60}Co) in air or in any medium such as water. However, it is recommended that a current calibration protocol such as AAPM TG-51 or IAEA Report 398 should be used in a clinical setting.

BRAGG-GRAY CAVITY THEORY

- The principle of Bragg-Gray (B-G) cavity theory is that the ionization produced in a gas-filled cavity placed in a medium is related to the energy absorbed in the medium surrounding the cavity. Figure 8A.2 shows an air cavity embedded in a medium.

- When the cavity is sufficiently small so that its introduction into the medium does not alter the number or distribution of the electrons that would exist in the medium without

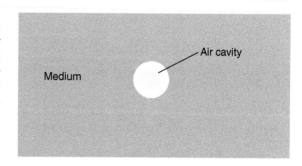

Figure 8A.2. Illustration of an air cavity placed in a medium.

the cavity, then the following relationship (Spencer-Attix formulation of the B-G theory) holds:

$$D_{med} = J_g \cdot \frac{\overline{W}}{e} \cdot \left(\frac{\overline{L}}{\rho} \right)_g^{med}$$

where D_{med} is the absorbed dose in the medium (in the absence of the cavity), J_g the ionization charge of one sign produced per unit mass of the cavity gas, and $(\overline{L}/\rho)_g^{med}$ a weighted mean ratio of the restricted mass stopping power of the medium to that of the gas for the electrons crossing the cavity. The product $J_g \left(\dfrac{\overline{W}}{e} \right)$ is the energy absorbed per unit mass of the cavity gas.

- Whereas exposure in roentgens cannot be measured accurately for photon beams of energy above 3 MeV (practically not above ^{60}Co), the B-G cavity theory has no limitation of energy or the type of ionizing radiation in the measurement of absorbed dose.

CHAMBER AS A BRAGG-GRAY CAVITY

An ion chamber placed in a medium (e.g., water) may be considered as a B-G cavity. Because the chamber cavity is of finite size, the Spencer-Attix formulation of the B-G theory applies but with additional corrections to account for perturbation of the electron fluence as a result of the chamber cavity and the nonequivalence of the chamber wall to the surrounding medium. If the chamber cavity has air, then the following relationship applies:

$$D_{med} = D_{air} \cdot \left(\frac{\overline{L}}{\rho} \right)_{air}^{med} \cdot P_{repl} \cdot P_{wall}$$

where D_{air} is the dose to the air of the cavity, P_{repl} the replacement factor that corrects for perturbation in the electron and photon fluences at point P as a result of insertion of the cavity in the medium, and P_{wall} the factor that accounts for perturbation caused by the wall material being different from the medium. The above equation forms the basis of TG-21 calibration protocol.

- All recent calibration protocols (TG-21, TG-51, and IAEA TRS-398) use B-G cavity theory with a varying degree of refinements to convert the ionization charge measured by an ion chamber in a water phantom to absorbed dose to water in the absence of the chamber.

DOSE CALIBRATION PROTOCOLS

TG-21

This AAPM calibration protocol (published in 1983) has been superseded by the AAPM TG-51 protocol.

- TG-21 requires chamber calibration in terms of air kerma or N_x (exposure calibration factor for ^{60}Co beam). N_{gas} (dose to cavity air per unit charge of ionization) is calculated from N_x and other factors related to chamber design.
- Basic equations for the calibration of photon and electron beams are given by Eq. 8.57 and Eq. 8.66 in the Textbook, respectively.

TG-51

- Major difference between TG-51 and TG-21 is the chamber calibration, which is based on absorbed dose to water in the case of TG-51 and air kerma or exposure in the case of TG-21. In the TG-51 protocol, the chamber calibration factor ($N_{D,w}$), provided by the calibration laboratory (National Institute of Standards and Technology (NIST) or Accredited Dose Calibration Laboratory (ADCL)), is in terms of absorbed-dose-to-water in a ^{60}Co beam measured under reference conditions.

- The basic TG-51 equation for absorbed calibration is as follows:

$$D_w^Q = M k_Q N_{D,w}^{^{60}Co}$$

where D_w^Q is the absorbed dose to water at the reference point of measurement in a beam of quality Q; M the electrometer reading that has been fully corrected for ion recombination, environmental temperature and pressure, electrometer calibration and chamber polarity effects; k_Q the quality conversion factor that converts the absorbed-dose-to-water calibration factor for a ^{60}Co beam into the calibration factor for an arbitrary beam of quality Q, and $N_{D,w}^{^{60}Co}$ the absorbed-dose-to-water calibration factor for the chamber in a ^{60}Co beam under reference conditions.

- The NIST's primary standard for $N_{D,w}^{^{60}Co}$ is currently based on absolute dosimetry with a calorimeter. Transfer ion chambers are used at the ADCLs to provide NIST traceable chamber calibrations.

- Beam quality for the purpose of photon beam calibration is specified by percentage depth dose for the photon component of the beam at 10 cm depth in water ($\%dd(10)_x$) for a 10×10 cm^2 field at 100 cm source-surface distance (SSD).

- Beam quality for the purpose of electron beam calibration is specified by the depth of 50% dose in water (R_{50}) for a broad beam of field size 10×10 cm^2 ($\geq 20 \times 20$ cm^2 for $R_{50} > 8.5$ cm).

- Calibration of a photon beam is performed at 10 cm depth in water. The measured dose can then be converted to dose at the reference depth of maximum dose (d_{max}) by using percentage depth dose or tissue-maximum ratio (TMR) at 10 cm depth. Sensitivity of monitor chambers in the accelerator is adjusted to give D_{max}/MU close to unity for a 10×10 cm field size at SSD = 100 cm (SSD-type calibration) or source-to-axis distance (SAD) = 100 cm (SAD-type calibration).

- Calibration of an electron beam is performed at a reference depth, d_{ref}, given by: $d_{ref} = 0.6R_{50} - 0.1$. It is then converted to dose at d_{max} by using percentage depth dose at d_{ref}. Calibration is set to give D_{max}/MU equal to unity for a 10×10 cm field size (reference applicator) at SSD = 100 cm.

- The difference in measured dose between TG-21 and TG-51 has been shown to be less than 2% for photons but it can be as much as 5% for electron beams.

IAEA TRS-398

- There are minor differences between TG-51 and IAEA TRS-398. The main difference is in the beam quality parameter k_Q, which in TRS-398 is specified by TPR$_{20,10}$ instead of $\%dd(10)_x$. The TPR$_{20,10}$ is determined by the ratio of ionization at 20 cm depth to that at 10 cm depth at the same source-to-chamber distance of 100 cm. The field size at the chamber position is 10×10 cm.

- Basic equation for the calibration of megavoltage photon and electron beams is the same as for TG-51 except for notation.

- The accuracy of absorbed dose calibration for the IAEA TRS-398 is comparable to that for the AAPM TG-51.

EXPOSURE RATE CONSTANT FOR RADIOACTIVE SOURCES

- Exposure rate constant is defined as exposure rate from a radioactive source of point size and unit activity at a unit distance. Its special unit is: $Rm^2 h^{-1} Ci^{-1}$, which stands for roentgens per hour at a distance of 1 meter from a point source of activity of 1 Ci.

- Exposure rate constant is unique to every radioactive source. It depends on the photon energies emitted in the decay scheme, their energy absorption coefficients in air, and the no. of photons/decay of respective energies.

- The exposure rate constant (Γ_δ) is given by:

$$\Gamma_\delta = 193.8 \sum_i^N f_i E_i \left(\frac{\mu_{en}}{\rho}\right)_{air,\, i} \quad Rm^2\ h^{-1}\ Ci^{-1}$$

where δ stands for a suitable cutoff for minimum photon energies emitted, f_i the number of photons emitted/decay of energy E_i, and $\left(\dfrac{\mu_{en}}{\rho}\right)_{air,\, i}$ the mass energy absorption coefficient in air for photon of energy E_i. In this equation, energy E_i is expressed in MeV and $\left(\dfrac{\mu_{en}}{\rho}\right)_{air,\, i}$ in m^2/kg.

- Exposure rate constant assumes a point source located in free air. It does not include effects of source filtration (unless specified), source design, or photon fluence attenuation or scattering in the medium. It assumes that the photon fluence (or exposure rate) changes with distance strictly in accordance with the inverse square law.

Dosimeters

 TOPIC OUTLINE

The following topics will be discussed in this lecture:

➤ Absolute dosimeters
  • Calorimeter
  • Ferrous sulfate (Fricke) dosimeter
➤ Secondary dosimeters
  • Thermoluminescent dosimeters
  • Silicon diodes
  • Radiographic films
  • Radiochromic films

ABSOLUTE DOSIMETERS

- Absolute dosimetry means that the dose is determined from the first principles—without reference to another dosimeter.

- Free-air ionization chamber, specially designed spherical chambers of known volume (e.g., at NIST), calorimeter, and ferrous sulfate (Fricke) dosimeter are examples of absolute dosimeters. They are also called as primary standards.

CALORIMETER

Calorimetry is based on the principle that the energy absorbed in a medium from radiation appears ultimately as heat energy while a small amount may appear in the form of a chemical change. This results in a small increase in temperature of the absorbing medium which, if measured accurately, can be related to the energy absorbed per unit mass or the absorbed dose.

Neglecting heat change (positive or negative) due to chemical change (called *heat defect*), one can calculate the rise in temperature of water by the absorption of 1 Gy of dose:

$$1\,Gy = 1\,J\,kg^{-1} = \frac{1}{4.18}\,cal\,kg^{-1}$$

where 4.18 is the mechanical equivalent of heat (4.18 J of energy = 1 cal of heat). Because the specific heat of water is 1 cal/g/°C or 10^3 cal/kg/°C, the increase in temperature (ΔT) produced by 1 Gy is:

$$\Delta T = \frac{1}{4.18}\,(cal\,kg^{-1}) \cdot \frac{1}{10^3}\,(kg\,cal^{-1}{}^\circ C)$$

$$= 2.39 \times 10^{-4}\,{}^\circ C$$

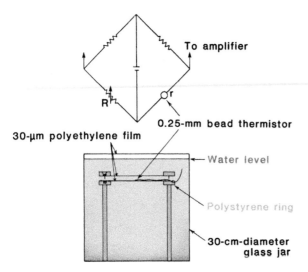

Figure 8B.1. Schematic diagram of Domen's calorimeter. (Redrawn from Domen SR. Absorbed dose water calorimeter. *Med Phys.* 1980;7:157.)

- To measure such a small temperature rise, *thermistors* are most commonly used.
- Thermistors are semiconductors that show a large change in electrical resistance with a small change in temperature (approximately 5% per 1°C).
- Change in resistance is measured by an apparatus called the Wheatstone bridge. It is then correlated with rise in temperature and hence the dose.
- Domen's calorimeter (Figure 8B.1) measures dose rates in water of about 4 Gy/min with a precision (reproducibility of measurements) of 0.5%.

FERROUS SULFATE (FRICKE) DOSIMETER

This dosimeter consists of a solution containing 1 mmol/L ferrous sulfate (or ferrous ammonium sulfate), 1 mmol/L NaCl, and 0.4 mol/L sulfuric acid. The reason for NaCl in the solution is to counteract the effects of organic impurities present despite all the necessary precautions. When the solution is irradiated, the ferrous ions, Fe^{2+}, are oxidized by radiation to ferric ions, Fe^{3+}. The ferric ion concentration is determined by spectrophotometry of the dosimeter solution, which shows absorption peaks in the ultraviolet light at wavelengths of 224 and 304 nm.

- G value is the radiation chemical yield defined as the number of molecules produced per 100 eV of energy absorbed. Thus, if the yield of ferric ions is measured for a given beam, the energy absorbed can be calculated when the G value is known.
- The G value ranges from 15.3 to 15.7/100 eV for photon beams from ^{137}Cs gamma ray energy to 30 MeV. A constant G value of 15.7 ± 0.6/100 eV is recommended for electrons in the energy range of 1 to 30 MeV for 0.4 mol/L H_2SO_4 dosimeter solution.

SECONDARY DOSIMETERS

Secondary dosimeters require calibration against a primary standard. EXAMPLE: thimble chambers and plane-parallel ion chambers (discussed in Lecture 6B).

Thermoluminescent dosimeters (TLDs), diodes, and films are also secondary dosimeters but are used primarily for relative dosimetry. They require calibration against a calibrated ion chamber and may require additional corrections for energy dependence and other conditions that may affect their dose–response characteristics.

THERMOLUMINESCENT DOSIMETERS

The most commonly used TLD consists of lithium fluoride (LiF) with a trace amount of impurities (magnesium). It is available in many forms and sizes for use in special dosimetry situations (e.g., powder capsules, extruded rods or chips, and crystals embedded in Teflon or silicon discs). It is reusable if properly annealed and recalibrated in terms of its dose–response curve.

- Density of TLD phosphor is 2.6 g/cm^3 and its effective atomic number is about 8.2 (compared to effective Z of about 7.6 for muscle and 7.5 for water). In most clinical dosimetry applications, however, TLD is assumed to be tissue equivalent.

- TLD response is almost independent of energy in the megavoltage range of photon and electron beams used clinically. However, the dosimeter's form and size may affect accuracy for certain beams and irradiation conditions due to fluence perturbation.

- Fading of thermoluminescence (TL) after irradiation is small, less than 5% for 12 weeks. Thus, the irradiated samples can be read off at leisure.

- The useful range of TLD for measuring dose is approximately 10^{-5} Gy to 10^3 Gy.

- Being a secondary dosimeter, TLDs must be calibrated against a calibrated ion chamber to determine their dose–response curve. A typical dose–response curve is shown in Figure 8B.2.

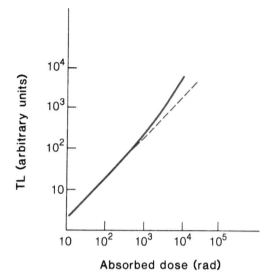

Figure 8B.2. An example of thermoluminescence (TL) versus absorbed dose curve for TLD-100 powder (schematic).

- The dose–response curve is generally linear up to about 10 Gy but becomes supralinear beyond that.

- With considerable care and quality control, a precision of approximately 3% can be obtained using TLDs.

- Because TLD material is available in many forms and sizes, it can be used for special dosimetry situations, such as for measuring dose distribution in the buildup region, around brachytherapy sources, and for personnel dose monitoring.

SILICON DIODES

Figure 8B.3 shows schematically a radiation diode detector that essentially consists of a silicon p–n junction diode connected to a coaxial cable and encased in epoxy potting material. This design is intended for the radiation beam to be incident perpendicularly at the long axis of the detector. Although the collecting or sensitive volume (depletion zone) is not known precisely, it is on the order of 0.2 to 0.3 mm^3. It is located within a depth of 0.5 mm from the front surface of the detector, unless electronic buildup is provided by encasing the diode in a buildup material.

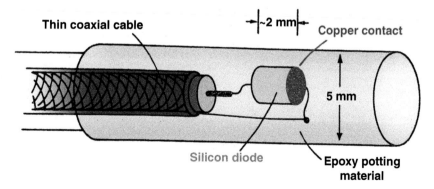

Figure 8B.3. Schematic diagrams showing (A) silicon p–n junction diode. (From Attix FH. *Introduction to Radiological Physics and Radiation Dosimetry.* New York: John Wiley & Sons; 1986.)

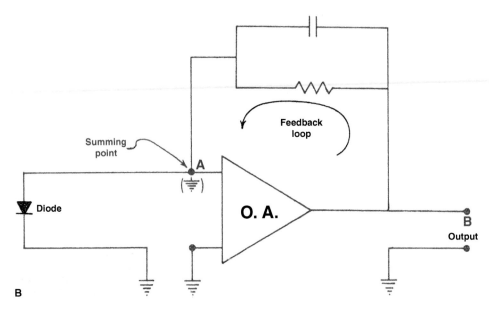

Figure 8B.4. Schematic diagram showing basic electronic circuit using operational amplifier with a feedback loop. (From Gager LD, Wright AE, Almond PR. Silicon diode detectors used in radiobiological physics measurements. Part I: development of an energy compensating shield. *Med Phys.* 1977;4:494–498.)

Figure 8B.4 shows the diode connected to an operational amplifier with a feedback loop to measure radiation induced current. There is no bias voltage applied.

- A p–n junction diode is designed with one part of a p-silicon disc doped with an n-type material. The p-region of the diode is deficient in electrons (or contains "holes") while the n-region has an excess of electrons.

- At the interface between p- and n-type materials, a small region, called the *depletion zone*, is created because of initial diffusion of electrons from the n-region and holes from the p-region across the junction, until equilibrium is established. The depletion zone develops an electric field, which opposes further diffusion of majority carriers once equilibrium has been achieved.

- When a diode is irradiated, electron-hole pairs are produced within the depletion zone. They are immediately separated and swept out by the existing electric field in the depletion zone. This gives rise to a radiation-induced current.

- The direction of electronic current flow is from the n- to the p-region (which is opposite to the direction of conventional current).

- Silicon p–n junction diodes are well suited for relative dosimetry of electron beams, output constancy checks, and in vivo patient dose monitoring.

- Their higher sensitivity, instantaneous response, small size (~0.2–0.3 mm^3), and ruggedness offer special advantages over ionization chambers in certain situations.

- Their major limitations as dosimeters include energy dependence in photon beams, directional dependence, thermal effects, and radiation-induced damage with prolonged use. Modern diodes minimize these effects.

- Unlike ion chambers, diodes do not require high voltage bias to collect ions.

RADIOGRAPHIC FILMS

A radiographic film consists of a transparent film base (cellulose acetate or polyester resin) coated with an emulsion containing very small crystals of silver bromide. When the film is exposed to ionizing radiation or visible light, a chemical change takes place within the exposed crystals to form what is referred to as a *latent image*. When the film is developed, the affected crystals are reduced to small grains of metallic silver. The film is then *fixed*. The unaffected granules are removed by the fixing solution, leaving a clear film in their place. The metallic silver, which is not affected by the fixer, causes darkening of the film. Thus, the degree of blackening of an area of the film depends on the amount of free silver deposited and, consequently, on the radiation energy absorbed.

- The degree of blackening of the film is measured by determining *optical density* with a densitometer. This instrument consists of a light source, a tiny aperture through which the light is directed, and a light detector (photocell) to measure the light intensity transmitted through the film.

- The optical density, OD, is defined as:

$$OD = \log\frac{I_0}{I_t}$$

where I_0 is the amount of light collected without film and I_t the amount of light transmitted through the film.

- Sensitivity of film depends on the size of emulsion grains (crystals of silver bromide) and the quality and type of radiation.

- Slow-speed films (small grain size) such as Kodak XV-2 and Kodak RPM-2 are suitable for relative dosimetry provided their sensitometric curve is predetermined in comparison with a calibrated ion chamber. Figure 8B.5 shows examples of characteristic curves for two commonly used dosimetry films.

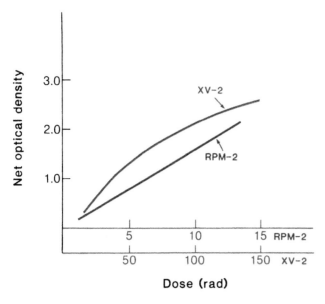

Figure 8B.5. Sensitometric curve of Kodak XV-2 film and Kodak RPM-2 (Type M) film.

- Processing conditions must be standardized. Any air pockets between film and its jacket must be eliminated to avoid artifacts.

- Film is well suited for relative dosimetry of electron beams (shows practically no energy dependence).

- In photon beams, however, it shows significant energy dependence and therefore it is used mostly for portal imaging and QA procedures such as checking beam alignment, isocentric accuracy, and beam flatness.

- For measuring dose distributions, photon energy dependence must be taken into account.

RADIOCHROMIC FILMS

Radiochromic film consists of an ultrathin (7- to 23-μm thick), colorless, radiosensitive leuco dye bonded onto a 100-μm thick Mylar base. Other varieties include thin layers of radiosensitive dye sandwiched between two pieces of polyester base.

- The unexposed film is colorless and changes to shades of blue as a result of a polymerization process induced by ionizing radiation.

- No physical, chemical, or thermal processing is required to bring out or stabilize this color.

- The degree of coloring is usually measured with a spectrophotometer using a narrow spectral wavelength (nominal 610–670 nm).

- Commercially available laser scanners and charge-coupled device microdensitometer cameras can also be used to scan the films. These measurements are expressed in terms of optical density as defined by the equation above for radiographic films.

- Radiochromic films are almost tissue equivalent with effective Z of 6.0 to 6.5.

- Post-irradiation color stability occurs after approximately 24 hours.

- Energy dependence is much lower than the silver halide (radiographic) films.

- Although radiochromic films are insensitive to visible light, they exhibit some sensitivity to ultraviolet light and temperature. They need to be stored in a dry and dark environment at the temperature and humidity not too different from those at which they will be used for dosimetry.

- Because radiochromic films are sensitive to ultraviolet light, they should not be exposed to fluorescent light or to sunlight. They may be read and handled in normal incandescent light.

- Radiochromic films must be calibrated before they can be used for dosimetry. The sensitometric curve shows a linear relationship up to a certain dose level beyond which its response levels off with increase in dose (see Figure 8B.6).

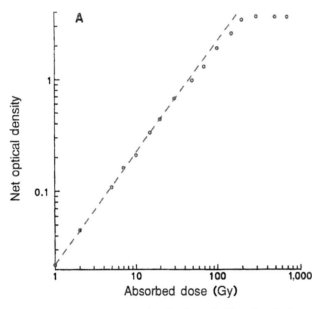

Figure 8B.6. A plot of net optical density as a function of dose for MD-55-2 radiochromic film. (From AAPM. Radiochromic film dosimetry: recommendations of AAPM Radiation Therapy Committee Task Group 55. *Med Phys.* 1998;25:3093–2115.)

- The most commonly used radiochromic films for dosimetry that are commercially available are GafChromic EBT film (International Specialty Product (ISP), Wayne, NJ) and Double-layer GafChromic MD-55-2 film (ISP or other vendor(s); Nuclear Associates, Carle Place, NY).

- Whereas HD-810 films are mainly used in the dose range of 50 to 2,500 Gy, MD-55-2 are useful in the range of 3 to 100 Gy. EBT films have a useful range of 1 to 800 cGy.

- Major advantages of radiochromic film dosimeters include:
  - ➤ Tissue equivalence
  - ➤ High spatial resolution
  - ➤ Large dynamic range (10^{-2}–10^6 Gy)
  - ➤ Relatively low spectral sensitivity variation (or energy dependence)
  - ➤ Insensitivity to visible light
  - ➤ No need for chemical processing

REVIEW QUESTIONS • Chapter 8

In multiple choice questions, more than one option may be correct.

✔ **TEST YOURSELF**

Review questions for this chapter are provided online.

1. A uniform dose is delivered to a volume of tissue. If the dose to 1 g of tissue is 2 Gy, what is the dose to 5 g of tissue?
    a) 0.4 Gy
    b) 1 Gy
    c) 2 Gy
    d) 10 Gy

2. A 20 MV x-ray beam is incident on a water phantom. The absorbed dose is:
    a) Less than kerma at the surface
    b) Equal to kerma in the buildup region
    c) Greater than kerma beyond the depth of maximum dose
    d) Less than kerma at all depths

3. Which of the following statements is (are) true? [$\overline{W}$ is the mean energy required to produce an ion pair in dry air.]
    a) $\overline{W}$ in eV/ion pair is 33.97.
    b) $\dfrac{W}{e}$ in J/C, where e is the electronic charge, is 33.97.
    c) Dose to air in cGy/R for orthovoltage beams is 0.876.
    d) Dose to air in cGy/R for a ^{60}Co beam 0.957.

4. In a megavoltage photon beam, the ionization charge measured by a thimble chamber is produced primarily by:
    a) Photon interactions with the cavity air
    b) Electron interactions with the cavity air
    c) Photon interactions with the central electrode
    d) Electron interactions with the central electrode

5. According to the Bragg-Gray cavity theory, the ratio of dose to the surrounding medium to the dose to cavity air is given by: [Assume cavity size to be infinitesimally small.]
    a) The ratio of mass absorption coefficient of medium to that of air for the photons crossing the cavity
    b) The ratio of mass stopping power of medium to that of air for the electrons crossing the cavity
    c) The ratio of electron density of medium to that of air
    d) Roentgen-to-cGy conversion factor for the medium

6. Which of the following detectors is (are) correctly matched with its (their) most appropriate use?
    a) Farmer-type ion chamber → Surface dose measurements
    b) Plane-parallel chamber → Beam calibration
    c) Calorimeter → Calibration of secondary chambers
    d) Radiographic film → Photon beam dosimetry
    e) Radiochromic film → Brachytherapy dosimetry
    f) Silicon diodes → Instantaneous patient dose monitoring
    g) Cutie Pie survey meter → Detection of a missing brachytherapy source

7. A ^{60}Co beam ($E = 1.25$ MeV) has an energy fluence of 500 J/m^2 at a point in a water phantom. What is K^{col} for this beam? [Consult Appendix A of the Textbook for pertinent data]

    a) 1.25×10^{-2} J/kg
    b) 1.5 J/kg
    c) 3.2 J/kg
    d) 4.0 J/m^2 MeV
    e) 500 cGy

8. Which of the following statements is/are true about radiation dosimeters?

    a) Radiographic film is more suitable for relative depth dose measurements for electron beams than for photon beams.
    b) LiF TLDs have a linear dose response until about 10 Gy, where the response saturates.
    c) Diodes have higher spatial resolution and larger energy dependence than ion chambers for photon beams.
    d) Radiochromic films are self-processing, but possess the same energy dependency that radiographic films have.
    e) An ADCL-calibrated ion chamber is an example of an absolute dosimeter.

9. If only 1 of every 100 photons incident on an exposed film is not absorbed by the film, what is the OD?

    a) 0.01
    b) 0.1
    c) 1
    d) 2
    e) 100

10. Which of the following statements is/are true about the AAPM TG-51 calibration protocol?

    a) Photon beam quality is specified by TPR$_{20,10}$ (the ratio of ionization at 20 cm depth to that at 10 cm depth at the same source-to-chamber distance of 100 cm).
    b) Electron beam quality is specified by the practical range, R_p.
    c) The reference depth for photon beam calibration measurement is d_m.
    d) The reference depth for electron beam calibration measurement is d_m.
    e) The protocol uses an absorbed dose to water calibration factor, provided by an ADCL.

11. In a 6 MV linear accelerator calibration measurement, the measured charge per unit mass of air in an ion chamber (J_g) is 0.35 C/kg. Neglecting chamber perturbation factors (i.e., P_{ion}, P_{wall}, P_{repl}), what is the measured dose to the medium (water)? [Assume the average, restricted stopping power for a 6 MV photon beam, $(\bar{L}/\rho)_{air}^{med}$ is 1.127.]

    a) 37.9 cGy
    b) 39.5 cGy
    c) 12.9 Gy
    d) 13.4 Gy

12. For 1 MeV photons incident on an Al slab the mass absorption coefficient is 0.0270 cm^2/g and the mass energy transfer coefficient is 0.0271 cm^2/g. What fraction of initial kinetic energy transfer to the electrons in the slab is emitted as bremsstrahlung?

    a) 4%
    b) 0.04%
    c) 0.4%
    d) 40%

13. A ^{137}Cs source ($E_\gamma = 0.662$ MeV) gives a photon fluence rate in air at a point away from the source of 6.25×10^7 m^{-2} s^{-1}. Calculate the dose rate in air at that point.

    a) 7.1 Gy/h
    b) 0.71 Gy/h
    c) 7.1 mGy/h
    d) 0.071 mGy/h

14. Compared to soft tissue, dose to bone [assuming the same photon energy fluence] is:
    a) More than 4 times higher when irradiated by 90 kV$_p$ x-rays.
    b) Less when irradiated by ^{60}Co γ-rays.
    c) Less when irradiated by 20 MV x-rays.
    d) Higher when irradiated by 40 MV x-rays.

15. The exposure rate constant of a radioactive source depends on:
    a) Energy of emitted photons.
    b) Half-life of the radioactive source.
    c) Activity of the source.
    d) Energy absorption coefficient of emitted photons in air.
    e) Energy fluence of emitted photons.

9

DOSE DISTRIBUTION AND SCATTER ANALYSIS

REFERENCE
Khan FM. *The Physics of Radiation Therapy*, 4th edition, 2009. Chapter 9 "Dose Distribution and Scatter Analysis"

Depth Dose and Tissue-Air Ratios

 TOPIC OUTLINE

The following topics will be discussed in this lecture:
- ➤ Dosimetry phantoms
- ➤ Depth dose distribution in photon beams
  - • Percent depth dose
  - • Tissue-air ratio
  - • Scatter-air ratio
- ➤ Dosimetry of irregular fields—Clarkson technique
- ➤ Dose calculation in rotation therapy

DOSIMETRY PHANTOMS

Basic dose distribution data are usually measured in a water phantom, which approximates the radiation absorption and scattering properties of muscle and other soft tissues. Since it is not always possible or convenient to put radiation detectors in water, solid dry phantoms have been developed as substitutes for water.

- • Ideally, for a given material to be tissue or water equivalent, it must have the same effective atomic number, number of electrons per gram, and mass density.
- • Because of Compton effect being the most predominant mode of interaction for megavoltage photon beams (in the clinical range), the necessary condition for water equivalence for such beams is for the phantom to have the same electron density (number of electrons per cubic centimeter) as that of water.
- • The electron density (ρ_e) of a material may be calculated from its mass density (ρ_m) and its atomic composition according to the formula:

$$\rho_e = \rho_m \times N_A \times \left(\frac{Z}{A}\right)$$

where

$$\frac{Z}{A} = \sum_i a_i \times \left(\frac{Z_i}{A_i}\right)$$

N_A is Avogadro's number and a_i is the fraction by weight of the ith element of atomic number Z_i and atomic weight A_i.

125

- The most commonly used dosimetry phantoms and their electron densities relative to water are the following:

Water	1
Polystyrene	~1.02
Acrylic	~1.15
Solid water	~1.00

DEPTH DOSE DISTRIBUTION IN PHOTON BEAMS

As the beam is incident on a patient (or a phantom), the absorbed dose in the patient varies with depth. This variation depends on many conditions: beam energy, depth, field size, distance from source, and beam collimation system. Thus, the calculation of dose in the patient involves considerations in regard to these parameters and others as they affect depth dose distribution. A number of dosimetric quantities have been defined for this purpose, major among these being percentage depth dose (PDD), tissue-air ratios (TARs), tissue-phantom ratios (TPRs), and tissue-maximum ratios (TMRs).

PERCENT DEPTH DOSE

The quantity *percentage* (or simply *percent*) *depth dose* may be defined as the quotient, expressed as a percentage, of the absorbed dose at any depth, d, to the absorbed dose at a fixed reference depth d_0, along the central axis of the beam (Figure 9.1).

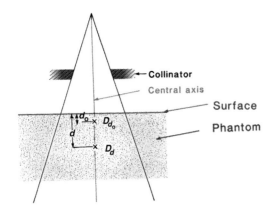

Figure 9.1. Percentage depth dose is (D_d / D_{d_0}) × 100, where d is any depth and d_0 is reference depth of maximum dose.

Mathematically, percentage depth dose (P) is given by:

$$P = \frac{D_d}{D_{d_0}} \times 100$$

- In clinical practice, the reference depth d_0 is chosen to be the reference depth of maximum dose (or peak dose).
- The reference depth of maximum dose is measured at a point on central axis for a small field (e.g., 5×5 cm or less).
- Because the depth of maximum dose decreases somewhat with increase in field size, the reference depth d_0 is kept constant for a given energy beam irrespective of field size.
- Variation of PDD with depth and beam quality is shown in Figure 9.2.

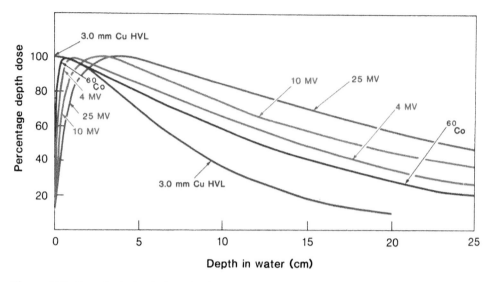

Figure 9.2. Central axis depth dose distribution for different-quality photon beams. Field size, 10×10 cm; source-to-surface distance (SSD) = 100 cm for all beams except for 3.0 mm Cu half-value layer (HVL), SSD = 50 cm (Data from Hospital Physicists' Association. Central axis depth dose data for use in radiotherapy. *Br J Radiol.* 1978; [suppl 110]; and the Appendix).

- *Properties*: the properties of PDD are summarized below:
  - ➤ After the initial buildup, PDD decreases with depth almost exponentially with depth.
  - ➤ The depth of maximum dose increases with increase in beam energy.
  - ➤ The higher the beam energy, the more gradual is the fall off of the depth dose curve beyond the depth of maximum dose.
  - ➤ PDD has two dose components: a) the primary dose contributed by primary photons–the photons that have traversed the overlying medium without interacting; and b) the scattered dose contributed by scattered photons.
  - ➤ PDD increases with increase in field size due to increase in the scattered component of dose.
  - ➤ The primary component of dose is independent of field size (provided the field dimensions are not less than the range of laterally scattered secondary electrons).
  - ➤ Field dimensions as well as shape (e.g., square, rectangular, or irregular) affect the PDD because of changes in the scatter contribution.
  - ➤ The magnitude of increase in PDD due to increase in field size depends on beam quality. The field size dependence of PDD is less pronounced for the higher-energy than for the lower-energy beams.
- *Field equivalence*: for central axis depth dose distribution, a rectangular field may be approximated by an equivalent square or circle. Tables of calculated equivalent squares and circles are available in the published literature (e.g., Table 9.2 in the Textbook.)
  - ➤ A simple rule of thumb has also been developed for approximate field equivalence. According to this rule, a rectangular field is equivalent to a square field if they have the same area/perimeter (A/P).
  - ➤ The following formulas are useful for quick calculation of the equivalent field parameter:
    For rectangular fields,

$$A/P = \frac{a \times b}{2(a+b)}$$

where a is the field width and b the field length.

For square fields, since $a = b$,

$$A/P = \frac{a}{4}$$

where a is the side of the square. From the above equations, it is evident that the side of an equivalent square of a rectangular field is $4 \times A/P$.

EXAMPLE: A 10×15-cm field has an A/P of 3.0. Its equivalent square is approximately 12×12 cm.

➤ Radii of equivalent circles may be obtained by the relationship:

$$r = \frac{4}{\sqrt{\pi}} \cdot A/P$$

The above equation is derived by assuming that the equivalent circle is the one that has the same area as the equivalent square.

• *Dependence on source-to-surface distance (SSD)*:

➤ Percent depth dose increases with SSD for all depths greater than the reference depth d_0 because of the effects of inverse square law.

➤ Although the actual dose rate at a point decreases with increase in distance from the source, the PDD, which is a relative dose with respect to a reference point at depth d_0, increases with SSD for depths greater than d_0.

➤ PDD for a standard SSD (e.g., 100 cm) can be converted to PDD for another SSD by multiplying it by an approximate factor, known as the *Mayneord F factor*.

➤ Mayneord F factor is based on a strict application of the inverse square law, without considering changes in scatter, as the SSD is changed.

➤ The Mayneord *F* factor is given by:

$$F = \left(\frac{f_2 + d_m}{f_1 + d_m} \right)^2 \cdot \left(\frac{f_1 + d}{f_2 + d} \right)^2$$

where f_1 is the SSD for which PDD is known, f_2 the SSD for which PDD is to be calculated, d_m the reference depth of maximum dose, and d the given depth. The field size projected at the depth d is kept the same for both SSDs. The geometry is illustrated in Figure 9.3.

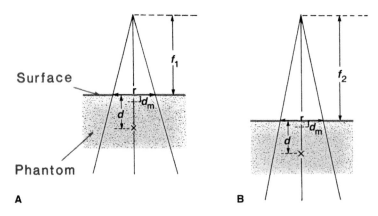

Figure 9.3. Change of percent depth dose with source-to-surface distance (SSD). Irradiation condition (**A**) has **SSD** = f_1 and condition (**B**) has SSD = f_2. For both the conditions, field size on the phantom surface, $r \times r$, and depth, d, are the same.

➤ It can be shown that the *F* factor is greater than 1 for $f_2 > f_1$ and less than 1 for $f_2 < f_1$. Thus, it may be restated that the PDD increases with increase in SSD.

➤ The Mayneord F factor method works reasonably well for small fields since the scattering is minimal under these conditions. However, the method can give rise to significant errors under extreme conditions such as lower energy, large field, large depth, and large SSD change.

➤ In general, the Mayneord F factor overestimates the increase in PDD with increase in SSD.

TISSUE-AIR RATIO

Tissue-air ratio may be defined as the ratio of the dose (D_d) at a given point in the phantom to the *dose in free space* (D_{fs}) at the same point.

• The term "dose in free space" stands for dose at the center of an equilibrium mass of tissue located in free air (i.e., a spherical tissue mass of radius large enough to provide electronic equilibrium at the center). This is illustrated in Figure 9.4.

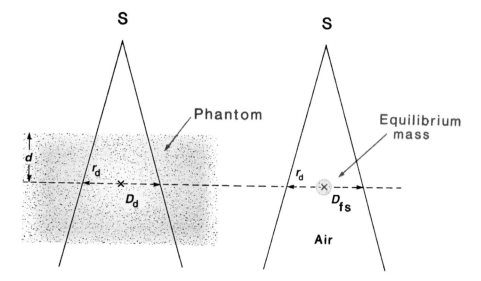

Figure 9.4. Illustration of the definition of tissue-air ratio (TAR). TAR (d, r_d) = D_d/D_{fs}.

• For a given quality beam, TAR depends on depth *d* and field size r_d at that depth:

$$\text{TAR}(d, r_d) = \frac{D_d}{D_{fs}}$$

• TAR, like the PDD, depends on depth, beam energy, field size, and field shape.

• TAR is almost independent of SSD.

• TARs have traditionally been used for dose calculation involving low-energy beams (up to ^{60}Co) and isocentric beam geometry (e.g., rotation therapy or stationary SAD techniques). Current methods of dose calculation use TPRs or TMRs, which have no limitation of beam energy and involve dosimetric measurements in phantom rather than in air (discussed in Chapter 10).

Backscatter Factor

Backscatter factor (BSF) or peak scatter factor (PSF) is a special case of TAR. It is the TAR at the reference depth of maximum dose on central axis of the beam. Mathematically,

$$\text{BSF} = \frac{D_{\max}}{D_{fs}}$$

or

$$\text{BSF} = \text{TAR}(d_{\text{m}}, r_{d_{\text{m}}})$$

where $r_{d_{\text{m}}}$ is the field size at the reference depth d_{m} of maximum dose.

- BSF is a substantial factor for beams in the orthovoltage range of energies (highest values are for beams of approximately 0.6 mm Cu HVL and can be as much as 1.20 to 1.24 (or 20%–40%), depending on field size). BSF decreases to a few percents for ^{60}Co and approaches unity (0%) for higher-energy x-ray beams.
- BSF, like the TAR, is no longer used in the dosimetry of megavoltage beams except for a few institutions where it is still used as a "dummy variable" in dose calculation formalisms (discussed in Chapter 10).

> *Relationship between TAR and PDD*: TAR and PDD are interrelated. Mathematically,

$$P(d, r, f) = \text{TAR}(d, r_d) \times \frac{1}{\text{BSF}(r)} \times \left(\frac{f + d_{\text{m}}}{f + d}\right)^2 \times 100$$

where $P(d, r, f)$ is the percent depth dose at depth d for a field size r at the surface and SSD f. $\text{TAR}(d, r_d)$ is the TAR at depth d for the field size r_d projected at depth d.

SCATTER-AIR RATIO

Scatter-air ratio (SAR) represents the scatter component of TAR. It is a useful concept for the dosimetry of irregularly shaped fields (e.g., Clarkson technique). SAR may be defined as the ratio of the scattered dose at a given point in the phantom to the dose in free space at the same point.

- The SAR is mathematically given by the difference between the TAR for the given field and the TAR for a 0×0 field (representing a small field containing no scattered radiation).

$$\text{SAR}(d, r_d) = \text{TAR}(d, r_d) - \text{TAR}(d, 0)$$

where $\text{TAR}(d, 0)$ represents TAR for 0×0 field (the primary component of TAR).

- Like the TARs, SARs may be used for ^{60}Co or lower energy beams. A more universal quantity is the SPR (the scatter component of TPR) or the SMR (the scatter component of TMR) (discussed in Chapter 10).

DOSIMETRY OF IRREGULAR FIELDS—CLARKSON TECHNIQUE

Clarkson method is based on the principle that the scattered component of the dose, which depends on the field size and shape, can be calculated separately from the primary component which is independent of the field size and shape. A special quantity, SAR, is used to calculate the scattered dose.

- The Clarkson technique involves dividing the field cross section into elementary sectors by drawing radii from the point of calculation to the boundary of the field at equal angular intervals (e.g., $\Delta\theta = 10°$), as illustrated in Figure 9.5.
- SAR values for the sectors are summed to give the average scatter-air ratio ($\overline{\text{SAR}}$) for the irregular field at the calculation point. The $\overline{\text{SAR}}$ thus computed is converted to average tissue-air ratio $\overline{\text{TAR}}$ by the equation:

$$\overline{\text{TAR}} = \text{TAR}(0) + \overline{\text{SAR}}$$

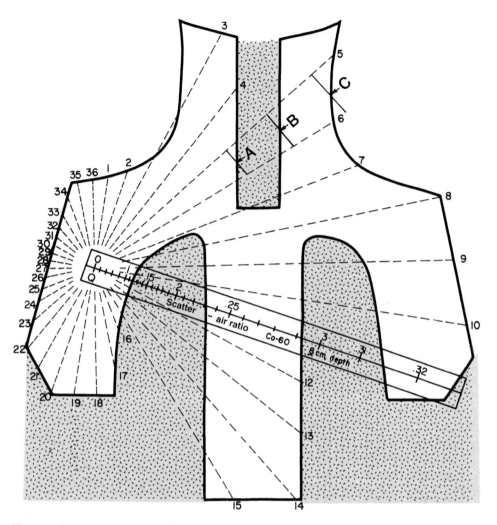

Figure 9.5. Outline of mantle field in a plane perpendicular to the beam axis and at a specified depth. Radii are drawn from point Q, the point of calculation. Sector angle = 10°. (Redrawn from American Association of Physicist in Medicine. Dosimetry workshop: Hodgkin's disease. Chicago, IL, MD Anderson Hospital, Houston, TX. Radiological Physics Center, 1970.)

where TAR(0) is the tissue-air ratio for 0×0 field and is given by:

$$\text{TAR}(0) = e^{-\bar{\mu}(d-d_m)}$$

where $\bar{\mu}$ is the average linear attenuation coefficient for the primary beam and d is depth of point of calculation. $\overline{\text{TAR}}$ can be converted to PDD, if needed, for an SSD technique.

- SARs have been traditionally used for ^{60}Co beams. For cobalt or higher-energy beams, SPRs or SMRs are more appropriate quantities to be used for the Clarkson integration technique.

DOSE CALCULATION IN ROTATION THERAPY

Calculation of depth dose in rotation therapy involves the determination of average TAR at the isocenter. The contour of the patient is drawn in a plane containing the axis of rotation. The isocenter is then placed within the contour (usually in the middle of the tumor or a few centimeters beyond it) and radii are drawn from this point at selected angular intervals (e.g., 20°) (Figure 9.6).

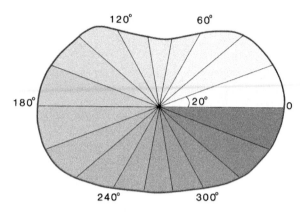

Figure 9.6. Contour of patient with radii drawn from the isocenter of rotation at 20° intervals. Length of each radius represents a depth for which tissue-air ratio is determined for the field size at the isocenter (see table in the Textbook).

Each radius represents a depth for which TAR can be obtained from the TAR table, for the given beam energy and field size defined at the isocenter. The TARs are then summed and averaged to determine $\overline{\text{TAR}}$.

- For beam energies greater than ^{60}Co, the dosimetric quantity used for dose calculation is TPR (or TMR) instead of TAR.

REVIEW QUESTIONS • Chapter 9

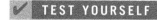

✔ TEST YOURSELF

Review questions for this chapter are provided online.

In multiple choice questions, more than one option may be correct.

1. For a phantom to be nearly tissue equivalent for measuring depth dose distribution in megavoltage photon beams, which one of the following properties should it have approximately the same as soft tissue?
   a) Number of electrons per unit mass
   b) Number of electrons per unit volume
   c) Mass per unit volume
   d) Effective atomic number

2. Which quantities are almost independent of SSD?
   a) Tissueair–ratio
   b) Scatter–air ratio
   c) Backscatter (or peakscatter) factor
   d) Mayneord F factor

3. Which of the following quality beams would have the largest backscatter factor for a 20×20 cm field?
   a) 20 keV photon beam
   b) 1.8 mm Al HVL x-rays
   c) 0.6 mm Cu HVL x-rays
   d) ^{60}C γ-rays

4. What is the dose in cGy to the spinal cord (point P, depth = 5 cm) when 180 cGy is delivered at the isocenter (point Q, depth = 10 cm) using a single 10×10 cm ^{60}Co field? [Assume SAD = 80 cm and TARs at points P and Q to be 0.900 and 0.709, respectively.]
   a) 228
   b) 252
   c) 260
   d) 293

5. In the above problem, what would be the dose to the spinal cord if the percentage depth doses at 5 and 10 cm depths obtained from a percentage depth dose table for 80 cm SSD are 78.0% and 54.8%, respectively?
   a) 228
   b) 252
   c) 260
   d) 293

6. A dense bone insert for a CT density phantom has the following chemical composition (by weight):

Element	Z	A	Chemical Composition
Hydrogen	1	1.0	4.45%
Carbon	6	12.0	39.11%
Nitrogen	7	14.0	0.87%
Oxygen	8	16.0	33.72%
Chlorine	17	35.4	0.05%
Calcium	20	40.1	21.77%

If the physical density of the insert is 1.61 g/cm^3, what is the electron density?
   a) 1.61×10^{23} electrons/cm^3
   b) 6.02×10^{23} electrons/cm^3

   c) 4.85×10^{23} electrons/cm^3

   d) 5.06×10^{23} electrons/cm^3

   e) 1.61×10^{23} electrons/g

7. Using the area/perimeter rule of thumb, what is the equivalent square of a rectangular field of size 10×20 cm^2?

   a) 12 cm^2

   b) 13.3 cm^2

   c) 14.0 cm^2

   d) 15.0 cm^2

   e) 16.7 cm^2

8. In the above problem, what is the radius of an equivalent circle?

   a) 3.8 cm

   b) 4.2 cm

   c) 6.5 cm

   d) 7.5 cm

9. Given the same equivalent area of a square and a rectangular ^{60}Co field, the central axis percent depth dose is:

   a) Greater for the rectangular field

   b) Greater for the square field

   c) Same for both fields

   d) Not dependent on field shape

10. The percentage depth dose at a depth of 10 cm for a 10×10 cm^2 6 MV beam at 100 cm SSD is 67.0%. Using the Mayneord F factor, and reference depth $d_m = 1.5$ cm, what is the percentage depth dose for the same field size and depth at 120 cm SSD?

   a) 65.3%

   b) 66.1%

   c) 67.9%

   d) 68.7%

   e) 69.6%

11. Which of the following statements is/are true?

   a) For all depths (greater than the reference depth) and field sizes, the Mayneord F factor is always ≥ 1, for increasing SSDs (i.e., $f_2 > f_1$).

   b) For rotational therapy, the average TAR is computed by computing the average radius over the area of rotation.

   c) The backscatter factor corrects for photons and electrons that backscatter into the monitor chamber from the collimating jaws.

   d) The peak of the backscatter factor occurs around 0.6 to 0.8 mm Cu, depending on the field size.

   e) TAR at depth d_m equals BSF.

12. The dose in free space for a ^{60}Co unit is 150 cGy/min at 80.5 cm for a field size of 10×10 cm^2, SSD = 80 cm. If the percentage depth dose is 64.7% at depth of 8 cm, what is the treatment time required to deliver 100 cGy for a 10×10 cm^2 field size at a depth of 8 cm at 100 cm SSD?

   a) 0.75 min

   b) 1.00 min

   c) 1.25 min

   d) 1.55 min

   e) 2.00 min

13. When treating with orthovoltage x-rays, the percentage depth dose will increase with increase in:

   a) Field size
   b) kV_p
   c) Tube mA
   d) Filtration

14. The depth of maximum dose in a megavoltage beam:

   a) Increases with field size
   b) Decreases with SSD
   c) Increases with beam energy
   d) Increases with dose rate

10

A SYSTEM OF DOSIMETRIC CALCULATIONS

LECTURE

10

REFERENCE

Khan FM. *The Physics of Radiation Therapy*, 4th edition, 2009. Chapter 10 "A System of Dosimetric Calculations"

Formalism for Monitor Units Calculation

 TOPIC OUTLINE

The following topics will be discussed in this lecture:

➤ Depth dose components
  • Primary dose
  • Scattered dose
➤ Dosimetric quantities
  • Collimator (head scatter) factor (S_c)
  • Total scatter factor ($S_{c,p}$)
  • Phantom scatter factor (S_p)
  • Tissue–phantom ratio (TPR)
  • Tissue–maximum ratio (TMR)
➤ Monitor unit calculation formalism
  • Isocentric and non-isocentric fields
  • Irregular fields
  • Asymmetric fields
➤ Appendix
  • Effect of buildup cap on S_c measurement

DEPTH DOSE COMPONENTS

The dose to a point in a medium may be analyzed into primary and scattered components. Mathematically:

$$D_T = D_p + D_s$$

where D_T is the total dose, D_p the primary dose, and D_s the scattered dose.

PRIMARY DOSE

The primary component of dose is the dose due to photons that have not experienced scatter.

• Primary dose in a phantom is represented by the dose in a hypothetical 0×0 cm^2 field which is obtained by extrapolation of the depth dose versus field size data. In practice, this extrapolation is performed for small fields, down to a field size just small enough to provide lateral scatter electronic equilibrium (e.g., field sizes in the range of 3×3 to 5×5 cm^2 for most energies) to a 0×0 cm^2 field size. Smaller field sizes where lateral electronic equilibrium may not exist are not included in this extrapolation.

- The representation of primary beam by a 0×0 cm^2 field, with the implicit assumption that lateral electronic equilibrium exists at all points, is a practical concept used for separating primary from scatter in a phantom under conditions of lateral electronic equilibrium. Strictly speaking, it is not valid for the absolute determination of primary or scattered dose in a phantom.
- For megavoltage photon beams, it is reasonable to consider collimator scatter as part of the primary beam so that the phantom scatter could be calculated separately. We, therefore, define an *effective primary dose* in phantom as the dose due to the primary photons as well as those scattered from the collimating system. The effective primary dose in a phantom may be thought of as the dose at depth minus the dose due to phantom scatter. Alternatively, the effective primary dose may be defined as the depth dose expected in the field when scattering volume is reduced to zero, while keeping the collimator opening constant.

SCATTERED DOSE

The scattered dose in a phantom is contributed by photons that have been scattered in the phantom (called phantom scatter).

- Phantom scatter increases with increase in field size irradiating the phantom.
- Collimator scatter increases with increase in the collimator opening. It is contributed by photon scatter from the target, primary collimator (fixed), flattening filter, monitor chambers, and movable collimators (jaws). Of the field size-dependent components of collimator scatter, the greatest contribution is from the flattening filter.

DOSIMETRIC QUANTITIES

In Chapter 9, we discussed dose calculation methods involving percentage depth dose (PDD) and tissue–air ratio (TAR). The beam output was represented by exposure rate or dose rate in free space. The problem with a dose calculation formalism based on these functions is that some of these parameters involve dose measurements in air or "free space". For high-energy beams (i.e., energy > ^{60}Co), for example, beam output in air in terms of exposure rate or dose rate in free space cannot be measured accurately. Thus, the use of TARs, scatter-air ratios (SARs), and backscatter factors is not suitable for high-energy linac x-ray beams. A formalism based on tissue-phantom ratios (TPRs), however, has no such limitations and is, therefore, recommended for photon beams of any energy. Essential features of this formalism are discussed below.

COLLIMATOR (HEAD SCATTER) FACTOR

The *collimator scatter factor* (S_c) is commonly called the *in air output ratio* and may be defined as the ratio of the output (photon energy fluence) in air for a given field to that for a reference field (e.g., 10×10 cm^2) at the same point.

- S_c may be measured in air with an ion chamber using a buildup cap of a size large enough to provide maximum dose buildup for the given energy beam. The measurement setup and the plot of data to determine S_c are shown in Figure 10.1A.
- Because S_c is a ratio of two ionization measurements in air with the same buildup cap and beam geometry, the attenuation and scatter effects of the buildup cap (i.e., fraction of fluence attenuated or scattered) cancel out. The ionization ratio thus measured represents the ratio of energy fluences in air that would exist at the point of measurement in the absence of the buildup cap. This is shown mathematically in the Appendix.
- In the measurement of S_c, the field must fully cover the buildup cap (without penumbral effects) for all field sizes. A lateral margin of at least 1 cm between the field edge and the buildup cap is considered adequate.
- Normally, the collimator scatter factors are measured at the source-to-axis distance (SAD). However, larger distances may be used provided the field sizes are all defined at the SAD.

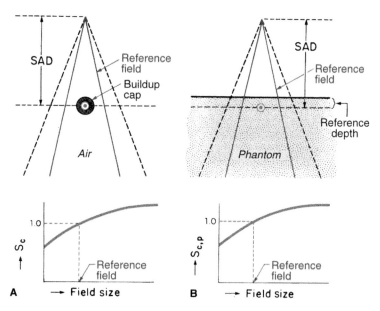

Figure 10.1. A,B. Arrangement for measuring S_c and $S_{c,p}$ **A:** Chamber with buildup cap in air to measure output relative to a reference field, for determining S_c versus field size. **B:** Measurements in a phantom at a fixed reference depth for determining $S_{c,p}$ versus field size. SAD, source-to-axis distance. (From Khan FM, Sewchand W, Lee J, et al. Revision of tissue–maximum ratio and scatter-maximum ratio and scatter-maximum ratio concepts for ^{60}Co and higher energy x-ray beams. *Med Phys.* 1980;7:230.)

- For small fields, one may take the output measurements (including those for the reference field) at distances larger than the SAD so that the smallest field covers the buildup cap with a suitable margin. Since the measurements for the given field and the reference field are made at the same distance, the effect of distance or the intervening air (assuming negligible photon scatter by air) is canceled out.

TOTAL SCATTER FACTOR

The *total scatter factor* ($S_{c,p}$) is defined as the dose rate (or dose per monitor unit [MU]) for a given field at a reference depth in a phantom divided by the dose rate at the same point and depth for the reference field (10×10 cm^2). The measurement geometry and the plot of data to determine $S_{c,p}$ are shown in Figure 10.1B.

- $S_{c,p}$ is a factor that combines both the collimator scatter and phantom scatter at the reference depth.

PHANTOM SCATTER FACTOR

The *phantom scatter factor* (S_p) may be defined as the ratio of dose rate (or dose per MU) for a given field at a reference depth to the dose rate at the same point and depth for the reference field (e.g., 10×10 cm) with the same collimator opening (same incident energy fluence) (see Figure 10.2).

- S_p may be measured using the geometry shown in Figure 10.2 or indirectly using the following equation:

$$s_p(r) = \frac{s_{c,p}(r)}{s_c(r)}$$

where r is the side of the equivalent square field at the reference depth.

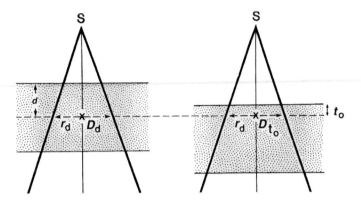

Figure 10.2. Diagram illustrating the definitions of tissue–phantom ratio (TPR) and tissue–maximum ratio (TMR). $\text{TPR}(d, r_\text{d}) = D_\text{d}/D_{t_\text{o}}$, where t_o is a reference depth. If t_o is the reference depth of maximum dose, then $\text{TMR}(d, r_\text{d}) = \text{TPR}(d, r_\text{d})$.

TISSUE–PHANTOM RATIO

The quantity TPR is defined as the ratio of the dose rate at a given point at depth in a phantom to the dose rate at the same point and distance at a reference depth.

- TPRs have the same properties as TARs, namely, they depend on energy, depth and field size, and are almost independent of SSD.

- The corresponding quantity for the scattered dose is called the scatter–phantom ratio (SPR), which is analogous in use to the SAR discussed in the previous chapter.

- The advantage of TPR over TAR is the fact that the former is determined from measurements in a phantom rather than in air, thus avoiding the limitations of measuring TAR for high-energy photon beams.

REFERENCE DEPTH

For the quantities discussed above, any reference depth may be chosen, provided:

- It is equal to or greater than the depth of maximum dose for all field sizes.
- It is fixed for all field sizes.

Reference Depth of Maximum Dose

- Since the depth of maximum dose is, in general, field-size dependent (because of changes in electron contamination with field size), it should be determined for a small field size (e.g., 3×3 cm^2) for which the electron contamination is negligibly small, or for a 0×0 cm^2 field size by extrapolation of the depths of maximum dose as a function of field size.

- The reference depth determined for a given energy beam should be kept the same for all field sizes and all dosimetric quantities involving reference depth, for example, PDD, TPRs, phantom scatter factors, and the depth at which the dose per MU is set for the accelerator calibration.

Reference Depth of 10 cm

- TPR may be normalized to a 10 cm depth, in which case the problem of electron contamination is eliminated.

- Formalism for MU calculations must ensure that all relevant dosimetric parameters, TPR, PDD, S_p, and the calibration dose/MU, are normalized to the same reference depth.

TISSUE–MAXIMUM RATIO

Tissue–maximum ratio (TMR) is a special case of TPR in which the reference depth is set at maximum dose. It is defined as the ratio of the dose at a given point in phantom to the dose at the same point and distance at the reference depth of maximum dose (see Figure 10.2).

• TMRs have the same properties as TPRs and TARs, namely, they depend on energy, depth, and field size, and are almost independent of SSD.

• Figure 10.3 shows TMR data for a 10-MV x-ray beam, as an example.

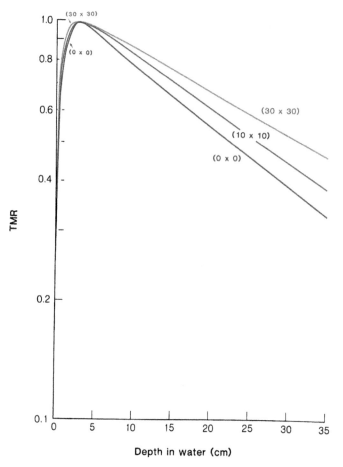

Figure 10.3. Plot of tissue–maximum ratio (TMR) for 10-MV x-rays as a function of depth for a selection of field sizes.

• The curve for 0×0 cm^2 field size represents the primary beam and shows the steepest drop-off with depth because of the lack of scatter.

• TMR and PDD are interrelated by the following equation:

$$TMR(d,r_\mathrm{d}) = \left[\frac{P(d,r,f)}{100}\right]\left[\frac{f+d}{f+t_0}\right]^2\left[\frac{S_p+(r_{t_0})}{S_p+r_\mathrm{d}}\right]$$

where P is the percent depth dose, d is the depth, t_0 the reference depth of maximum dose, and r the field size at the surface.

$$f = \mathrm{SSD}, \quad r_d = r\left(\frac{f+d}{f}\right)$$

$$r_{t_0} = r\left(\frac{f+t_0}{f}\right)$$

The PDD *P* is referenced against the dose at depth t_0 so that $P(t_0, r, f) = 100$ for all field sizes and SSDs.

- Although TMRs can be measured directly, they can be calculated from PDD by using the above equation.
- The above equation for TMR may be generalized to TPR for any reference depth (d_{ref}) (e.g., 10 cm):

$$TPR(d,r_d) = \left[\frac{P_N(d,r,f)}{100}\right]\left[\frac{f+d}{f+d_0}\right]\left[\frac{S_p(r_{d_0})}{S_p(r_d)}\right]$$

where d_0 is the reference depth and P_N the normalized percentage depth dose.

$$r_{d_0} = r \cdot \left(\frac{f+t_0}{f}\right)$$

- P_N is the ratio, expressed as a percentage, of the dose rate at depth d to the dose rate at the normalization depth, d_0, for a given field size r at the surface.
- The normalized PDDs (P_N) can be obtained from the regular PDDs (P) (which are normalized to a reference depth of maximum dose, t_0) by using the following equation:

$$P_N(d,r,f) = \frac{P(d,r,f)}{P(d_0,r,f)} \times 100$$

MONITOR UNIT CALCULATION FORMALISM

Radiotherapy institutions vary in their treatment techniques and calibration practices. For example, some rely exclusively on the SAD (isocentric)-type techniques, while others use both the SSD- and SAD-type techniques. Accordingly, units are calibrated in phantom at a reference depth for the standard SSD (SSD-type calibration) or at the isocenter (SAD-type calibration). Although most institutions use a reference depth of maximum dose, some prefer 10-cm depth as the reference depth. In addition, clinical fields, although basically rectangular or square, are more often than not shaped to protect critical or normal regions of the body. Thus, a calculation system must be generally applicable to the above practices, with acceptable accuracy and simplicity for routine use.

GENERAL EQUATIONS

The following general equations cover most of the clinical situations involving MU calculations.

FOR ISOCENTRIC FIELDS

$$MU = \frac{D}{D_{cal} \cdot S_c(r_c) \cdot S_p(r_d) \cdot TPR(d,r_d) \cdot WF(d,r_d,x) \cdot TF \cdot OAR(d,x) \cdot \left[\frac{SCD}{SPD}\right]^2}$$

Or,

$$MU = \frac{D}{D_{cal} \cdot S_c(r_c) \cdot S_p(r_d) \cdot TMR(d,r_d) \cdot WF(d,r_d,x) \cdot TF \cdot OAR(d,x) \cdot \left[\frac{SCD}{SPD}\right]^2}$$

FOR NON-ISOCENTRIC FIELDS

$$MU = \frac{D}{D_{cal} \cdot S_c(r_c) \cdot S_p(r) \cdot \frac{P}{100}(d,r,f) \cdot WF(d,r_d,x) \cdot TF \cdot OAR(d,x) \cdot \left[\frac{SCD}{f+t_0}\right]^2}$$

Or,

$$MU = \frac{D}{D_{cal} \cdot S_c(r_c) \cdot S_p(r) \cdot \frac{P_N}{100}(d,r,f) \cdot WF(d,r_d,x) \cdot TF \cdot OAR(d,x) \cdot \left[\frac{SCD}{f+d_0}\right]^2}$$

where:

D = dose to be delivered at the point of interest;

D_{cal} = calibration dose per MU at d_{ref} under reference conditions;

$S_c(r_c)$ = collimator scatter (or head scatter) factor for the collimator-defined field size r_c;

$S_p(r)$ = phantom scatter factor at d_{ref} for the field size r at the surface;

$S_p(r_d)$ = phantom scatter factor at d_{ref} for the field size r_d at depth d;

$WF(d, r_d, x)$ = wedge factor at depth, d; field size, r_d; and off-axis distance, x;

TF = Tray factor;

$OAR(d,x)$ = off-axis ratio at depth d and off-axis distance x;

SCD = source-to-calibration point distance at which D_{cal} is specified;

SPD = source-to-point of interest distance at which D is delivered;

d_0 = d_{ref} for TPR and PDD$_N$;

t_0 = d_{ref} of maximum dose for TMR and PDD.

- The above MU equations assume that:

  ➤ The calibration dose per MU, D_{cal}, is specified at the source-to-calibration point distance, *SCD*, for the reference field size and at the reference depth.

  ➤ d_{ref} for D_{cal} and S_p is the same as for the respective dosimetric quantity (TPR, TMR, PDD, or PDD$_N$) in conjunction with which they are used.

  ➤ Tray factor, TF, is a transmission factor for the blocking tray, independent of field size and depth.

  ➤ Inverse-square law holds good for change in photon energy fluence in air as a function of distance from the source.

IRREGULAR FIELDS

Clarkson technique (described in Chapter 9) may be used to calculate dose in an irregular field using SPRs—in the same way as with SARs for low-energy beams. A field of any shape projected at depth d is divided into n elementary sectors with radii emanating from the point of interest. Integration of SPRs, $SPR(d, r_d)$, is performed to give average $\overline{SPR}(d, r_d)$:

$$\overline{SPR}(d, r_d) = \frac{1}{n}\sum_{i=1}^{n} SPR(d, r_i)$$

where r_i is the radius of the ith sector at depth d and n the total number of sectors ($n = 2\pi/\Delta\theta$, where $\Delta\theta$ is the sector angle). $\overline{TPR}(d, r_d)$ is given by:

$$\overline{TPR}(d, r_d) = [K_p \cdot TPR(d,0) + \overline{SPR}(d, r_d)] \times \frac{S_p(0)}{\overline{S}_p(r_d)}$$

where K_p is the off-axis ratio at the point of interest for the primary beam, and $\overline{S}_p(r_d)$ is the average S_p for the irregular field.

- Clarkson technique is a general method of calculating depth dose distribution in an irregularly shaped field, but it is not practical for routine manual calculations.

- Reasonably accurate calculations can be made for most blocked fields using an approximate method. An approximate method is illustrated in Figure 10.4.

- In this method, approximate rectangles may be drawn containing the point of calculation to include most of the irradiated area surrounding the point and exclude only those areas that are remote to the point. In doing so, a blocked area may be included in the rectangle, provided this area is small and is remotely located relative to that point. The rectangle thus formed may be called the *effective field* irradiating the phantom while the unblocked field, defined by the collimator, may be called the *collimator field*.

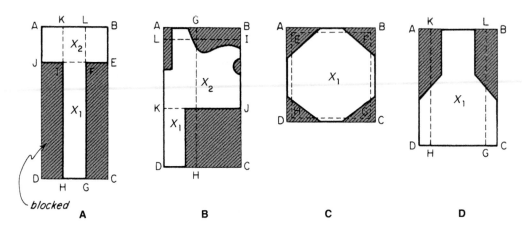

Figure 10.4. Examples of irregularly shaped fields. Equivalent rectangles for dose at points of interest are shown by dashed lines. Points versus equivalent rectangles are **(A)** 1, *GHKL*; 2, *ABFJ*. **(B)** 1, *AGHD*; 2, *LIJK*. **(C)** 1, *EFGH*. **(D)** 1, *KLGH*. (From Levitt SH, Khan FM, Potish RA, eds. *Technological Basis of Radiation Therapy: Practical and Clinical Applications.* 2nd ed. Philadelphia, PA: Lea & Febiger; 1992:73.)

- Once the effective field has been determined, one may proceed with the usual MU calculations as discussed above.
- Whereas S_c pertains to the collimator-defined field, S_p and the dosimetric function involving TPR, TMR, or PDD correspond to the effective field irradiating the patient.

ASYMMETRIC FIELDS

When a field is collimated asymmetrically, one needs to take into account changes in:

- Collimator scatter
- Phantom scatter
- Off-axis depth dose distribution
  - ➤ For a point at the center of an asymmetric field and a lateral distance *x* away from the beam central axis, the collimator scatter factor, S_c, may be approximated by the S_c for a symmetric field of the same collimator opening as that of the given asymmetric field.
  - ➤ The phantom scatter can also be assumed to be the same for an asymmetric field as for a symmetric field of the same dimensions and shape, provided the point of calculation is located away from the field edges (absence of penumbral effects).
  - ➤ An appropriate off-axis ratio, OAR(d,x), is required to take into account the change in off-axis depth dose distribution. This factor, if derived from beam profiles measured in a large symmetric field, may be unsuitable for asymmetric fields collimated at large off-axis distances. Primary off-axis ratios, POAR(d,x), would be more suitable. The latter are either calculated by using a treatment planning system or measured by using small asymmetric fields and various thickness absorbers under good geometry conditions.

APPENDIX

EFFECT OF BUILDUP CAP ON S_C MEASUREMENT

Suppose the buildup cap is of a sufficiently large diameter so that there is a maximum electronic buildup and negligible electron contamination at the chamber position.

Let: ψ_1 and ψ_2 be the energy fluence rates in air at the point of measurement (in the absence of buildup cap) for the given field and the reference field, respectively. Let I_1 and I_2 be the respective ionization currents measured using the buildup cap. Let f_a be the fraction of fluence attenuated and f_s be the fraction of fluence added due to scatter by the buildup cap. Then:

$$S_c = \frac{I_1}{I_2} = \frac{\psi_1(1 - f_a + f_s)}{\psi_2(1 - f_a + f_s)} = \frac{\psi_1}{\psi_2}$$

Thus the attenuation and scatter effects of the buildup cap cancel out in the measurement of S_c.

REVIEW QUESTIONS • Chapter 10

In multiple choice questions, more than one option may be correct.

1. The collimator scatter (or head scatter) factor (S_c):
   a) Is independent of SSD.
   b) Decreases as the field is reduced by inserting secondary blocks.
   c) Increases with increase in the collimator-defined field size.
   d) Is the same as the normalized backscatter factor.

2. Phantom scatter factor (S_p):
   a) Is independent of SSD.
   b) Is the same as the peak scatter factor for megavoltage beams.
   c) Depends on the extent of field blocking.
   d) Is unity at the depth of maximum dose for megavoltage beams.

3. A 4-MV linear accelerator is calibrated to give 1 cGy (10^{-2} Gy) per MU in phantom at a reference depth of maximum dose of 1 cm, 100-cm SSD, and 10×10 cm field size. Determine the MU values to deliver 100 cGy to a patient at 100-cm SSD, 10-cm depth, and 15×15 cm field size, given S_c (15×15 cm) = 1.02. [Use data given in TABLE A.10.1, page A-15, Textbook Appendix].
   a) 141
   b) 146
   c) 150
   d) 154

4. Calculate MU values for the above problem using TMR instead of PDD. [Use data from TABLE A.10.2, page A-16, Textbook Appendix].
   a) 141
   b) 146
   c) 150
   d) 154

5. In problem 3, what is the dose at 5-cm depth?
   a) 124.3 cGy
   b) 128.0 cGy
   c) 134.5 cGy
   d) 141.6 cGy

6. In problem 4, what is the dose at 5-cm depth?
   a) 124.3 cGy
   b) 128.0 cGy
   c) 134.5 cGy
   d) 141.6 cGy

7. Tissue–phantom ratios (TPRs) are:
   a) The same as TMRs if the reference depth for both quantities is the reference depth of maximum dose.
   b) Independent of field blocking as long as the collimator opening remains the same.
   c) Less than TMRs at all corresponding depths if the reference depth for TPRs is 10 cm.
   d) Less than the (PDD/100) at all corresponding depths.

8. Which quantity would likely be least affected by choice of reference depth:
   a) S_c
   b) S_p
   c) TPR(d, r_d)
   d) $PDD_N(d, r, f)$

Use the following dosimetric data for problems 9 to 12:

* 6 MV Linac;
* D_{cal} = 0.8 cGy/MU for 10×10 cm^2, depth = 10 cm, 100 cm SAD;
* Normalization depth: 10 cm

Measured output factors

Field Size (cm)	S_c	S_{cp}
8×8	0.991	0.962
10×10	1.000	1.000
12×12	1.007	1.028
15×15	1.014	1.045

Normalized Percent Depth Dose (SSD = 100)

Depth (cm)	8×8	9×9	10×10	11×11	12×12
1.5	153.6	151.9	150.4	149.5	148.7
5	131.1	130.1	129.3	128.8	128.4
10	100.0	100.0	100.0	100.0	100.0
20	56.4	56.9	57.3	57.7	58.2

9. The phantom scatter factor for a 5×20 cm^2 field size is:
   a) 0.991
   b) 0.962
   c) 1.030
   d) 1.035
   e) 0.971

10. The TPR for a 10×15 cm^2 field size at $d = 5$ cm is:
    a) 0.991
    b) 1.012
    c) 1.176
    d) 0.912
    e) 1.107

11. The monitor units (MUs) necessary to deliver 100 cGy to a 12×12 cm^2 field size, $d = 5$ cm, 100 cm SAD are:
    a) 95
    b) 103
    c) 109
    d) 91
    e) 83

12. The MU necessary to deliver 100 cGy to a 12×12 cm^2 field size, $d = 5$ cm, 100 cm SSD are:
    a) 114
    b) 121
    c) 103
    d) 97
    e) 136

11

TREATMENT PLANNING I: ISODOSE DISTRIBUTIONS

REFERENCE
Khan FM. *The Physics
of Radiation Therapy*,
4th edition, 2009.
Chapter 11 "Treatment
Planning I: Isodose
Distributions"

Isodose Distribution and Plan Evaluation

 TOPIC OUTLINE

The following topics will be discussed in this lecture:
- ➤ Isodose distributions and parameters
- ➤ Measurement of isodose curves
- ➤ Wedge filters
- ➤ Multiple field combinations
- ➤ Wedge field techniques
- ➤ ICRU volumes for treatment planning
- ➤ Dose specification and reporting
- ➤ Plan evaluation

ISODOSE DISTRIBUTIONS AND PARAMETERS

Isodose curves in a radiation field are lines passing through points of equal dose. The curves are usually drawn at regular intervals of absorbed dose and expressed as a percentage of the dose at a reference point. Thus, the isodose curves represent levels of absorbed dose in the same manner that isotherms are used for heat and isobars for pressure.

GENERAL PROPERTIES

An *isodose chart* for a given beam consists of a family of isodose curves usually drawn at equal increments of percentage depth dose (PDD), representing the variation in dose as a function of depth and transverse distance from the central axis. The depth-dose values of the curves are normalized either at the reference point of maximum dose on the central axis or at a fixed distance along the central axis in the irradiated medium (Figure 11.1).

Examination of isodose charts reveals some general properties of x- and γ-ray dose distributions.

- Dose in a radiation field varies as a function of depth and lateral distance from the central axis.
- Dose variation along central axis is not linear with depth. Beyond the depth of maximum dose buildup, it varies almost exponentially, governed by an effective attenuation coefficient that depends on beam energy (spectral distribution) and field size (scatter distribution).
- Uniformity of lateral dose distribution depends on the inherent field flatness (uniformity of energy fluence across the beam), lateral scatter distribution (influenced by beam energy, field size, and depth), and penumbra (Figure 11.2).

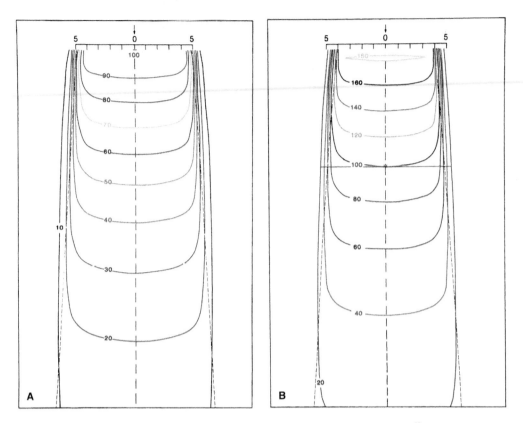

Figure 11.1. Example of an isodose chart. **A:** Source-to-surface distance (SSD) type, ^{60}Co beam, SSD = 80 cm, field size = 10 × 10 cm at surface. **B:** Source-to-axis distance (SAD) type, ^{60}Co beam, SAD = 100 cm, depth of isocenter = 10 cm, field size at isocenter = 10 × 10 cm. (Data from University of Minnesota Hospitals, Eldorado 8 Cobalt Unit, source size = 2 cm.)

- In general, the dose at any depth is greatest on the central axis of the beam and gradually decreases toward the edges of the beam, with the exception of some linac x-ray beams, which exhibit areas of high dose or "horns" near the surface in the periphery of the field. These horns are created by the flattening filter, which may overcompensate near the surface to obtain flat isodose curves at greater depths.

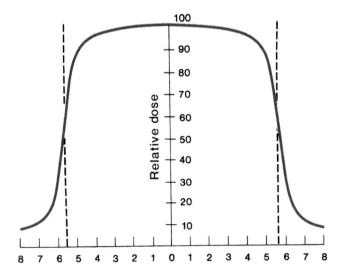

Figure 11.2. Dose profile at depth showing variation of dose across the field. ^{60}Co beam, source-to-surface distance = 80 cm, depth = 10 cm, field size at surface = 10 × 10 cm. Dotted line indicates geometric field boundary at a 10-cm depth.

- Flatness of the isodose curves within the central 80% of the field is described by a parameter called *field flatness*. For the linac x-ray beams, field flatness depends on the flattening filter in the head of the machine, as well as energy (lateral scatter characteristics).

- Flatness is derived from a lateral dose profile measured in a phantom in a plane perpendicular to central axis of the beam at a specified depth (e.g., 10 cm) (Figure 11.3).

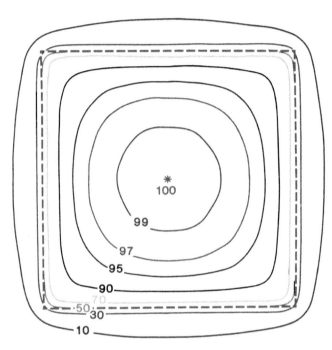

Figure 11.3. Cross-sectional isodose distribution in a plane perpendicular to the central axis of the beam. Isodose values are normalized to 100% at the center of the field. The dotted line shows the boundary of the geometric field.

- The American Association of Physicists in Medicine Task Group 45 specifies flatness in terms of maximum percentage variation from average dose across the central 80% of the full width at half maximum of the profile in a plane transverse to the beam axis. This variation or flatness *F* is mathematically given by:

$$F = \frac{M - m}{M + m} \times 100\%$$

where *M* and *m* are the maximum and minimum dose values in the central 80% of the profile. A dose variation of ±3% is considered acceptable.

- Near the beam edge, falloff of the beam is caused not only by the geometric penumbra but also by the reduced side scatter of photons and the lateral transport of secondary electrons. The penumbra that shows the composite effect is called *physical penumbra*.

- The physical penumbra width is defined as the lateral distance between two specified isodose curves at a specified depth (e.g., lateral distance between 90% and 10% isodose lines at the depth of D_{max}).

- Outside the geometric penumbra, the dose and its falloff is the result of:
  - ➤ Side scatter of photons from the field
  - ➤ Side scatter of secondary electrons from the field
  - ➤ Leakage and scatter from the collimator
  - ➤ Leakage and scatter from the head of the machine (also called *source housing*)

MEASUREMENT OF ISODOSE CURVES

- Ion chamber is the most suitable detector for measuring isodose curves, mainly because of its relatively flat energy response and precision.

- Water is the phantom of choice. The chamber can be made waterproof by a thin plastic sleeve that covers the chamber as well as the portion of the cable immersed in the water.

- The ionization chamber used for isodose measurements should be small so that measurements can be made in regions of high-dose gradient, such as wedged fields or near the edges of the beam. It is recommended that the sensitive volume of the chamber be less than 15 mm long and have an inside diameter of 5 mm or less.

- Basically, the apparatus consists of a water tank with two ionization chambers, referred to as the detector A (or probe) and the monitor B. Whereas the probe is arranged to move in the tank of water to sample the instantaneous ionization current (assumed proportional to dose rate) at various points, the monitor is fixed at some point in the field to monitor the instantaneous beam intensity. The ratio of the detector to the monitor response (A/B) is recorded as the probe is moved in the phantom.

- Isodose curves are synthesized from dose profiles measured at regular intervals of depth using the computer software provided with the water phantom. The isodose values may be normalized to the dose at a reference depth (e.g., the reference depth of maximum dose) or another specified depth (e.g., 10 cm).

- Sample isodose curves for a number of field sizes and treatment conditions (e.g., open fields, wedged fields, asymmetric fields, and fields with a central block) are obtained at the time of commissioning. These data are used as benchmark to test dose distributions generated by a treatment planning system under similar conditions.

WEDGE FILTERS

There are two classes of wedge filters: a) physical wedge filters and b) nonphysical wedge filters.

- A physical wedge filter is a wedge-shaped absorber that causes a progressive decrease in the intensity across the beam from its thin end to the thick end. This differential attenuation of photon fluence across the field results in a tilt of the isodose curves from their normal positions. Figure 11.4 shows an example of wedged isodose curves for a ^{60}Co beam.

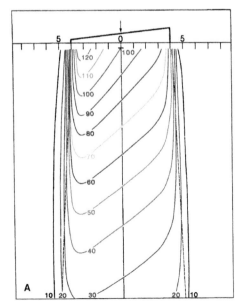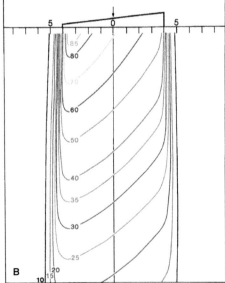

Figure 11.4. Isodose curves for a wedge filter. **A:** Normalized to D_{max}. **B:** normalized to D_{max} without the wedge. ^{60}Co, wedge angle = 45°, field size = 8 × 10 cm, source-to-surface distance = 80 cm.

• A nonphysical wedge filter is an electronic filter that generates a tilted dose distribution profile similar to a physical wedge by moving one of the collimating jaws from one end of the field to the other.

PHYSICAL WEDGE FILTERS

• A physical wedge is usually made of a dense material, such as lead, steel, or brass, and is mounted on a transparent plastic tray or a frame that can be inserted in the designated slot in the head of the machine (Figure 11.5).

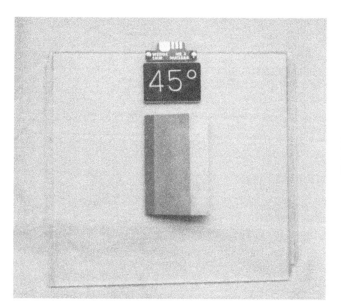

Figure 11.5. Photograph of a 45° wedge filter for a 4-MV x-ray linac (ATC-400).

• In most accelerators, physical wedges are placed at least 50 cm from the isocenter (it is usually less in a cobalt units). However, in isocentric treatments, the distance of the wedge filter from the patient surface varies, depending on the treatment source-to-surface distance. It is important to ensure that the wedge (or the blocking tray below it) is at a sufficiently large distance from the skin surface so that the electron contamination produced by the absorber facing the surface does not destroy the skin-sparing effect of the megavoltage photon beam. As a rule of thumb, the minimum distance of approximately 15 cm is required between any absorber in the beam and the surface to keep the skin dose below 50% of D_{max} (details in Chapter 13).

• *Wedge isodose angle* (or simply *wedge angle*) refers to the angle of the isodose tilt at a specified depth (e.g., 10 cm). It is defined as the angle between the isodose curve at the specified depth and a line perpendicular to the central axis. Most commonly, the wedges are designed to provide wedge isodose angles of approximately 15°, 30°, 45°, and 60°.

• *Wedge transmission factor* (or simply *wedge factor*) is defined as the ratio of doses with and without the wedge, at a point in phantom. For symmetric fields, it is usually defined at central axis at 10 cm depth.

  ➤ The wedge factor changes drastically as a function of lateral (off-axis) distance along the wedged direction because of differential attenuation. It does not vary significantly in the unwedged direction because there is no change in wedge thickness or attenuation along that direction.

  ➤ The wedge factor increases slightly (a few percents) with increase in depth (due to beam hardening and photon scatter produced by the wedge) and with field size because of increased photon scatter in the transmitted beam.

➤ Although the wedge produces some change in beam quality (e.g., beam hardening), the effect is not large enough to warrant new tables of dosimetric functions such as S_c, S_p, PDD, and TPR. These quantities may be assumed to be the same as for open beams when used in the monitor unit (MU) calculation formalism.

NONPHYSICAL WEDGE FILTERS

Nonphysical wedges are available with most accelerators.
EXAMPLES: The Varian's enhanced dynamic wedge, Siemens' Virtual Wedge.

- The main advantage of nonphysical wedges is the automation of treatment delivery. The other often-cited advantage is the less peripheral dose compared to the physical wedge filter, for example, less dose to the contralateral breast when using tangential breast irradiation technique with nonphysical wedges.

- The disadvantage is the greater dosimetric complexity in the acquisition of commissioning data, beam modeling for a treatment planning system, and monitor unit calculations for various field sizes and configurations. Consequently, the quality assurance procedures for nonphysical wedges are more elaborate and the chances of a major error are greater in a busy department.

- Wedges and compensators, which are basically intensity-modulating devices, are superseded by intensity-modulated radiation therapy technology (discussed in Chapter 20).

MULTIPLE FIELD COMBINATIONS

Treatment by a single photon beam is seldom used except in some cases in which the tumor is superficial. Examples of a few treatments that use single megavoltage beams include the supraclavicular nodes (anterior field), internal mammary nodes (anterior field), and the spinal cord (posterior field).

For treatment of most tumors, however, a combination of two or more beams is required for an acceptable distribution of dose within the tumor and the surrounding normal tissues.

PARALLEL OPPOSED FIELDS

The simplest combination of two fields is a pair of fields directed along the same axis from opposite sides of the treatment volume. A composite isodose distribution for a pair of parallel opposed fields is shown in Figure 11.6.

- A treatment using equally weighted pair of parallel opposed beams gives rise to *tissue lateral effect* (i.e., greater dose at superficial depths than at the midpoint). The ratio of maximum peripheral dose to midpoint dose is much higher for lower energy beams than for the higher energy beams. This is seen in Figure 11.7.

- The magnitude of tissue lateral effect depends on the patient thickness, beam energy, and beam flatness (Figure 11.8).

- Biologically, it is better to treat all fields the same day than one field a day. For example, for parallel opposed fields, it has been shown that the biologic effect on normal tissue is greater if it receives alternating high- and low-dose fractions compared with equal but medium-sized dose fractions resulting from treating both fields daily. This phenomenon has been called the *edge effect*, or the *tissue lateral damage*.

INTEGRAL DOSE

One of the most important criteria in the choice of a particular treatment technique is to deliver a sterilizing dose to tumor while minimizing dose to critical organs. In addition, it is desirable to minimize the *integral dose* to the patient.

- The quantity integral dose is the total energy imparted to the patient and is given by the product of the mass of tissue and the dose it receives. The unit of integral dose is the joule or kilogram-gray (kg-Gy).

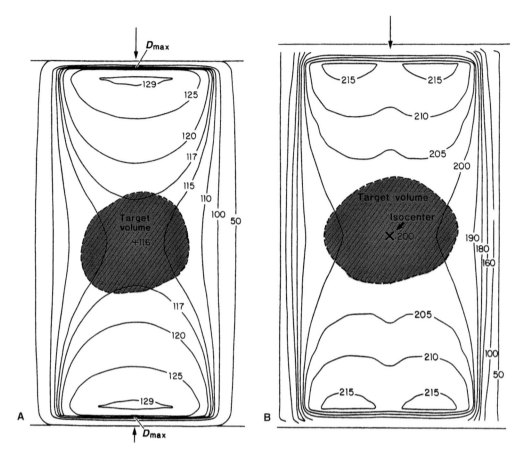

Figure 11.6. Composite isodose distribution for a pair of parallel opposed fields. **A:** Each beam is given a weight of 100 at the depth of D_{max}. **B:** Isocentric plan with each beam weighted 100 at the isocenter.

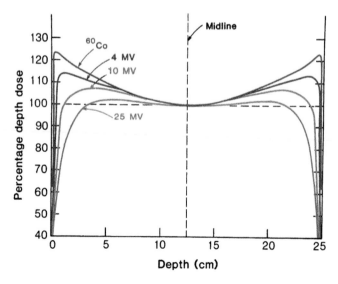

Figure 11.7. Depth dose curves for parallel opposed fields normalized to midpoint value. Patient thickness = 25 cm, field size = 10 × 10 cm, source-to-surface distance = 100 cm.

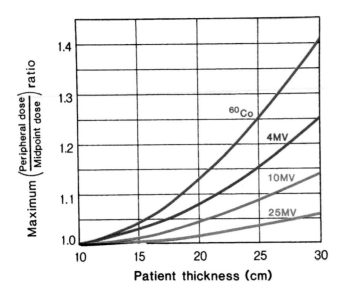

Figure 11.8. Ratio of maximum peripheral dose to the midpoint dose plotted as a function of patient thickness for different beam qualities. Parallel opposed fields, field size = 10 × 10 cm, source-to-surface distance = 100 cm.

- For an equally weighted parallel opposed field treatment, the integral dose decreases with increase in beam energy (Figure 11.9).

- Integral dose is an interesting concept but so far it has not been correlated precisely to treatment outcomes.

- Although minimizing the integral dose is not an overriding criterion in treatment plan evaluation, it is an important consideration, especially for younger and pediatric patients. Higher integral dose to normal tissue carries a greater risk of radiation-induced secondary malignancies.

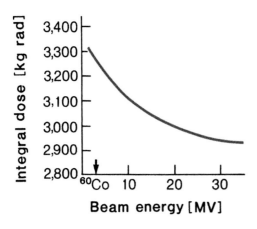

Figure 11.9. Integral dose as a function of photon beam energy, when 1,000 rad (10 Gy) are delivered at a midpoint of a 25-cm-thick patient. Field size, 10-cm diameter at a source-to-surface distance of 100 cm. (Redrawn from Podgorsak EB, Rawlinson JA, Johns HE. X-ray depth doses for linear accelerators in the energy range from 10 to 32 MeV. *Am J Roentgenol.* 1975;123:182.)

MULTIPLE STATIONARY FIELDS

Achieving dose uniformity within the tumor volume and sparing of critical organs are important considerations in developing a treatment plan. Some of the strategies useful in achieving these goals are the following:

   a) Using fields of appropriate size and shape.

   b) Increasing the number of fields directed at the tumor.

   c) Selecting an appropriate beam direction for each field.

   d) Adjusting beam weights (relative dose contribution from individual fields).

   e) Using beam modifiers such as wedge filters and compensators or delivering beams of nonuniform profiles (e.g., intensity modulation).

   f) Using appropriate beam modality and energy.

ROTATION THERAPY

Rotation therapy is an isocentric technique in which the beam moves continuously about the patient. The isocenter is placed at the center of the tumor (for a full 360° rotation) or at a suitable distance beyond the tumor center for a partial arc. The latter technique is referred to as *past pointing*. Figure 11.10 shows three examples of isodose distribution for rotation therapy: (A) 100° arc rotation; (B) 180° arc rotation; and (C) full 360° rotation. Past pointing is used in (A) and (B).

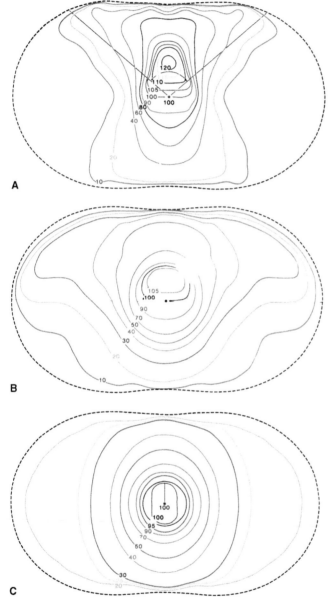

Figure 11.10. Examples of isodose distribution for rotation therapy. **A:** Arc angle = 100°. **B:** Arc angle = 180°. **C:** Full 360° rotation; 4 MV, field size = 7 × 12 cm at isocenter, source-to-axis distance = 100 cm.

- Rotation therapy is best suited for small, deep-seated tumors. If the tumor is confined within a region extending not more than halfway from the center of the contour cross section, rotation therapy may be a proper choice.

- Rotation therapy is not indicated if (a) volume to be irradiated is too large, (b) the external surface differs markedly from a cylinder, and (c) the tumor is too far off center relative to the surface contour.

WEDGE FIELD TECHNIQUES

Wedges (physical or nonphysical) are used to deliberately skew the isodose curves of individual fields so that the composite dose distribution gives a region of acceptable dose uniformity to the target volume and minimizes dose to the surrounding normal tissue.

- *Wedge-pair* technique is suitable for relatively superficial tumors (approximately 0–7 cm deep). In this technique, the target volume is irradiated by two "wedged" beams directed from the same side of the patient.

  ➤ By inserting appropriate wedge filters in each of the angled beams and positioning them with the thick ends adjacent to each other, the composite dose distribution can be made fairly uniform (Figure 11.11).

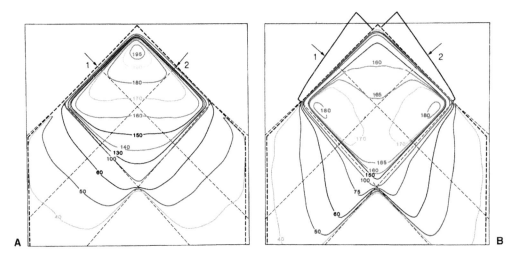

Figure 11.11. Isodose distribution for two angled beams. **A:** Without wedges. **B:** With wedges; 4 MV, field size = 10 × 10 cm, source-to-surface distance = 100 cm, wedge angle = 45°, and each beam weighted 100 at the depth of D_{max}. (*Prefer isocentric plan.*)

- ➤ The region of uniform dose (within plus or minus a few percents) lies within the volume where the two beams overlap. This region is called the "plateau" region.

- ➤ Because wedge pair techniques are normally used for treating small, superficial tumor volumes, a high-dose region (*hot spot*) of up to +10% within the treatment volume is usually acceptable.

- ➤ These hot spots in a wedge-pair technique usually occur under the thin ends of the wedges and their magnitude increases with field size and wedge angle. This effect is related to the differential attenuation of the beam under the thick end relative to the thin end.

- ➤ There are three parameters that affect the plateau region in terms of its depth, shape, and dose distribution: θ, φ, and S, where θ is the wedge angle, φ the hinge angle, and S the separation. These parameters are illustrated in Figure 11.12.

- ➤ There is an optimum relationship between the wedge angle θ and the hinge angle φ, which provides the most uniform distribution of radiation dose in the plateau:

$$\theta = 90° - \phi/2$$

This equation is based on the principle that for a given hinge angle the wedge angle should be such that the isodose curves from each field are parallel to the bisector of the hinge angle, as illustrated in Figure 11.12.

- ➤ The above relationship also assumes that each beam is incident perpendicularly on a flat surface and, therefore, the wedge isodose curves are not modified by the surface contour. In an actual patient, however, this may not be the case. So, the choice of wedge angle may be

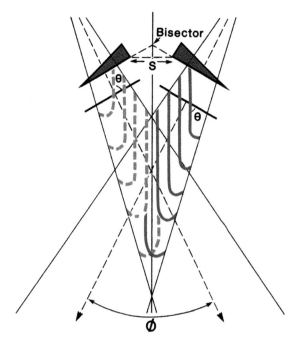

Figure 11.12. Parameters of the wedge beams: θ is wedge angle, Φ the hinge angle, and S the separation. Isodose curves for each wedge field are parallel to the bisector.

different depending on the contour shape. The above equation may be used as a starting point and modified, as needed, based on the given patient contour.

OPEN AND WEDGED FIELD COMBINATION

Although wedge filters were originally designed for use in conjunction with the wedge-pair arrangement, it is possible to combine open and wedged beams with appropriate weights to obtain a particular dose distribution. Two of such arrangements are shown in Figure 11.13A and B.

- In modern radiation therapy, complex treatment techniques are frequently used, which may involve one or more wedge filters, compensators, field blocking, and field reductions, all for the same patient. Complex treatments, including wedged fields, must be planned using an appropriate computer treatment planning system, as a matter of standard practice.

ICRU VOLUMES FOR TREATMENT PLANNING

Figure 11.14 is a schematic representation of various volumes that the International Commission on Radiation Units and Measurements (ICRU) (Report 62) recommends to be identified in a treatment plan. Delineation of these volumes is greatly facilitated by 3D imaging but the concept is independent of the methodology used for their determination.

- *Gross tumor volume*: The gross tumor volume (GTV) is the gross demonstrable extent and location of the tumor. Delineation of GTV is possible if the tumor is visible, palpable, or demonstrable through imaging. GTV cannot be defined if the tumor has been surgically removed, although an outline of the tumor bed may be substituted by examining preoperative and postoperative images.
- *Clinical target volume*: The CTV consists of the demonstrated tumor(s) if present and any other tissue with presumed tumor. It represents, therefore, the true extent and location of the tumor. Delineation of CTV assumes that there are no tumor cells outside this volume. The CTV must receive adequate dose to achieve the therapeutic aim.
- *Internal target volume*: ICRU Report recommends that an internal margin be added to CTV to compensate for internal physiological movements and variation in size, shape, and position of the CTV during therapy in relation to an internal reference point and its corresponding coordinate system. The volume that includes CTV with these margins is called the *internal target volume.*

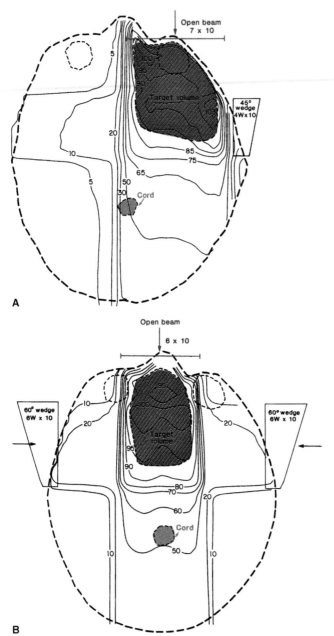

Figure 11.13. Treatment plans using open and wedged field combinations. **A:** Isocentric plan with anterior open field weighted 100 and lateral wedged field weighted 15 at the isocenter. **B:** A combination of anterior open beam and two lateral wedged beams; 4 MV x-ray beam from ATC-400 linac.

- *Planning target volume:* The volume that includes CTV with an internal margin as well as a setup margin for patient movement and setup uncertainties is called the *planning target volume* (PTV). The margin around CTV in any direction must be large enough to compensate for internal movements as well as patient-motion and setup uncertainties.

- *Planning organ at risk volume:* The organ(s) at risk (OR) needs adequate protection just as CTV needs adequate treatment. Once the OR is identified, margins need to be added to compensate for its movements, internal as well as setup. Thus, in analogy to the PTV, one needs to outline planning organ at risk volume to protect OR effectively.

- *Treated volume:* Additional margins must be provided around PTV to allow for limitations of the treatment technique. Thus, the minimum target dose should be represented by an isodose surface that adequately covers the PTV to provide that margin. The volume enclosed by this isodose surface is called the *treated volume.* The treated volume is, in general, larger than the planning target volume and depends on a particular treatment technique.

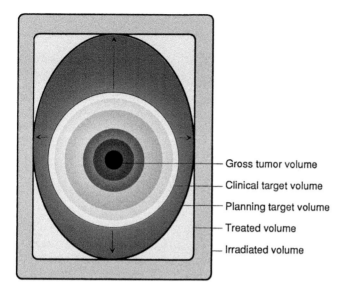

Figure 11.14. Schematic illustration of International Commission of Radiation Units and Measurements volumes. (From International Commission of Radiation Units and Measurements. *Prescribing, Recording, and Reporting Photon Beam Therapy.* ICRU Report 50. Bethesda, MD: International Commission of Radiation Units and Measurements; 1993.)

— Gross tumor volume

— Clinical target volume

— Planning target volume

— Treated volume

— Irradiated volume

- *Irradiated volume*: The volume of tissue receiving a significant dose (e.g., ≥50% of the specified target dose) is called the *irradiated volume*. The irradiated volume is larger than the treated volume and depends on the treatment technique used.

Schematic illustration of the process of delineating ICRU volumes is shown in Figure 11.15.

DOSE SPECIFICATION AND REPORTING

The ICRU recommends that an internationally standardized system of dose specification (e.g., ICRU Reports 50 and 62) should be followed in specifying and reporting dosages in the patient's chart as well as in the literature. The main objectives of a dose specification and reporting system are to achieve uniformity of dose reporting among institutions, to provide meaningful data for assessing the results of treatments, and to enable the treatment to be repeated elsewhere without having recourse to the original institution for further information.

TARGET DOSE STATISTICS

- *Maximum target dose*: The highest dose in the target area is called the maximum target dose, provided this dose covers a minimum area of 2 cm^2. Higher dose areas of less than 2 cm^2 may be ignored in designating the value of maximum target dose.

- *Minimum target dose*: The minimum target dose is the lowest dose in the target area.

- *Mean target dose*: If the dose is calculated at a large number of discrete points uniformly distributed in the target area, the mean target dose is the mean of the absorbed dose values at these points. Mathematically:

$$\text{Mean target dose} = \frac{1}{N} \Sigma_{A_T} D_{i,j}$$

  where N is the number of points in the matrix and $D_{i,j}$ the dose at lattice point i, j located inside the target area (A_T).

- *Median target dose*: The median target dose is the middle value in the ordered values of dose matrix within the target.

- *Modal target dose*: The modal target dose is the absorbed dose that occurs most frequently within the target area. If the dose distribution over a grid of points covering the target area is plotted as a frequency histogram, the dose value showing the highest frequency is called the modal dose.

- *Hot spots*: A hot spot is an area outside the target that receives a higher dose than the specified target dose. Like the maximum target dose, a hot spot is considered clinically meaningful only if it covers an area of at least 2 cm^2.

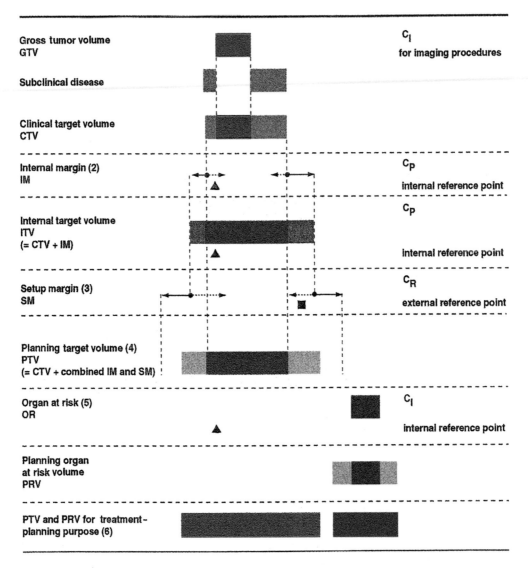

Figure 11.15. Schematic representation of International Commission of Radiation Units and Measurements (ICRU) volumes and margins. (From International Commission of Radiation Units and Measurements. *Prescribing, Recording and Reporting Photon Beam Therapy [supplement to ICRU Report 50].* ICRU Report 62. Bethesda, MD: International Commission on Radiation Units and Measurements; 1999.)

REFERENCE POINT FOR DOSE SPECIFICATION

Stationary Photon Beams

- For a single beam, the target absorbed dose should be specified on the central axis of the beam placed within the PTV.
- For parallel opposed, equally weighted beams, the point of target dose specification should be on the central axis midway between the beam entrances.
- For parallel opposed, unequally weighted beams, the target dose should be specified on the central axis placed within the PTV.
- For any other arrangement of two or more intersecting beams, the point of target dose specification should be at the intersection of the central axes of the beams placed within the PTV.

Rotation Therapy

For full rotation or arcs of at least 270°, the target dose should be specified at the center of rotation in the principal plane. For smaller arcs, the target dose should be stated in the principal plane; first, at the center of rotation and, second, at the center of the target volume. This dual-point specification is required because in a small arc therapy, *past-pointing* techniques are used that give maximum absorbed dose close to the center of the target area. The dose at the isocenter in these cases, although important to specify, is somewhat less.

PLAN EVALUATION

Essential tools for plan evaluation are: a) isodose curves, b) isodose surfaces, and c) dose-volume histograms.

- *Isodose curves*: Dose distributions of competing plans are evaluated by viewing isodose curves in individual slices and in orthogonal planes (e.g., transverse, sagittal, and coronal).

- *Isodose surfaces*: Isodose surfaces are isodose curves in three dimensions. They represent surfaces of a designated dose value covering a volume.

- *Dose–volume histograms*: The DVH may be represented in two forms: the cumulative integral DVH and the differential DVH.

  ➤ The cumulative DVH is a plot of the volume of a given structure receiving a *certain dose or higher* as a function of dose. Any point on the cumulative DVH curve shows the volume that receives the indicated dose or higher.

  ➤ The differential DVH is a plot of volume receiving a dose within a specified dose interval (or dose bin) as a function of dose. The differential form of DVH shows the extent of dose variation within a given structure. For example, the differential DVH of a uniformly irradiated structure is a single bar of 100% volume at the stated dose.

  ➤ Of the two forms of DVH, the cumulative DVH has been found to be more useful and is more commonly used than the differential form.

  Figure 11.16 shows an isodose and DVH representation of a treatment plan.

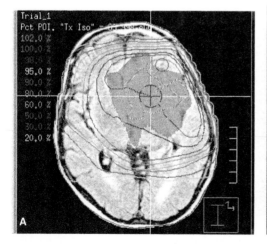
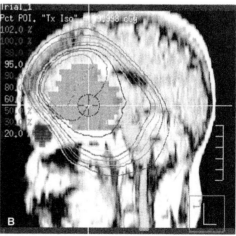

Figure 11.16. A three-dimensional plan for the treatment of glioblastoma is displayed. Isodose curves in **A:** transverse, **B:** lateral, and **C:** coronal planes are used to evaluate the plan. **D:** Cumulative dose-volume histogram (DVH) is also useful in the evaluation process. **E:** Differential DVH shown here for the tumor only, is more of an academic interest. (*continued*)

*Textbook below means *The Physics of Radiation Therapy* by Khan, 4th ed.

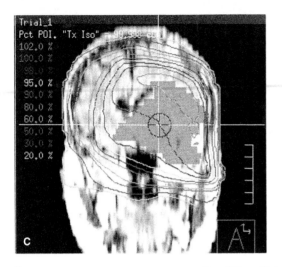

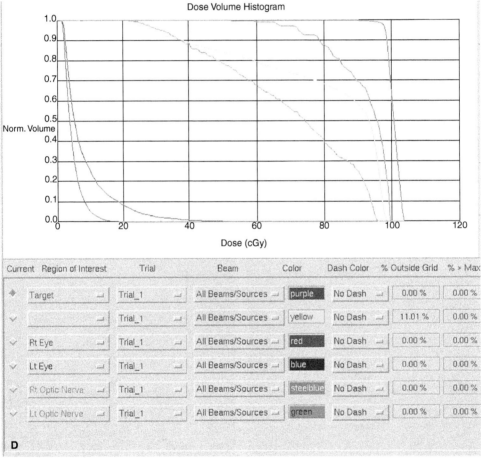

Figure 11.16. (*Continued*)

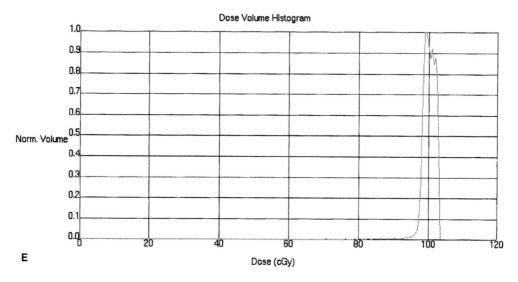

E

Figure 11.16. (*Continued*)

REVIEW QUESTIONS • Chapter 11

✔ **TEST YOURSELF**

Review questions for this chapter are provided online.

In multiple choice questions, more than one option may be correct.

1. Dose distribution outside the field boundaries is significantly affected by:
   a) Flattening filter
   b) Geometric penumbra
   c) Depth
   d) Leakage radiation through collimators

2. Compared to the dose at central axis, the dose at the geometric field border at the same depth is approximately:
   a) $100 \pm 3\%$
   b) 95%
   c) 80%
   d) 50%
   e) 2%

3. For a wedged beam:
   a) The wedge angle is defined as the angle of the physical wedge filter
   b) The wedge factor generally increases with field size and depth
   c) The central axis percent depth dose generally increases compared to the open beam of the same dimensions
   d) The isodose curves are tilted through the same angle at all depths

4. Integral dose:
   a) Is measured in units of Gy/kg
   b) Decreases with increase in beam energy for the same target dose delivered by equally weighted parallel opposed beams
   c) Should be maximized as much as possible to sterilize the tumor
   d) Should be minimized in treating pediatric patients

5. In a wedge-pair technique:
   a) Thin ends of the wedges must be placed adjacent.
   b) Wedge angle of each wedge must be half the hinge angle.
   c) Hot spots generally occur under the thin ends.
   d) The dose within the target volume is uniform within $\pm 5\%$.

6. A point on the cumulative dose-volume histogram (DVH) curve represents:
   a) The volume that receives the indicated dose.
   b) The volume that receives the indicated dose or higher.
   c) The volume that receives the indicated dose or lower.
   d) The volume that receives the indicated dose on the average.

7. Select an arrangement in the increasing order of volume (CTV = clinical target volume, GTV = gross tumor volume, ITV = internal target volume, PTV = planning target volume):
   a) CTV, GTV, ITV, PTV
   b) ITV, GTV, CTV, PTV
   c) GTV, CTV, PTV, ITV
   d) GTV, CTV, ITV, PTV

8. Which of the following statements is/are true? An isodose curve can:
   a) Have a concavity
   b) Cross another curve of a different value
   c) Cover the entire patient
   d) Exceed 100%
   e) Have more than one incidence (e.g., two separate 95% isodose lines) on a single plane

9. Which of the following statements is/are true regarding wedge filters?

    a) The wedge angle is equivalent to the angle of the wedge, when converted to water-equivalent thickness.

    b) The wedge angle is defined as the angle of the wedge profile measured at depth of 10 cm in water.

    c) Physical wedge factors vary only slightly with field size, depth, and lateral distance.

    d) The surface dose for wedge filters increases the skin dose beyond 50% of D_{max}, due to electron contamination produced in the filter.

    e) The wedge angle is defined the same for physical and nonphysical wedges.

10. For treatment plans involving multiple treatment fields:

    a) The prescription point is defined by the maximum dose in the composite dose distribution.

    b) The magnitude of tissue lateral effect is dependent on energy and depth, but primarily on the beam flatness.

    c) The sum of all the dose points contained in the calculation dose grid is the integral dose.

    d) For rotational fields, the isocenter is sometimes placed beyond the tumor center for partial arcs.

11. Calculate the optimal wedge angle for a wedged-pair plan with beams directed at 60° from one another:

    a) 15°
    b) 30°
    c) 45°
    d) 60°

12. Which of the following statement(s) is/are true regarding target volume delineation according to ICRU 62:

    a) Treatment fields are blocked to the PTV, which includes the CTV plus uncertainties in daily patient setup.

    b) The treated volume is larger than the CTV volume, but smaller than the irradiated volume.

    c) The minimum target dose is defined as the lower dose within the PTV, provided this dose covers a minimum area of 2 cm^2.

    d) The margins assigned to CTV to create a PTV are not necessarily the same as those assigned to OR to generate a PRV.

13. According to ICRU specifications, the wedge angle is defined at:

    a) Depth of 50% isodose line
    b) Depth of 80% isodose line
    c) Depth of D_{max}
    d) 10 cm depth

14. Using a lateral dose profile taken at depth of D_{max}, the distance between the 90% and the 10% dose values is the description of the:

    a) Geometric penumbra
    b) Effective field size
    c) Treatment field size
    d) Physical penumbra

15. Rotational x-ray beam therapy is acceptable (choose all that apply):

    a) When the external contour of the patient is fairly cylindrical
    b) When blocking is required to shield sensitive structures
    c) When target volume is small
    d) When target volume is centrally located

16. Per ICRU specifications (select all that apply):
    a) For multibeam arrangements the dose should be specified at the intersection point of the central axes of the beam.
    b) The target dose should be specified at the deepest region of the target, for a single SSD photon beam.
    c) For rotational photon therapy involving arcs of 270° and larger, the dose should be specified at the center of rotation of the beam.
    d) The dose for parallel opposed photon beams should be specified midway between the beam entrance points.

17. For isocentric parallel opposed equally weighted photon fields (select all that apply):
    a) The target dose specification point is the depth of D_{max}.
    b) There is reproducibility of setup with less chance of geometric miss.
    c) Treating one field per day is less harmful to normal tissues than treating both fields per day.
    d) The peripheral dose increases with increasing energy for constant midline dose.

18. For a single photon field, the integral dose depends on (select all that apply):
    a) Dose delivered at D_{max}.
    b) Beam energy
    c) Field size
    d) Depth of the 50% dose

19. The following factors affect the isodose distribution of rotational photon therapy (select all that apply):
    a) The shape of patient contour
    b) The velocity of rotation
    c) The beam energy
    d) The location of isocenter in the contour

20. If the hinge angle of an "ideal" treatment situation of two wedged fields is 90°, select the appropriate wedge angle:
    a) 60°
    b) 45°
    c) 30°
    d) 15°

21. Regarding the photon beam isodose curves (select all that apply):
    a) For ^{60}Co, the isodose curves become more rounded with increasing field size.
    b) Beam flatness is usually specified at D_{max} in water and should be ±3% of the central axis value over 80% of the width of the largest field.
    c) The flattening filter causes the photon beam to be less penetrating at the central axis and results in horns at the edges of the field.
    d) The depth of a given isodose line increases with energy.

22. For two parallel opposed fields the ratio of maximum peripheral dose to midpoint dose increases with increase in:
    a) Beam energy
    b) Field size
    c) Patient thickness
    d) Geometric penumbra

12

TREATMENT PLANNING II: PATIENT DATA, CORRECTIONS, AND SETUP

12A

REFERENCE

Khan FM. *The Physics of Radiation Therapy*, 4th edition, 2009. Chapter 12 "Treatment Planning II: Patient Data, Corrections, and Setup"

Patient Data Acquisition, Simulation, and Treatment Verification

 TOPIC OUTLINE

The following topics will be discussed in this lecture:
- ➤ Patient data acquisition
- ➤ Treatment simulation
- ➤ Treatment verification

PATIENT DATA ACQUISITION

Accurate patient dosimetry is only possible when sufficiently accurate patient data are available. Such data include body surface contours, images of internal anatomy, density of relevant internal structures, and localization of target volume and organs at risk.

- *Surface contours*: Acquisition of body contours and internal structures is best accomplished by imaging (e.g., computed tomography). Important points must be considered in regard to the accuracy of image-based contours:

  - ➤ The patient must be in the same position as used in the actual treatment.

  - ➤ Beam entry points/laser intersection points should be marked with radio-opaque markers or other markers depending on the image modality used.

- *Internal structures*: Localization of internal structures must be obtained under conditions similar to those of the actual treatment position and on a couch similar to the treatment couch. The following devices are used for the localization of internal structures and tissue densities.

  - ➤ *Computed tomography (CT)*: In a CT scanner, a narrow beam of x-rays scans across a patient in synchrony with a radiation detector on the opposite side of the patient. This is accomplished by an x-ray tube that rotates axially or helically around the patient (Figure 12A.1).

  From the transmission measurements taken at different orientations of the x-ray source and detector, the distribution of attenuation coefficients within a layer is determined. By assigning different levels to different attenuation coefficients, an image is reconstructed that represents various structures with different attenuation properties. Such a representation of attenuation coefficients constitutes a CT image.

Slice-by-slice scan

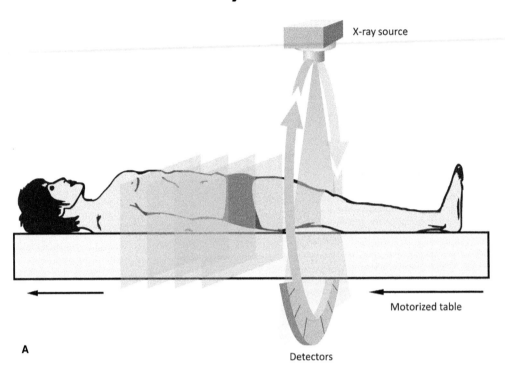

A

Helical scan

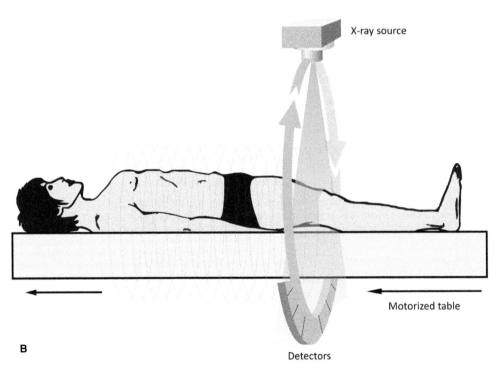

B

Figure 12A.1. Illustration of computed tomography (CT) scanning. **A:** Slice-by-slice CT scanning. **B:** Helical CT scanning.

- The reconstruction algorithm generates what is known as *CT numbers*, which are related to attenuation coefficients.
- The CT numbers start at −1,000 for vacuum and pass through 0 for water. The CT number for bone is approximately +1,000, depending on the bone type and energy of the CT beam. The CT numbers normalized in this manner are called Hounsfield numbers (*H*).

$$H = \frac{\mu_{\text{tissue}} - \mu_{\text{water}}}{\mu_{\text{water}}} \times 1,000$$

where μ is the linear attenuation coefficient. Thus, a Hounsfield unit represents a change of 0.1% in the attenuation coefficient of water.

- CT numbers bear a linear relationship with attenuation coefficients.
- CT numbers depend on electron density (electrons/cm^3) as well as atomic number, if the scanning beam used is kilovoltage x-rays as in conventional CT scanners.
- Although CT numbers can be correlated with electron density, the relationship is not linear in the entire range of tissue densities.
- The nonlinearity is caused by the change in atomic number of tissues, which affects the proportion of beam attenuation by Compton versus photoelectric interactions.
- Correlation between CT numbers and electron density of various tissues can be established by scanning phantoms of known electron densities in the range that includes lung, muscle, and bone.

Figure 12A.2 shows a relationship that is linear between lung and soft tissue but nonlinear between soft tissue and bone.

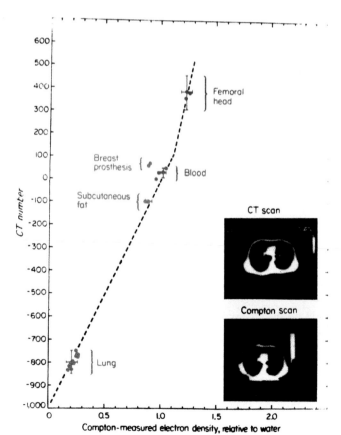

Figure 12A.2. Computed tomography numbers plotted as a function of electron density relative to water. (From Battista JJ, Rider WD, Van Dyk J. Computed tomography for radiotherapy planning. *Int J Radiat Oncol Biol Phys.* 1980; 6:99, with permission.)

➤ *Magnetic resonance imaging (MRI)*: Basic physics of MRI involves a phenomenon known as nuclear magnetic resonance. It is a resonance transition between nuclear spin states of certain atomic nuclei when subjected to a radio frequency signal of a specific frequency in the presence of an external magnetic field.

- The signal source in an MRI can be any nucleus with nonzero spin or angular momentum. However, certain nuclei give larger signal than others.

- Hydrogen nuclei (protons), because of their high intrinsic sensitivity and high concentration in tissues, produce signals of sufficient strength for imaging.

- On the scan: dark area means low signal collected and bright area means high signal collected.

- MRI is used primarily for soft tissue imaging. EXAMPLES: brain imaging, soft tissue sarcomas, and images for stereotactic radiosurgery.

- Although a CT scan provides the primary image data set for treatment planning, MRI scans are often fused with CT images.

➤ *Ultrasound*: An ultrasound (or ultrasonic) wave is a sound wave having a frequency greater than 20,000 cycles per sec or hertz (Hz). At this frequency, the sound is inaudible to the human ear. Ultrasound waves of frequencies 1 to 20 MHz are used for imaging.

- Ultrasonic waves are generated as well as detected by an *ultrasonic probe* or *transducer*.

- An ultrasonic transducer converts electrical energy into ultrasound energy, and vice versa. This is accomplished by a process known as the *piezoelectric effect*.

- Piezoelectric effect is exhibited by certain crystals in which a variation of an electric field across the crystal causes it to oscillate mechanically, thus generating acoustic waves.

- Ultrasound may be used to produce images by means of either transmission or reflection. However, in most clinical applications, ultrasonic waves reflected from different tissue interfaces are used.

- These reflections or echoes are caused by variations in *acoustic impedance* of materials on opposite sides of the interfaces. The acoustic impedance (Z) of a medium is defined as the product of the density of the medium and the velocity of ultrasound in the medium.

- The larger the difference in Z between the two media, the greater is the fraction of ultrasound energy reflected at the interface. For example, strong reflections of ultrasound occur at the air–tissue, tissue–bone, and chest wall–lung interfaces because of high impedance mismatch.

- Because lung contains millions of air–tissue interfaces, strong reflections at the numerous interfaces prevent the use of ultrasound in lung imaging.

- Ultrasound can provide useful information in localizing many malignancy-prone structures in the lower pelvis, retroperitoneum, upper abdomen, breast, and chest wall.

- *Positron emission tomography (PET)*: PET provides functional images that can differentiate between malignant tumors and the surrounding normal tissues. The physics of PET involves positron-electron annihilation into photons. The imaging procedure consists of injecting patient with positron-emitting radionuclide (e.g., ^{18}F, ^{15}O, ^{11}C) and detecting two annihilation photons (511 keV) emitted simultaneously in opposite directions. The image is reconstructed by detection of coincidence photons by a ring of detectors positioned around the patient.

➤ PET is useful in providing a physiological image of the internal structures.

➤ PET images may allow differentiation between benign and malignant lesions well enough in some cases to permit tumor staging.

➤ PET image reconstruction requires CT data to apply an attenuation correction. Attenuation correction is made to account for different distances in tissue annihilation photons must travel before reaching the detectors.

TREATMENT SIMULATION

- *Radiographic simulator*: A radiographic simulator (Figure 12A.3) is an apparatus that uses a diagnostic x-ray tube but duplicates a radiation treatment unit in terms of its geometrical, mechanical, and optical properties.

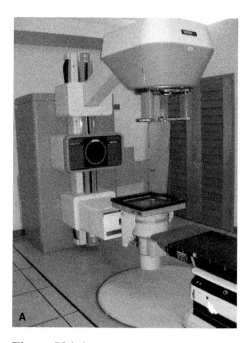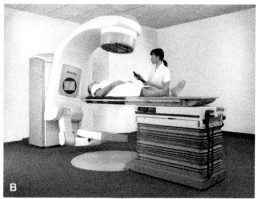

Figure 12A.3. A: Photograph of Varian Ximatron CDX simulator at the University of Minnesota. **B:** Varian Acuity Simulator that has superseded the Ximatron. (Courtesy of Varian Associates, Palo Alto, CA.)

➤ Most commercially available simulators have fluoroscopic capability for dynamic visualization before a hard copy is obtained in terms of radiographs.

➤ Modern simulators combine the capabilities of radiographic simulation, planning, and verification in one system. These systems provide commonality in hardware and software of the treatment machine including 2D and 3D imaging, accessory mounts, treatment couch, and multileaf collimator. EXAMPLE: Varian's Acuity Simulator (Figure 12A.3B).

• *CT simulator*: A dedicated radiation therapy CT scanner with simulation accessories (e.g., flat table, laser lights for positioning, immobilization and image registration devices, and appropriate software for virtual simulation) is called a *CT simulator*. Many types of such units are commercially available. Figure 12A.4 shows one example.

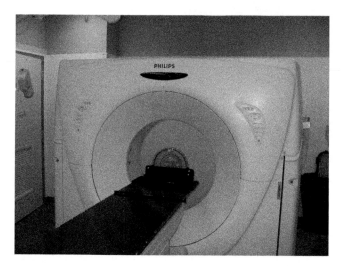

Figure 12A.4. Photograph of Phillips computed tomography simulator at the University of Minnesota.

➤ The nomenclature of *virtual simulation* arises out of the fact that both the patient and the treatment machine are virtual—patient is represented by CT images and the treatment machine is modeled by its beam geometry.

➤ The simulation film in this case is a reconstructed image called the digitally reconstructed radiograph (DRR) that has the appearance of a standard 2D simulation radiograph but is actually generated from CT scan data by mapping average CT values computed along ray lines drawn from a "virtual source" of radiation to the location of a "virtual film."

➤ The quality of the DRR image is not as good as the simulation radiograph but it contains additional useful information such as the outlined target area, critical structures, and beam aperture defined by blocks or multileaf collimator. Figure 12A.5 shows an anterior field DRR (A) and a posterior oblique field DRR (B), as examples.

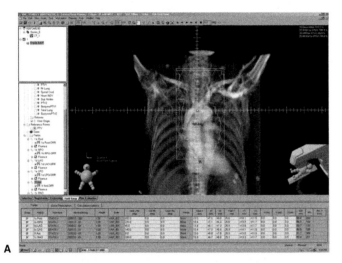

A

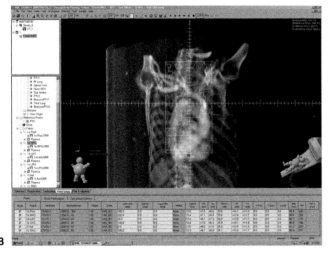

B

Figure 12A.5. A: Digitally reconstructed radiograph (DRR) anterior field. **B:** DRR posterior oblique.

➤ A DRR can substitute for a simulator radiograph by itself, but it is preferable to additionally obtain final verification by comparing it with a radiographic simulation film.

• *PET/CT*: A PET/CT unit consists of PET and CT scanners combined together with a common patient couch (Figure 12A.6).

➤ Because the patient position on the couch is kept constant for both the PET and the CT scanning procedures, it is possible to fuse the information together from the two scanners.

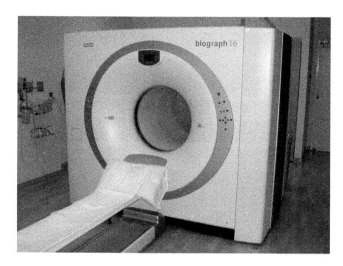

Figure 12A.6. Photograph of Siemens positron emission tomography/computed tomography at the University of Minnesota.

➤ Although PET provides physiologic information about the tumor, it lacks correlative anatomy and is inherently limited in resolution. CT, however, lacks physiologic information but provides superior images of anatomy and localization.

➤ PET requires CT data to perform attenuation correction. These data are readily available with PET/CT scanners.

➤ PET/CT provides images that when combined through image fusion yield images that are superior to the either PET or CT images alone.

TREATMENT VERIFICATION

• *Port films*: The primary purpose of port filming is to verify the treatment volume under actual conditions of treatment.

➤ The image quality of a film exposed to megavoltage x-ray beam is poorer than that of a diagnostic or simulator film.

➤ For port filming with megavoltage beams, a single emulsion film with the emulsion adjacent to a single high-atomic number intensifying screen between the film and the patient is preferable to a double emulsion film or a film with more than one screen.

➤ For optimum resolution, one needs a single emulsion film with a front lead screen and no rear screen. Conventional nonmetallic screens are not recommended at megavoltage energies.

➤ Certain slow-speed films (e.g., Kodak XV-2), ready packed but without a screen, can be exposed during the entire treatment duration. In addition to providing a port film record of the treatment, such films can be used to construct compensators for both the contour surface and tissue heterogeneities.

• *Electronic portal imaging*: Electronic portal imaging it possible to view the portal images instantaneously, that is, images can be displayed on computer screen before initiating a treatment or in real-time during the treatment. Portal images can also be stored on computer discs for later viewing or archiving.

➤ A modern electronic portal imaging device consists of a flat panel of x-ray detectors mounted on the accelerator gantry opposite the x-ray target. The mounting arm swings into position for imaging and swings out of the way when not needed.

➤ The detector system may consist of a matrix of ion chambers or solid-state detectors. An example of the later class of detectors is an array of amorphous silicon (a-Si) scintillating crystals. A scintillator converts the radiation beam into visible photons. The light is detected by an array of photodiodes implanted in the detector panel.

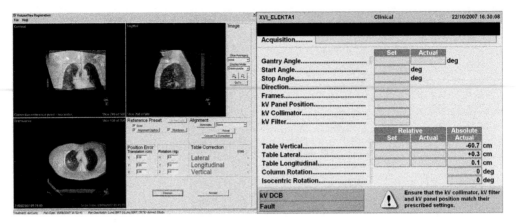

Figure 12A.7. Example of kilovoltage cone-beam computed tomography images of a lung cancer patient.

- *Cone-beam CT*: It is possible to perform CT scans with detectors embedded in a flat panel instead of a circular ring (as in a CT scanner). CT scanning that uses this type of geometry is known as *cone-beam computed tomography (CBCT)*.

  a. In CBCT, planar projection images are obtained from multiple directions as the source with the opposing detector panel rotates around the patient through 180° or more. These multi-directional images provide sufficient information to reconstruct patient anatomy in 3D, including cross-sectional, sagittal, and coronal planes.

  b. A filtered back-projection algorithm is used to reconstruct the volumetric images.

  ➤ *Kilovoltage CBCT*: Kilovoltage x-rays for a kVCBCT system are generated by a conventional x-ray tube that is mounted on a retractable arm at 90° to the therapy beam direction. A flat panel of x-ray detectors is mounted opposite the x-ray tube.

    • The imaging system for kVCBCT is capable of CBCT as well 2D radiography and fluoroscopy. An example of kVCBCT images is shown in Figure 12A.7.

    • The advantages of a kVCBCT system are its ability to:

      1. Produce volumetric CT images with good contrast and submillimeter spatial resolution.

      2. Acquire images in therapy room coordinates.

      3. Use 2D radiographic and fluoroscopic modes to verify portal accuracy, management of patient motion, and making positional and dosimetric adjustments before and during treatment.

  ➤ *Megavoltage CBCT*: Megavoltage cone-beam CT (MVCBCT) uses the megavoltage x-ray beam of the linear accelerator and its portal electronic imaging device mounted opposite the source.

    • MVCBCT is useful for online or pretreatment verification of patient positioning, anatomical matching of planning CT and pretreatment CT, avoidance of critical structures such as spinal cord, and identification of implanted metal markers, if used for patient setup.

    • Although kVCBCT has better image quality (resolution and contrast), MVCBCT has the following potential advantages over kVCBCT:

      1. Less susceptibility to artifacts due to high Z (atomic number) objects such as metallic markers in the target, metallic hip implants, and dental fillings;

      2. No need for extrapolating attenuation coefficients from kV to megavoltage photon energies for dosimetric corrections.

LECTURE

12B

REFERENCE
Khan FM. *The Physics of Radiation Therapy*, 4th edition, 2009. Chapter 12 "Treatment Planning II: Patient Data, Corrections, and Setup"

Corrections for Irregular Surface and Tissue Inhomogeneities

 TOPIC OUTLINE

The following topics will be discussed in this lecture:
- ➤ Corrections for contour irregularities
- ➤ Corrections for tissue inhomogeneities
- ➤ Absorbed dose within bone
- ➤ Dose to lung
- ➤ Dose at the surface of air cavities
- ➤ Tissue compensators

CORRECTIONS FOR CONTOUR IRREGULARITIES

Basic dose distribution data are obtained under standard conditions, which include homogeneous unit density phantom (e.g., water), perpendicular beam incidence, and a flat surface. For an actual treatment, however, the beam may be obliquely incident with respect to the surface and, in addition, the surface may be curved or irregular in shape. Under such conditions, the standard dose distributions cannot be applied without proper modifications or corrections.

- Contour corrections may be avoided by using a compensator (to be discussed later), but it is desirable to view the actual dose distribution before deciding on the need for a compensator.

- Manual methods of correcting isodose curves for contour irregularities (e.g., effective source-to-surface distance method, isodose shift method, and tissue–air ratios/tissue–maximum ratio [TAR/TMR] method) have given way to more accurate analytical methods incorporated into the computer treatment planning algorithms.

- Contour corrections made by a treatment planning system depend on the dose calculation algorithm (e.g., a semiempirical correction-based algorithm or a model-based algorithm simulating radiation transport). In either case, the point of calculation is assigned its actual depth along the ray line emanating from the radiation source position.

CORRECTIONS FOR TISSUE INHOMOGENEITIES

Manual methods of contour and tissue heterogeneity corrections are semiempirical and have given way to computer algorithms for treatment planning. These are collectively called correction-based algorithms. Currently, the most sophisticated algorithms are model based. EXAMPLE: pencil beam, convolution/superposition, and Monte Carlo techniques.

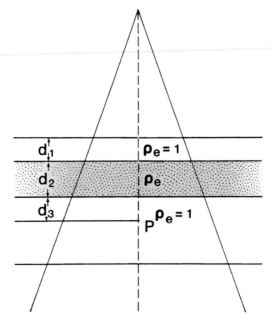

Figure 12B.1. Schematic diagram showing a water-equivalent phantom containing an inhomogeneity of electron density ρ_e relative to that of water. P is the point of dose calculation.

- The main difference between the correction-based and model-based algorithms is that the former reconstitutes the measured beam data before correcting them for the patient treatment situation whereas the latter simulates the treatment situation from first principles.

- *Correction-based algorithms*: Correction-based algorithms represent various methods ranging from those that simply interpolate measured depth-dose data to specially formulated analytic functions that predict the various correction factors under specified conditions. Figure 12B.1 is a general schematic diagram showing an inhomogeneity of electron density ρ_e relative to that of water. The material preceding and following the inhomogeneity is water equivalent (relative $\rho_e = 1$). Calculation is to be made at point P, which is located at a distance d_3 from the lower boundary, distance $(d_2 + d_3)$ from the front boundary of the inhomogeneity, and distance $d = d_1 + d_2 + d_3$ from the surface.

➤ *TAR (or TMR or TPR) method*: The correction factor, CF, is a multiplication factor applied to the dose at P expected if the entire phantom were water equivalent:

$$CF = \frac{T(d', r_d)}{T(d, r_d)}$$

where T is the tissue–air ratio (or TMR or tissue–phantom ratio [TPR]), d' the equivalent water depth, that is, $d' = d_1 + \rho_e d_2 + d_3$, and d the actual depth of P from the surface; r_d is the field size projected at point P.

- This correction method does not take into account the position of the inhomogeneity relative to point P. In other words, the correction factor will not change with d_3 as long as d and d' remain constant.

➤ *Batho's power law method*: In this method, the ratio of the TARs (or TMRs or TPRs) is raised to a power. Referring again to Figure 12B.1, the correction factor at point P is given by:

$$CF = \left[\frac{T(d_2 + d_3, r_d)}{T(d_3, r_d)} \right]^{\rho_e - 1}$$

where ρ_e is the electron density (number of electrons/cm^3) of the heterogeneity relative to that of water.

- As seen in the above equation, the correction factor does depend on the location of the inhomogeneity relative to point P but not relative to the surface.

- The above formulation is based on theoretical considerations that assume Compton interactions only.
- It does not apply to points inside the inhomogeneity or in the buildup region.

➤ *Generalized Batho's power law*: A more general form of the power law method, provided by Sontag and Cunningham, is given by:

$$CF = \frac{T(d_3, r_d)^{\rho_3 - \rho_2}}{T(d_2 + d_3, r_d)^{1 - \rho_2}}$$

where ρ_3 is the density of the material in which point P lies and d_3 its depth within this material. ρ_2 is the density of the overlying material, and $(d_2 + d_3)$ the depth below the upper surface of it.

- The generalized Batho's power law allows for correction of the dose to points within an inhomogeneity as well as below it.

➤ *Equivalent TAR (or TMR or TPR) method*: Sontag and Cunningham proposed a method using "equivalent" tissue–air ratios. The correction factor, CF, is given by:

$$CF = \frac{T(d', r')}{T(d, r)}$$

where d' is the water equivalent depth, d the actual depth, r the beam dimension at depth d, $r' = r \cdot \tilde{\rho} = $ scaled field size dimension, and $\tilde{\rho}$ the weighted density of the irradiated volume, given by:

$$\tilde{\rho} = \frac{\sum_i \sum_j \sum_k \rho_{ijk} \cdot W_{ijk}}{\sum_i \sum_j \sum_k W_{ijk}}$$

where ρ_{ijk} are the relative electron densities of scatter elements (e.g., pixels in a series of CT images of the irradiated volume) and W_{ijk} the weighting factors assigned to these elements in terms of their relative contribution to the scattered dose at the point of calculation.

- The equivalent TAR method is an attempt to better account for the effect of scatter from different scattering structures. This is done by scaling of the field size at depth according to the weighted densities of the surrounding structures.
- An alternative approach to the equivalent tissue–air ratio method is to calculate scattered dose separately from the primary dose by summation of the scatter contribution from individual scatter elements in the irradiated heterogeneous volume. EXAMPLES:
  - Differential scatter–air ratio method
  - Delta volume method
  - Dose spread array method
  - Differential pencil beam method

- *Model-based algorithms*: Two types of model-based algorithms are described below:
  ➤ *Convolution/Superposition method*: A convolution/superposition method involves a convolution equation that separately considers the transport of primary photons and that of the scatter photon and electron emerging from the primary photon interaction. The dose $D(\vec{r})$ at a point $\vec{r}$ is given by:

$$D(\vec{r}) = \int \frac{\mu}{\rho} \Psi_p(\vec{r}') A(\vec{r} - \vec{r}') d^3\vec{r}'$$
$$= \int T_p(\vec{r}') A(\vec{r} - \vec{r}') d^3\vec{r}'$$

where μ/ρ is the mass attenuation coefficient, $\Psi_p(\vec{r}')$ the primary photon energy fluence, and $A(\vec{r} - \vec{r}')$ the convolution kernel (a matrix of dose distribution deposited by scatter photons and electrons set in motion at the primary photon interaction site). Figure 12B.2 shows the geometry of the radiation transport.

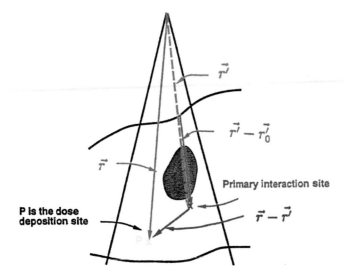

Figure 12B.2. Geometry of photon interaction and radiation transport from the site of interaction. (From Mackie TR, personal communication.)

- The product of mass attenuation coefficient and the primary energy fluence is called *terma*, $T_p(\vec{r}')$, which stands for total energy released per unit mass. Terma is analogous to kerma, that is, kerma = $(\mu_{tr}/\rho) \cdot \Psi$ and terma = $(\mu/\rho) \cdot \Psi$.

- Convolution kernel, $A(\vec{r} - \vec{r}')$, can be represented by a dose spread array obtained by calculation (e.g., Monte Carlo) or by direct measurement. EXAMPLE: Figure 12B.3 shows a 6-MeV photon kernel generated by a Monte Carlo program.

- The kernels are typically computed for monoenergetic beams using a Monte Carlo code. A kernel representing a polyenergetic beam (e.g., x-rays) can be computed by weighing the kernel with respect to the normalized incident energy fluence spectrum.

- Primary photon energy fluence at depth is calculated by ray tracing through the phantom, that is, along ray lines diverging from the source position.

- A convolution equation when modified for radiological path length (distance corrected for electron density relative to water) is called the convolution-superposition equation:

$$D(\vec{r}) = \int T_p(\rho_{\vec{r}} \cdot \vec{r}') A(\rho_{\vec{r}\text{-}\vec{r}'} \cdot (\vec{r} - \vec{r}')) \, d^3\vec{r}'$$

where $\rho_{\vec{r}} \cdot \vec{r}'$ is the radiologic path length from the source to the primary photon interaction site and $\rho_{\vec{r}\text{-}\vec{r}'} \cdot (\vec{r} - \vec{r}')$ the radiologic path length from the site of primary photon interaction to the site of dose deposition.

- The dose kernel $A(\rho_{\vec{r}\text{-}\vec{r}'} \cdot (\vec{r} - \vec{r}'))$ can be calculated by using range scaling by electron density of the Monte Carlo–generated kernel in water. Figure 12B.3 above shows that the kernel obtained with the range scaling method compares well with that generated by Monte Carlo directly for the heterogeneous medium.

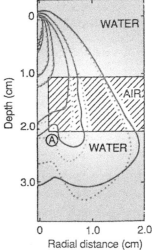

Figure 12B.3. Comparison of Monte Carlo–generated 6-MeV primary photon kernel in a water phantom containing a ring of air. The continuous line is a kernel computed expressly for the heterogeneous situation. The dotted line is a kernel modified for the heterogeneous phantom using range scaling. (From Woo MK, Cunningham JR. The validity of the density scaling method in primary electron transport for photon and electron beams. *Med Phys.* 1990;17:187–194, with permission.)

- *Direct Monte Carlo for treatment planning*: The Monte Carlo technique consists of a computer program (MC code) that simulates the transport of millions of photons and particles through matter. It uses fundamental laws of physics to determine probability distributions of individual interactions of photons and particles.

  ➤ The larger the number of simulated particles (histories), the greater the accuracy of predicting their distributions.

  ➤ It is estimated that the transport of a few hundred million to a billion histories will be required for radiation therapy treatment planning with adequate precision.

  ➤ Notwithstanding inordinate amounts of computational times, Monte Carlo is the most accurate method of calculating dose distribution in a patient.

ABSORBED DOSE WITHIN BONE

- For a given quality radiation and the energy fluence, the absorbed dose in bone mineral relative to absorbed dose in muscle is given by the ratio of F factors or mass energy absorption coefficients (Ch. 8, Section 8.3B of the Textbook):

$$\frac{f_{bone}}{f_{muscle}} \quad \text{or} \quad \left(\frac{\mu_{en}}{\rho}\right)^{bone}_{muscle}$$

- Of greater importance biologically is the dose to soft tissue embedded in bone (e.g., blood vessels or the Haversian canals, living cells called osteocytes and bone marrow). The ratio γ of dose to a soft tissue element embedded in bone to the dose in a homogeneous medium of soft tissue, for the same photon energy fluence, is given by:

$$\gamma = D_{STB}/D_{ST} = (\bar{\mu}_{en}/\rho)^{B}_{ST} \cdot (\bar{S}/\rho)^{ST}_{B}$$

  where D_{STB} is the dose to a small volume of soft tissue embedded in bone, D_{ST} the dose to homogeneous soft tissue, $(\bar{\mu}_{en}/\rho)^{B}_{ST}$ the ratio of mass energy absorption coefficient for bone to soft tissue, and $(\bar{S}/\rho)^{ST}_{B}$ the ratio of average mass collision stopping power of soft tissue to bone for the electrons.

- Because collision mass stopping power of electrons for lower atomic number materials is greater than that for the higher atomic number materials (Ch. 14, Section 14.1.A.1 of the Textbook), the factor $(\bar{S}/\rho)^{ST}_{B} > 1$. Consequently, dose to soft tissue within bone is greater than the dose to the surrounding bone mineral.

- Dose enhancement in soft tissue imbedded in bone is not considered in most treatment planning algorithms. However, it should be taken into account when critical bony structures (e.g., spine, femoral heads, ribs) are subjected to near-tolerance doses.

DOSE TO LUNG

Dose to lung or tissues beyond lung is primarily governed by lung density. Because of low density of normal lung (~0.25 g/cm^3), beam transmission is greater in a given thickness of lung than in the same thickness of water or soft tissue of unit density.

- Because of low lung density, the dose is reduced at the tissue–lung interface. The dose then increases, following the electronic buildup with depth.

- Under full electronic buildup conditions, the increase in transmitted dose per cm of normal lung is approximately: 10% for orthovoltage, 4% for ^{60}Co, 3% for 6-MV, 2% for 10-MV, and 1% for 20-MV x-rays.

- Because of low lung density, there can be a partial loss of lateral electronic equilibrium in small fields (<6 × 6 cm^2) and high-energy beams (>6 MV), resulting in dose reduction that may not be accurately predicted by treatment planning algorithms that assume full electronic buildup in lung.

DOSE AT THE SURFACE OF AIR CAVITIES

The most important effect of air cavities in megavoltage beam dosimetry is the partial loss of electronic equilibrium at the cavity surface.

- Dose to tissue immediately beyond and in front of the cavity may be appreciably lower than expected, depending on the beam energy, cavity dimensions, and field size.

- The most significant decrease in dose occurs at the surface beyond the cavity, for large cavities (4 cm deep) and the smallest field (4 × 4 cm).

- It is estimated that in the case of ^{60}Co the reduction in dose in practical cases, such as the lesions located in the upper respiratory air passages, is not greater than 10% unless field sizes smaller than 4 × 4 cm^2 are used. The underdosage is expected to be greater for higher-energy radiation.

- Underdosage at the air cavity surface is not accurately predicted by a treatment planning algorithm that assumes full electronic buildup at the air–tissue interface.

TISSUE COMPENSATORS

Compensators are used to compensate for missing tissue at the surface or internal inhomogeneities such as lung. Figure 12B.4 illustrates the design of a compensator for an irregular surface.

- The compensator design takes into account the extent of missing tissue, compensator-to-surface distance, and the density of the compensator material.

- A tissue equivalent compensator designed with the same thickness as that of the missing tissue will overcompensate, that is, the dose to the underlying tissues will be less than that expected if a compensating bolus was placed right on the surface. This reduction in dose is caused by the reduction in scatter reaching a point at depth as a result of the compensator bolus being farther away from the surface instead of being placed at surface.

- The decrease in depth dose due to the reduction in scatter reaching a point at depth depends on the distance of the compensator from the surface, field size, depth, and beam quality.

- For irregular surface compensation, the required thickness for compensation is reduced (to make up for reduction in scatter) so that the dose at a given depth is the same whether the missing tissue is replaced with an equivalent bolus at the surface or with the compensator at the given distance from the surface.

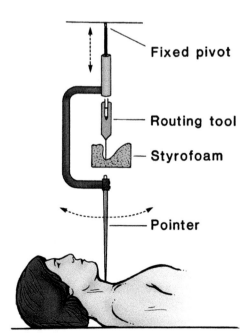

Figure 12B.4. Schematic diagram of a Styrofoam cutter fitted with a routing tool for constructing compensators. (Redrawn from Boge RJ, Edland RW, Mathes DC. Tissue compensators for megavoltage radiotherapy fabricated from hollowed Styrofoam filled with wax. *Radiology.* 1974;111:193.)

- The required thickness of a tissue-equivalent compensator along a ray divided by the missing tissue thickness along the same ray is called the *thickness ratio* (τ).

- In the actual design of the compensator, the thickness ratio is used to calculate compensator thickness (t_c) at a given point in the field:

$$t_c = \text{TD} \cdot (\tau / \rho_c)$$

where TD is the tissue deficit at the point considered, τ the thickness ratio, and ρ_c the density of the compensator material.

- The concept of thickness ratios also reveals that a compensator cannot be designed to provide dose compensation exactly at all depths. If, for given irradiation conditions, τ is chosen for a certain compensation depth, the compensator overcompensates at shallower depths and undercompensates at greater depths.

- A term *compensator ratio* (CR) has also been used in the literature to relate tissue deficit to the required compensator thickness. It is defined as the ratio of the missing tissue thickness to the compensator thickness necessary to give the required dose for a particular field size and depth. The concepts of compensator ratio and the thickness ratio are the same, except that the two quantities are inverse of each other, that is, $\text{CR} = \text{TD}/t_c = \rho_c/\tau$.

- Compensator ratio depends on beam energy, density of compensator material, compensator-to-surface distance, field size, and depth for which dose compensation is required.

REVIEW QUESTIONS • Chapter 12

In multiple choice questions, more than one option may be correct.

1. In kilovoltage cone-beam CT, CT numbers for all materials are proportional to:

   a) Mass density
   b) Electron density
   c) Atomic number
   d) Attenuation coefficients

2. What would the CT number be for tissue with an attenuation coefficient 25% of that for water?

   a) 0
   b) 250
   c) −250
   d) −750
   e) 25

3. Compared to CT, MRI provides better:

   a) Quality of images for bone or calcification
   b) Quality of images for soft tissue or tumors
   c) Spatial resolution
   d) Correlation with electron density

4. Compared to CT, PET images provide better:

   a) Geometric accuracy
   b) Differentiation of malignant tumor and normal tissue
   c) Correlation with electron density   .
   d) Spatial resolution

5. Compared to kilovoltage cone-beam CT, megavoltage cone-beam CT images provide:

   a) Better contrast
   b) Better resolution
   c) Less susceptibility to artifacts due to high-Z objects
   d) Better correlation with electron density

6. In ultrasound imaging:

   a) Strong reflection takes place at the interface of air–tissue because of large difference in acoustic impedance.
   b) The attenuation of ultrasound in tissue is due only to reflection.
   c) The ultrasonic transducer converts electromagnetic energy to mechanical energy in tissues.
   d) For radiotherapy planning, the ultrasonic cross-sectional image is of B mode.
   e) Common ultrasonic frequencies in medical imaging are 1 to 20 MHz.

7. A 10×10 cm^2 4-MV x-ray beam is incident on the phantom illustrated in Figure 12.B.1. Using the tissue–air ratio method and the data from appendix A.10.2, what is CF at point P, if $d_1 = d_2 = d_3 = 5$ cm, and ρ_e for the inhomogeneity is 0.4?

   a) 1.21
   b) 1.14
   c) 1.08
   d) 1.05
   e) 0.88

8. Repeat problem 7 above using the Batho's power law method:
   a) 1.23
   b) 1.18
   c) 1.12
   d) 1.02
   e) 0.91

9. Compared to homogeneous soft tissue, dose to soft tissue in bone is approximately: [Assume same photon energy fluence and complete electronic equilibrium]
   a) 3% less for ^{60}Co beam
   b) 3% higher for 6-MV x-rays
   c) 9% higher for 20-MV x-rays
   d) The same for all megavoltage photon beams

10. Which of the following is/are geometries that are <u>not</u> well accounted for in traditional (non–Monte Carlo) treatment planning algorithms:
    a) Dose at depths greater than 5 cm beyond a heterogeneity.
    b) Dose in lung for small field sizes and/or high energies.
    c) Dose in soft tissues embedded in bone.
    d) Dose at the exit surface of a heterogeneity.
    e) Dose for field sizes greater than 30×30 cm^2.

11. A compensator designed for irregular surface compensation:
    a) Has the same thickness (g/cm^3) along ray lines as the tissue deficit.
    b) Provides the same depth dose distribution as expected with flat surface.
    c) Has a compensator ratio that is independent of compensator-to-surface distance.
    d) Should be placed at compensator-to-surface distance of 20 cm or greater to maintain skin-sparing effect of megavoltage photon beams.

13

TREATMENT PLANNING III: FIELD SHAPING, SKIN DOSE, AND FIELD SEPARATION

REFERENCE

Khan FM. *The Physics of Radiation Therapy*, 4th edition, 2009. Chapter 13 "Treatment Planning III: Field Shaping, Skin Dose, and Field Separation"

Field Shaping, Surface Dose, and Field Separation

 TOPIC OUTLINE

The following topics will be discussed in this lecture:
- ➤ Field shaping
- ➤ Skin dose
- ➤ Separation of adjacent fields

FIELD SHAPING

A radiation field collimated by x-ray jaws is rectangular in shape. Fields of any shape can be created by secondary blocking (standard lead blocks or custom Cerrobend blocking) or multileaf collimators (MLCs).

- *Block thickness*: The thickness of lead required to provide adequate protection of the shielded areas depends on the beam quality and the allowed transmission through the block.

  - ➤ A primary beam transmission of 5% or less through the block is considered acceptable for most clinical situations.

  - ➤ If n is the number of half-value layers to achieve 5% transmission,

$$\frac{1}{2^n} = 0.05$$

  Or,

$$n = 4.32$$

  Thus, a thickness of lead of approximately 4.5 half-value layers would give less than 5% primary beam transmission and is, therefore, recommended for most clinical shielding.

- *Custom blocking*: Fields of complex shapes require custom blocking. The blocking material most commonly used for custom blocking in megavoltage beams is the Lipowitz metal (brand name, Cerrobend).

  - ➤ Cerrobend has a density of approximately 9.4 g/cm^3 at room temperature (~83% of lead density). This material consists of bismuth, lead, tin, and cadmium. (Cadmium-free Cerrobend is also available.)

  - ➤ The main advantage of Cerrobend over lead is that it melts at approximately 70°C (cad-free at 95°C) (compared with 327°C for lead) and, therefore, can be easily cast into any shape. At room temperature, it is harder than lead.

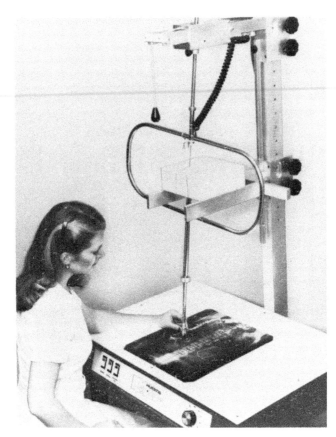

Figure 13.1. Photograph of block cutter. (Courtesy of Huestis Machine Corp., Bristol, RI, USA.)

➤ Unlike standard (straight) lead blocks, Cerrobend blocks are made divergent. As seen in Figure 13.1, an electrically heated wire pivots about a point simulating the source or the x-ray target. The simulation film with blocks drawn, the Styrofoam block, and the wire apparatus simulate the actual treatment geometry, that is, same source-to-film distance as for the simulator film and the same source-to-block distance as in the actual treatment. The lower end of the wire traces the block outline on the film while the heated wire cuts a divergent Styrofoam cavity.

• *Multileaf collimators*: An MLC for photon beams consists of a large number of collimating blocks or leaves that can be driven automatically and independently, to generate a field of any shape.

➤ Typical MLCs consist of 60 to 80 pairs, independently driven.

➤ Individual leaf typically has a width of 0.5 or 1 cm as projected at the isocenter.

➤ The leaf thickness is sufficient to provide primary x-ray transmission through the leaves of less than 2% (compared with about 1% for the jaws and 5% for the Cerrobend blocks).

➤ The interleaf (between adjacent leaves) transmission is usually less than 3%. The primary beam transmission may be further minimized by combining jaws with the MLC in shielded areas outside the MLC field opening.

➤ The physical penumbra with MLC is larger than that produced by the collimator jaws or the Cerrobend blocks. This is usually not a serious drawback except for the treatment of small fields or when blocking is required close to critical structures.

➤ Stair-step effect of the MLC field edges makes it difficult to match adjacent fields.

SKIN DOSE

Skin sparing is one of the most desirable characteristics of high-energy photon beams. In contrast to lower energy beams (e.g., superficial and orthovoltage x-rays), which produce maximum ionization at/or close to the skin surface, the megavoltage beams create an initial electronic buildup with depth. Consequently, the surface dose is less than the maximum dose that occurs at a depth downstream. The higher the energy, the deeper is the depth of maximum dose.

- Surface dose in megavoltage beams is predominantly due to electron contamination incident at the surface. These electrons are mostly Compton electrons produced by photon interactions with the collimators and other materials in the path of the beam such as the flattening filter, wedges, and shadow tray.

- If a shadow tray is the last absorber in the beam, it will absorb most of the electrons incident on it but, in turn, will generate its own Compton electrons. The tray is then the main contributor of contaminant electrons incident on the patient.

- Percentage surface dose ($\%D_s$) decreases with increase in shadow tray-to-surface distance because of divergence and scattering of the contaminant electrons in the air (Figure 13.2).

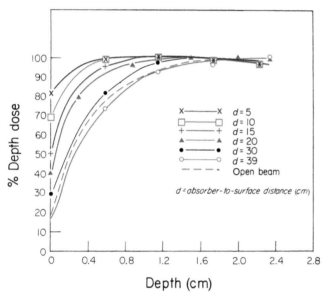

Figure 13.2. Effect of Lucite shadow tray on dose buildup for 10-MV x-rays. Percentage depth dose distribution is plotted for various tray to surface distances (d). 10-MV x-rays, tray thickness = 1.5 g/cm^2, field size = 15 × 15 cm, source-to-surface distance = 100 cm, and source-to-diaphragm distance = 50 cm. (From Khan FM, Moore VC, Levitt SH. Effect of various atomic number absorbers on skin dose for 10-MeV x-rays. *Radiology*. 1973; 109:209, with permission.)

- $\%D_s$ decreases with increase in photon energy because of relatively less photon interactions (i.e., less electron production). Remember that the Compton cross section decreases with increase in energy.

- $\%D_s$ increases with increase in field size because of greater electron contamination produced (Figure 13.3).

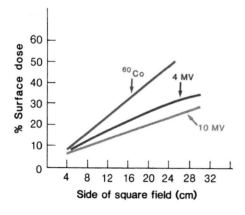

Figure 13.3. Percentage surface dose as a function of field size. ^{60}Co, Theratron 80, source-to-surface distance (SSD) = 80 cm, source-to-diaphragm distance (SDD) = 59 cm. 4 MV, Clinac 4, SSD = 80 cm. 10 MV, LMR 13, SSD = 100 cm, SDD = 50 cm. ^{60}Co and 4-MV. (Data are from Velkley DE, Manson DJ, Purdy JA, et al. Buildup region of megavoltage photon radiation sources. *Med Phys.* 1975;2:14. 10-MV data are from Khan FM, Moore VC, Levitt SH. Effect of various atomic number absorbers on skin dose for 10-MeV x-rays. *Radiology.* 1973;109:209.)

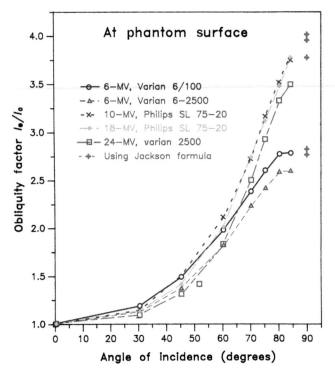

Figure 13.4. Obliquity factor at the surface plotted as a function of beam angle for various energy beams. Jackson formula for tangential beam incidence is based on Equation 13.1 in the Textbook. (From Gerbi BJ, Meigooni AS, Khan FM. Dose buildup for obliquely incident photon beams. *Med Phys.* 1987; 14:393, with permission.)

- $\%D_s$ increases with increase in beam obliquity (Figure 13.4) because of increased contribution of electrons generated by photon interactions with the phantom at oblique angles.

- For tangential beam incidence, $\%D_s$ is approximately given by:

$$\%D_s \text{ at tangential incidence} = \tfrac{1}{2}(100\% + \%D_s \text{ for perpendicular incidence})$$

- *Electron filters*: Electron filters are medium atomic number absorbers (Z = ~50) that reduce the surface dose by scattering out contaminant electrons more than the lower Z materials and producing secondary electrons less than in the higher Z materials (Figure 13.5).

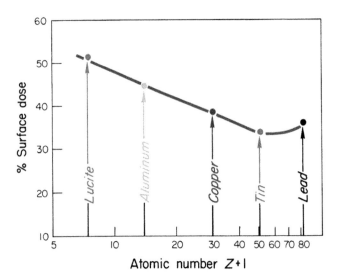

Figure 13.5. Variation of percentage surface dose with atomic number of absorber. Each absorber had a thickness of 1.5 g/cm² and was mounted underneath a Lucite shadow tray. 10-MV x-rays, field size = 15 × 15 cm and absorber-to-surface distance = 15 cm. (From Khan FM, Moore VC, Levitt SH. Effect of various atomic number absorbers on skin dose for 10-MeV x-rays. *Radiology.* 1973;109: 209, with permission.)

➤ The thickness of an electron filter should be at least equal to the maximum range of secondary electrons. This is approximately given by (d_m/ρ_e), where d_m is the depth of maximum dose for the given energy beam in water and ρ_e the electron density of the electron filter relative to water.

➤ As seen in Figure 13.5, the surface dose decreases with increase in Z of the absorber until tin and then increases slightly for lead. Although tin is the best electron filter, a lead filter may be preferable because of its greater availability in a radiation therapy department.

• *Measurement of surface/dose in the buildup region*: Because of the steep dose gradient, the size of the dosimeter along the beam direction should be as small as possible for surface or buildup dose measurements.

➤ Extrapolation chambers are the most accurate instruments for measuring surface dose or dose in the buildup region in a plastic phantom.

➤ Parallel-plate (also called plane-parallel) chambers are more practical than the extrapolation chambers and therefore more commonly used for the above measurements in a phantom.

➤ Thin TLD chips, film, and unshielded diodes may be used where ion chambers cannot be used, for example, patient skin dose or other in vivo measurements.

SEPARATION OF ADJACENT FIELDS

Adjacent treatment fields are commonly used in external beam radiation therapy, such as the "mantle" and "inverted-Y" fields, bilateral neck and supraclavicular fields, craniospinal fields, and fields for treating tumors close to previously treated areas.

• Separation of adjacent fields, when needed, may be accomplished geometrically or dosimetrically. Some of these techniques are listed below:

➤ Angling the adjacent beams away from each other

➤ Matching fields at depth (with calculated skin gap)

➤ Beam splitting at central axis to eliminate beam divergence

➤ Modifying penumbra at adjacent field edges

➤ Matching fields based on composite isodose distribution generated by a treatment planning system

These techniques are illustrated in Figure 13.6.

• If two adjacent fields are incident from one side only and are made to junction at a given depth, the required skin gap (field separation at the surface) is given by:

$$S = S_1 + S_2 = \frac{1}{2}L_1 \cdot \frac{d}{\text{SSD}_1} + \frac{1}{2}L_2 \cdot \frac{d}{\text{SSD}_2}$$

where S is total separation, S_1 the separation for field 1, S_2 the separation for field 2, L_1 and L_2 the field lengths, and SSD_1 and SSD_2 the source-to-surface distances. The geometry is illustrated in Figure 13.7.

• For an adjacent set of parallel opposed fields (e.g., mantle and para-aortic or inverted Y fields), the four fields are made to junction at the midline. If the adjacent fields have different lengths or SSDs, there is a problem of three-field overlap, as illustrated in Figure 13.8.

• To avoid the above three-field overlap, the field separation may be increased. Alternatively, the length and SSD of the smaller field (field 2) are made the same as for the larger field (field 1) and the resulting extra length of field 2 is blocked off on the side away from the junction (e.g., inferiorly for the spine field 2).

ORTHOGONAL FIELD JUNCTIONS

Orthogonal fields denote an arrangement in which the central axes of the adjacent fields are orthogonal (i.e., perpendicular to each other). EXAMPLES: craniospinal irradiation for medulloblastoma

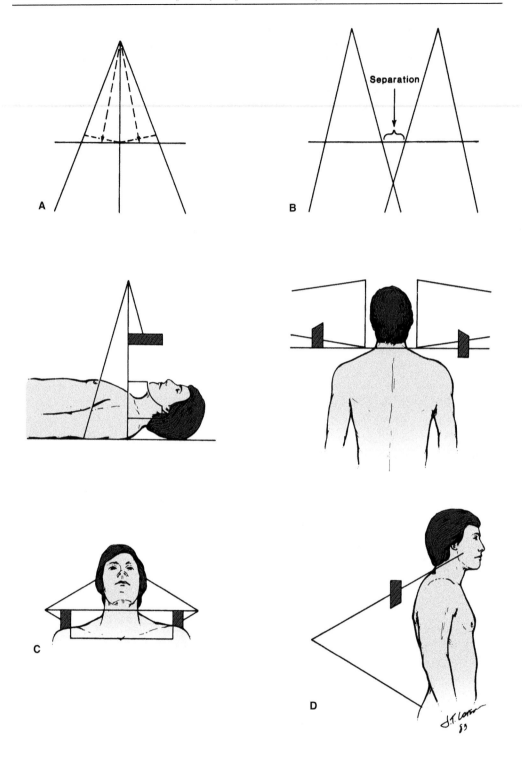

Figure 13.6. Schematic representation of various techniques used for field matching. **A:** Angling the beams away from each other so that the two beams abut and are aligned vertically. **B:** Fields separated at the skin surface. The junction point is at a depth where dose is uniform across the junction. **C:** Isocentric split-beam technique for head and neck tumors. (Redrawn from Williamson TJ. A technique for matching orthogonal megavoltage fields. *Int J Radiat Oncol Biol Phys.* 1979;5:111.) **D:** Craniospinal irradiation using penumbra generators. (Redrawn from Griffin TW, Schumacher D, Berry HC. A technique for cranial-spinal irradiation. *Br J Radiol.* 1976;49:887.)

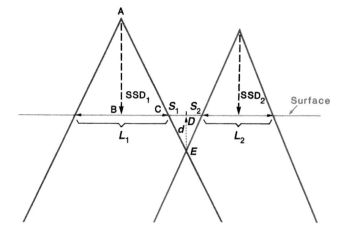

Figure 13.7. Geometry of two adjacent beams, separated by a distance $S_1 + S_2$ on the surface and junctioning at depth d. SSD, source-to-surface distance.

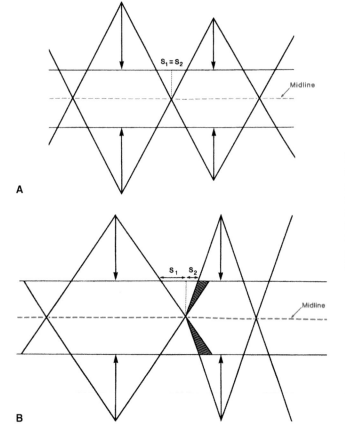

Figure 13.8. Two pairs of parallel opposed fields. Adjacent fields are separated on the surface so that they all join at a point on the midline. **A:** Ideal geometry in which there is no three-field overlap. **B:** Arrangement in which there are two regions (shaded) of three-field overlap.

(parallel–opposed brain fields + posterior spine field), and head and neck cancers (e.g., bilateral parallel–opposed neck fields + anterior supraclavicular field).

• *Craniospinal irradiation*: One of the techniques for craniospinal irradiation is illustrated in Figure 13.9.

Orthogonal field matching is accomplished by: (a) rotating the cranial fields through an angle θ_{coll} so that their caudad margins are parallel with the diverging cephalad margin of the spinal field; and (b) rotating the couch (also known as kicking the couch) through angle θ_{couch} to match the superior margin of the spinal field with the diverging cranial fields. Alternative to couch rotation is to

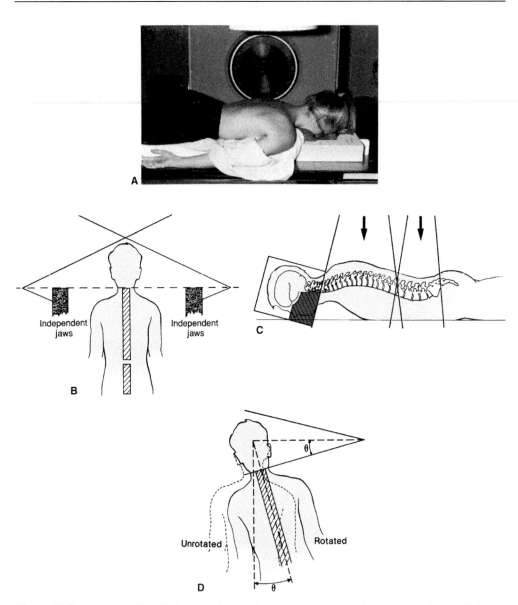

Figure 13.9. Craniospinal irradiation technique. **A:** Patient set-up showing Styrofoam blocks and Alpha Cradle mold to provide stable position for abdomen, chest, and head. **B:** Elimination of cranial field divergence by using an independent jaw as a beam splitter. **C:** Lateral view of fields showing cranial field rotated to align with the diverging border of the spinal field. **D:** Couch rotated to provide match between the spinal field and the diverging border of the cranial field. This provides an alternative to setup **B**.

split the cranial fields at their central axes using independent jaws. The collimator and couch angles are calculated geometrically as below.

$$\theta_{coll} = arc\tan\left(\frac{1}{2} \cdot L_1 \cdot \frac{1}{SSD}\right)$$

$$\theta_{couch} = arc\tan\left(\frac{1}{2} \cdot L_2 \cdot \frac{1}{SAD}\right)$$

where L_1 is the length of the posterior spinal field, L_2 the length of the lateral cranial fields, SSD the source-to-surface distance for the spinal field, and SAD the source-to-axis distance for the cranial fields, assuming the SSD technique is used for the spinal field and the SAD technique for the cranial fields. The couch is rotated toward the side the cranial field enters the head.

- **Guidelines for field matching:**

  1. The site of field matching should be chosen, insofar as possible, over an area that does not contain tumor or a critically sensitive organ.

  2. If the tumor is superficial at the junction site, the fields should not be separated because a cold spot on the tumor will risk recurrence. One may abut the fields at the surface but eliminate beam divergence using a beam splitter or by tilting the beams away to make them parallel to each other.

  3. The line of field matching must be drawn at each treatment session on the basis of the first field treated.

  4. A field matching must be verified by actual isodose distribution using a treatment planning system.

REVIEW QUESTIONS • Chapter 13

✔ **TEST YOURSELF**

Review questions for this chapter are provided online.

In multiple choice questions, more than one option may be correct.

1. How many HVLs are required to reduce the primary beam to 2% of its initial value?

    a) 3.76
    b) 4.32
    c) 5
    d) 5.64
    e) 7.5

2. Half-value layer (HVL) for a 6-MV x-ray beam is 13 mm of lead ($\rho = 13.5$ g/cm^3). What is the thickness of Cerrobend in centimeters to reduce the primary beam to 5% transmission? [Assume density of Cerrobend to be 83% of that of lead.]

    a) 5.2
    b) 6.7
    c) 7.8
    d) 9.9

3. A 12×12 cm^2 6-MV field is blocked to 10×10 cm^2 using a nondivergent lead block. The source-to-block tray distance is 65 cm. Assuming an HVL of 1.5 cm of lead for this beam, what is the resultant transmission penumbra (90%/10%) at 100 cm from the source?

    a) 0.10 cm
    b) 0.25 cm
    c) 0.36 cm
    d) 0.50 cm
    e) 0.75 cm

4. Surface dose would increase for what conditions in a megavoltage beam?

    a) Increasing field size
    b) Reducing shadow tray-to-surface distance
    c) Inserting a 1-mm-thick lead in the beam under the shadow tray
    d) Increasing beam obliquity

5. What are the possible causes for loss of skin sparing for MV photon beams?

    a) Secondary electron contamination of the photon beam.
    b) Larger SSDs.
    c) Larger field sizes.
    d) Solid materials in the beam positioned at less than 10 cm from the skin.
    e) MLCs instead of custom blocks.

6. The most suitable dosimeter for measuring surface dose in a phantom is:

    a) Farmer chamber
    b) Plane-parallel chamber
    c) Shielded diode
    d) TLD capsule

7. For a linear accelerator x-ray beam:

    a) X-ray jaws reduce the primary beam transmission to approximately 2% or less.
    b) Multileaf collimators (MLCs) reduce the primary beam transmission to 5% or less.
    c) MLCs have an interleaf transmission of 10% or less.
    d) Lead blocks are designed to reduce the primary beam transmission to 5% or less.
    e) Cerrobend blocks are designed to reduce the primary beam transmission to 5% or less.

8. Physical penumbra (lateral distance between 90% and 20% isodose curves) at 10-cm depth:

   a) Is larger with MLCs than with divergent Cerrobend blocks
   b) Increases with field size
   c) Decreases with decrease in source-to-collimator distance
   d) Decreases with increase in photon energy

9. A 10×10 cm field is abutted to a 20×20 cm field, both at 100 cm SSD. What skin gap is necessary if the fields are matched at a depth of 5 cm?

   a) 0.75 cm
   b) 0.89 cm
   c) 1.00 cm
   d) 1.21 cm
   e) 1.50 cm

10. Lateral whole brain fields of size 20×20 cm^2 (SAD = 100 cm) are used with an abutting 8×40 cm^2 posterior spine field (SSD = 100 cm). [Fields are defined as X × Y, with X the lateral and Y the longitudinal length.]. How many degrees should the couch be rotated to match the divergence of the whole brain fields?

   a) 3.8
   b) 5.7
   c) 8.5
   d) 11.3

14

ELECTRON BEAM THERAPY

REFERENCE
Khan FM. *The Physics of Radiation Therapy,* 4th edition, 2009. Chapter 14 "Electron Beam Therapy"

Electron Beam Interactions and Dosimetry

 TOPIC OUTLINE

The following topics will be discussed in this lecture:
- ➤ Electron interactions
- ➤ Stopping power
- ➤ Scattering power
- ➤ Absorbed dose calculation
- ➤ Energy specification and measurement
- ➤ Measurement of absorbed dose
- ➤ Electron dosimetry phantoms
- ➤ Clinical electron beam characteristics
- ➤ Field size dependence of depth dose
- ➤ Electron source position
- ➤ X-ray contamination

ELECTRON INTERACTIONS

As high-energy electrons travel through a medium, they interact with atoms by various processes owing to Coulomb force interactions. These interaction processes include the following:

a) **Inelastic collisions with atomic electrons** (ionization and excitation, secondary electron production or δ-rays)

b) **Inelastic collisions with atomic nuclei** (bremsstrahlung)

c) **Elastic collisions with atomic nuclei** (nuclear Coulomb scattering)

d) **Elastic collisions with atomic electrons** (electron–electron scattering)

   ➤ *Inelastic collisions* are Coulomb force interactions in which a part of the kinetic energy of the colliding particle is lost in producing ionization/excitation, bremsstrahlung, or occasionally a secondary electron.

   ➤ The secondary electron production is relatively a rare interaction compared to the ionization/excitation. In this collision process (also called knock-on collision) the stripped electron acquires enough kinetic energy to cause further ionization/excitation on its own.

   ➤ *Elastic collisions* are Coulomb force interactions in which there is no significant loss of electron energy but the trajectory is deflected from the original direction. The elastic collisions with nuclei are called nuclear Coulomb scattering and the elastic collisions with electrons are called electron–electron scattering.

➤ Multiple elastic collisions of a high-energy electron (multiple scattering) produce multiple small angle deflections. As a result the electron follows a tortuous (zigzag) path, while it continuously loses kinetic energy through inelastic collisions with atoms until all its kinetic energy is gone.

STOPPING POWER

The stopping power of a material for a charged particle is the rate of its energy loss per unit path length. The linear stopping power (S) is defined as dE/dl, where dE is the fraction of energy that the particle loses in traversing an increment of path length dl. The mass stopping power is given by (S/ρ), where ρ is the density of the medium. Because the energy losses of an electron can be collisional (ionization/excitation) as well as radiative (bremsstrahlung), the total mass stopping power $(S/\rho)_{tot}$ is given by:

$$(S/\rho)_{tot} = (S/\rho)_{col} + (S/\rho)_{rad}$$

where $(S/\rho)_{col}$ and $(S/\rho)_{rad}$ apply to collisional losses and radiative losses, respectively.

- The units of linear stopping power and mass stopping power are MeV/cm and MeV/g cm^{-2}, respectively.
- The linear stopping power depends on electron density of the medium (electrons/cm^3).
- The mass stopping power depends on number of electrons per gram. Because electrons per gram for low atomic number (Z) materials are greater than for high Z materials (see Table 5.1, page 63, of the Textbook), the mass stopping power is greater for low Z materials than for high Z materials. (Compare the water curve to the lead curve in Figure 14A.1.)

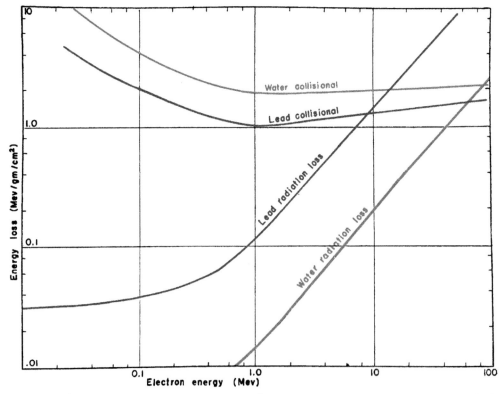

Figure 14A.1. Rate of energy loss in MeV per g/cm^2 as a function of electron energy for water and lead. (From Johns HE, Cunningham JR. *The Physics of Radiology*. 3rd ed. Springfield, IL: Charles C Thomas; 1969, with permission.)

- The mass stopping power is greater in a gas than in a denser medium of the same composition. This effect is due to *polarization* of the condensed medium in which atoms close to the electron track screen those remote from the track. In a dense medium, a screening electric field around atoms close to the track excludes distant atoms from participating in Coulomb interactions. This decreases the stopping power.
- The stopping power or the rate of energy loss depends on electron energy (Figure 14A.1). However, for electrons of energy 1 MeV and above, the rate of energy loss in water is almost constant and is roughly 2 MeV/cm.
- The rate of energy loss per centimeter in a medium due to bremsstrahlung is approximately proportional to the electron energy and to the square of the atomic number (Z^2).
- The probability of radiative loss relative to the collisional loss increases with increase in electron energy and with Z. That means that the efficiency of x-ray production is greater for higher energy electrons and higher atomic number absorbers.

SCATTERING POWER

When a pencil beam of electrons passes through a medium, the electrons suffer energy degradation as well as multiple scattering. As a result the beam becomes more heterogeneous in energy and acquires an angular spread that depends on the density and composition of the medium.

- By analogy with mass stopping power, the mass angular scattering power of the medium is defined as the quotient $\bar{\theta}^2/\rho l$, where $\bar{\theta}^2$ is the mean square scattering angle, ρ the density, and l the path length.
- The scattering power varies approximately as the square of the atomic number and inversely as the square of the kinetic energy.

ABSORBED DOSE CALCULATION

In calculating the absorbed dose (energy absorbed per unit mass) in a medium, one needs to know the electron fluence and the restricted mass collision stopping power. If Φ_E is the differential distribution of fluence with respect to energy $\left[\Phi_E = \dfrac{d\Phi(E)}{dE}\right]$, the absorbed dose D is closely approximated by:

$$D = \int_\Delta^{E_0} \Phi_E \cdot \left(\frac{L}{\rho}\right)_{col, \Delta} \cdot dE$$

where E_0 is the maximum electron energy and $\left(\dfrac{L}{\rho}\right)_{col,\Delta}$ the *restricted mass collision stopping power* with Δ as the cutoff energy.

ENERGY SPECIFICATION AND MEASUREMENT

Before exiting the accelerator window, the electron beam is a narrow pencil (2–3 mm in diameter) and almost monoenergetic. It suffers scattering and energy degradation as it passes through the exit window, scattering foil, monitor chambers, air, and other materials. This results in the beam acquiring an angular spread and taking on a spectral distribution of energies at the phantom surface. Further spatial spread and energy degradation of the beam take place with depth in the phantom (Figure 14A.2).

- In clinical practice, an electron beam energy is specified by the *most probable energy at the surface*, $(E_p)_0$. This is the kinetic energy possessed by most of the electrons incident at the surface.
- The average or mean energy is slightly less than the most probable energy. That means the energy spectrum is skewed more toward the lower energies.

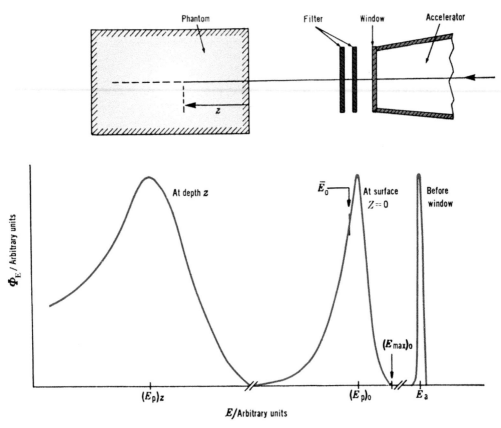

Figure 14A.2. Distribution of electron fluence in energy, Φ_E, as the beam passes through the collimation system of the accelerator and the phantom. (From International Commission on Radiation Units and Measurements. *Radiation Dosimetry: Electrons with Initial Energies between 1 and 50 MeV.* Report No. 21. Washington, DC: International Commission on Radiation Units and Measurements; 1972, with permission.)

- The most probable energy may be determined from a measured broad beam depth dose curve (Figure 14A.3).
- The parameter, R_p, of the depth dose curve is related to $(E_p)_0$ by the following equation:

$$(E_p)_0 = C_1 + C_2 R_p + C_3 R_p^2$$

where R_p is the practical range in centimeters as defined in Figure 14.3. For water, $C_1 = 0.22$ MeV, $C_2 = 1.98$ MeV cm^{-1}, and $C_3 = 0.0025$ MeV cm^{-2}.

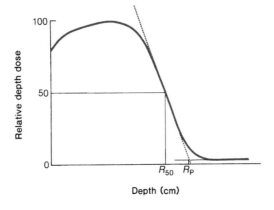

Figure 14A.3. Depth dose curve illustrating the definition of R_p and R_{50}.

- As a rough approximation, $(E_p)_0$ in MeV is numerically equal to $2 \times R_p$ in centimeters of water.
- The depth dose curve for the determination of R_p should be measured for a broad beam (e.g., 20×20 cm field size).
- The mean energy of the beam at the surface, $\bar{E}_0$, is related to R_{50} (the depth at which the dose is 50% of the maximum dose) by the following equation:

$$\bar{E}_0 = C_4 \cdot R_{50}$$

where $C_4 = 2.4$ MeV cm^{-1} for water.

ENERGY AT DEPTH

The most probable and the mean energies at depth z in a phantom decrease linearly with depth and are given by the following equations:

$$(E_p)_z = (E_p)_0 \left(1 - \frac{z}{R_p} \right)$$

and

$$\bar{E}_z = \bar{E}_0 \left(1 - \frac{z}{R_p} \right)$$

MEASUREMENT OF ABSORBED DOSE

Calorimetry and Fricke dosimetry are the most basic methods for measuring absorbed dose in a phantom, but the use of these instruments is not practical in a clinical setting. Calibrated ion chambers are used instead.

ABSORBED DOSE CALIBRATION

- The most current protocols for the calibration of absorbed dose are the AAPM TG-51 (1999) and the IAEA TRS-398 (2000) (discussed in Chapter 8 of the Textbook).
- For each electron energy available with the accelerator, the beam is calibrated to give 1 cGy/MU for the reference applicator (e.g., 10×10 cm), at the respective depth of maximum dose (d_{max}) on central axis and at the standard SSD (nominally, 100 cm).

OUTPUT FACTORS

- The output factor S_e for a particular beam energy, applicator or field size, and at the standard SSD is defined as the ratio of dose per monitor unit D/U, on central axis at d_{max} for that field, to the dose per monitor unit D_0/MU for the reference applicator or field size at d_{max} for the reference field on central axis at the standard SSD. Mathematically:

$$S_e = \frac{D/\text{MU}}{D_0/\text{MU}}$$

DEPTH DOSE DISTRIBUTION

The depth-dose and isodose distributions can be measured by ion chambers, diodes, or films. Automated beam scanning systems in a water phantom are useful in this regard and are available commercially.

- *Ionization chambers*: Cylindrical ionization chambers are most commonly used for the measurement of depth dose distribution. Depth ionization curves measured with an ion chamber need to be converted to depth dose curves by making the following corrections:

➤ Corrections for restricted mass stopping power ratio of water to air, $(L/\rho)_{air}^{w}$, as a function of mean electron energy at depth (d);

➤ Chamber replacement correction, P_{repl}. This factor is dependent on the air cavity diameter as well as the mean electron energy at the depth of measurement. P_{repl} has two components, namely, fluence correction and gradient correction (see Chapter 8, pages 107 and 108, of the Textbook).

• The following equation for the conversion of percentage depth ionization, $\%DI_{w}$, in water to percentage depth dose, $\%DD_{w}$, in water takes into account the above corrections:

$$\%DD_{w}(d) = \%DI_{w}(d) \times \frac{\left[(\bar{L}/\rho)_{air}^{w} \times P_{repl}\right]_{d}}{\left[(\bar{L}/\rho)_{air}^{w} \times P_{repl}\right]_{d_{max}}}$$

➤ The software for converting depth ionization curves to percentage depth dose curves for electron beams is usually available with the water phantom scanning systems.

• *Diodes*: Unshielded silicon *p–n* junction diodes may be used for measuring depth dose distribution in a water phantom. They offer some advantages in terms of small size and high sensitivity (Chapter 8 of the Textbook).

➤ Diodes show temperature and directional dependence and their sensitivity may change over time. Therefore, they are not suitable for determining an absolute value of dose.

➤ Because the variation of silicon-to-water stopping power ratio with electron energy is quite minimal (~5% between 1 and 20 MeV), measurements made with a diode may be used directly to give depth dose distribution without further correction.

➤ A sample depth dose distribution obtained with a diode should be checked by ion chamber measurements to ensure proper diode operation.

• *Film*: For electron beams, film dosimetry offers a convenient and rapid method of obtaining depth dose distribution or a complete set of isodose curves in the plane of the film.

➤ Unlike its response to photons, the film does not show significant energy dependence with electrons. This energy independence may be explained by the fact that the ratio of electron collision stopping power in the film emulsion to that in water varies slowly with electron energy. Thus, the optical density of the film can be converted to dose by using its sensitometric (H&D) curve determined at one energy with essentially no further corrections.

➤ Film cannot be used reliably for absolute dosimetry because the optical density of an exposed film depends on many variables such as emulsion, processing conditions, magnitude of absorbed dose, and some measurement conditions, which can give rise to serious artifacts. The use of film is, therefore, restricted to relative dosimetry.

➤ Film may be used for measuring output factors for small fields where an ion chamber cannot be used because of its large size.

ELECTRON DOSIMETRY PHANTOMS

Water is the standard medium for clinical dosimetry. However, plastic phantoms may be used where a detector cannot be placed in water.

• For a phantom to be water equivalent for electron beam dosimetry, it must have the same linear stopping power and the same linear angular scattering power as those for water. This may be approximately achieved in materials that have electron density and effective atomic number close to those of water.

• There are several commercially available phantoms for electron beam dosimetry, for example, polystyrene, acrylic, and electron solid water. These phantoms may be used by assigning an empirically determined effective density for scaling depth to make them water equivalent.

- The water equivalent depth d_w for a depth d_{med} in a phantom or its effective density (ρ_{eff}) may be estimated from the following relationship:

$$d_w = d_{med} \times \rho_{eff} = d_{med} \left(\frac{R_{50}^{water}}{R_{50}^{med}} \right)$$

where R_{50} is the depth of the 50% depth dose.

CLINICAL ELECTRON BEAM CHARACTERISTICS

The major attraction of the electron beam irradiation is the shape of the depth dose curve, especially in the energy range of 6 to 15 MeV. A region of more or less uniform dose followed by a rapid drop-off of dose offers a distinct clinical advantage over the conventional x-ray modalities. This advantage, however, tends to disappear with increasing energy.

- *Central axis depth dose distribution:* Figure 14A.4 shows an example of central axis depth dose curves for various energy electron beams.

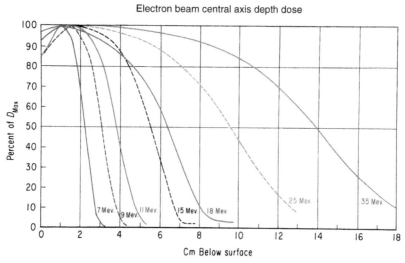

Figure 14A.4. Comparison of central axis depth dose distributions of the Sagittaire linear accelerator (*continuous curves*) and the Siemens betatron (*dashed curves*). (From Tapley N, ed. *Clinical Applications of the Electron Beam.* New York: John Wiley; 1976, with permission.)

➤ Electron beams have a modest skin-sparing effect that is energy dependent.

➤ Unlike photon beams, the percentage surface dose in electron beams increases with increase in beam energy (e.g., approximately in the range of 70% to 80% for 6 MeV, increasing to 95% to 100% for 25 MeV).

➤ The depth of D_{max} (d_{100}) does not follow a linear relationship with energy but it covers a broad region. Its value in centimeters of water for a broad beam may be approximated by $0.46E^{0.67}$, where E is the most probable beam energy at the surface in MeV.

➤ For a broad beam, the depths of other percentage depth dose values of clinical interest are approximately given by: $d_{90} = E/3.2$, $d_{80} = E/2.8$.

- *Isodose curves:* The energy, scattering foil, and collimation are important in determining beam flatness and the shape of the isodose curves. Figure 14A.5 shows sample isodose patterns for two different energy beams.
  From these curves, it may be noted that:

➤ The low-level isodose curves (<50%) bulge out beyond the field borders.

➤ The higher level isodose curves (>80%) tend to show lateral constriction, which becomes worse with increasing energy and depth.

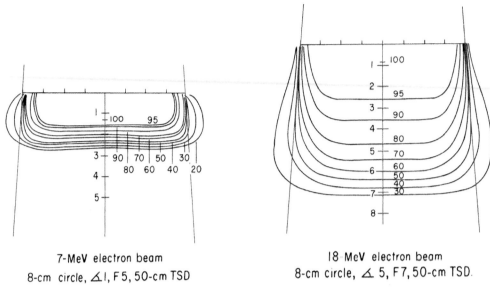

7-MeV electron beam

8-cm circle, ∡1, F5, 50-cm TSD

18 MeV electron beam

8-cm circle, ∡ 5, F7, 50-cm TSD.

Figure 14A.5. Comparison of isodose curves for different energy electron beams. (From Tapley N, ed. *Clinical Applications of the Electron Beam.* New York: John Wiley; 1976:86, with permission.)

- *Flatness and symmetry:* Uniformity of an electron beam is usually specified in a plane perpendicular to the beam axis and at a fixed depth.

  ➤ The AAPM TG-25 recommends the following criteria for acceptable beam flatness:

    • *Field flatness* of an electron beam should be specified in a reference plane perpendicular to the central axis, at the depth of the 95% dose beyond the depth of dose maximum.

    • In the reference plane, the lateral dose variation relative to the dose at central axis should not exceed ±5% (optimally to be within ±3%) over an area confined within lines 2 cm inside the geometric edge of fields of size equal to or larger than 10×10 cm^2.

    • *Beam symmetry* compares a dose profile on one side of the central axis to that on the other. The AAPM recommends that the cross-beam profile in the reference plane should not differ more than 2% at any pair of points located symmetrically on opposite sides of the central axis.

FIELD SIZE DEPENDENCE OF DEPTH DOSE

In general, the output and the central axis depth dose distribution are field size dependent. Figure 14A.6 shows the change in central axis depth dose distribution with field size.

- As the field size is increased, the percentage depth dose initially increases but becomes constant beyond a certain field size when the lateral scatter equilibrium is reached. Furthermore, the depth d_{max} shifts toward the surface for the smaller fields.

- The minimum field diameter for the establishment of lateral scatter equilibrium at all depths on central axis is given by the following approximate relationship:

$$D_{eq} \cong 1.76\sqrt{(E_p)_0}$$

where D_{eq} is the field diameter in cm and $(E_p)_0$ the most probable energy at the surface in MeV.

- *Field equivalence:* Field equivalence here is defined in terms of central axis percentage depth doses and not the output factors, which depend on particular jaw setting for the given applicator or other collimation conditions.

  ➤ All broad fields (in which the lateral scatter equilibrium exists by definition) are equivalent and their depth dose distribution is the same irrespective of their size. EXAMPLE: Field

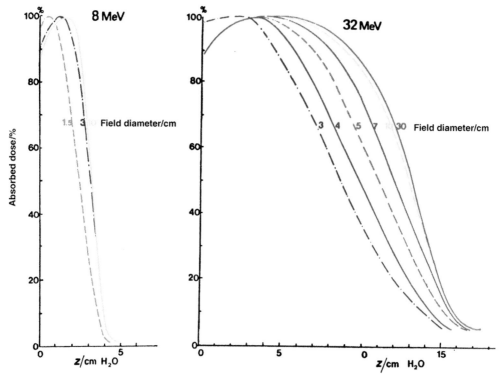

Figure 14A.6. Variation of depth dose distribution with field size. (From International Commission on Radiation Units and Measurements. Radiation Dosimetry: *Electron Beams with Energies between 1 and 50 MeV.* Report No. 35. Bethesda, MD: International Commission on Radiation Units and Measurements; 1984, with permission.)

sizes larger than 10×10 cm^2 are all broad fields for energies up to 30 MeV and hence are equivalent.

➤ Field equivalence is relevant only for small fields in which the lateral scatter equilibrium does not exist and consequently, the depth dose distribution is field size dependent.

➤ For a square field of dimensions $a \times a$, the equivalent circular field has a diameter D_{equiv}, given by:

$$D_{\text{equiv}} \cong 1.12a$$

➤ The depth dose for rectangular field sizes can be extracted from square field data by the following relationships:

$$D^{X,Y} = [D^{X,X} \cdot D^{Y,Y}]^{1/2}$$

where D is the central axis depth dose and X and Y the field dimensions.

ELECTRON SOURCE POSITION

Unlike an x-ray beam, an electron beam does not emanate from a physical source in the accelerator head.

• *Virtual source*:

➤ An electron beam *appears* to diverge from a point, called the *virtual source*.

➤ Virtual source may be defined as an intersection point of the back projections along the most probable directions of electron motion at the patient surface. This is illustrated in Figure 14A.7.

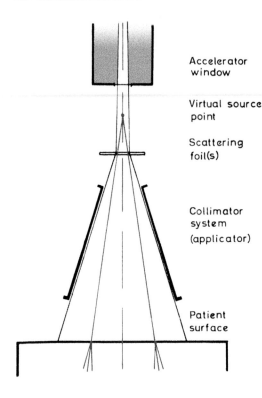

Figure 14A.7. Definition of virtual point source of an electron beam: the intersection point of the back projections along the most probable directions of motion of electrons at the patient surface. (From Schroeder-Babo P. Determination of the virtual electron source of a betatron. *Acta Radiol.* 1983;364[suppl]:7, with permission.)

- *Virtual SSD*:
  - ➤ Virtual SSD may be measured radiographically by exposing films to a broad field (e.g., 10×10 cm^2) at a number of extended distances and calculating the virtual SSD from the field magnification as a function of distance.
  - ➤ In general, the use of virtual source-to-surface distance does not give accurate inverse square law correction for output at extended SSDs under all clinical conditions. This is true especially for low energies and small field sizes.
  - ➤ Virtual source position is used primarily for modeling beam geometry in electron treatment planning algorithms.
- *Effective SSD*:
  - ➤ Effective SSD is an assumed SSD for which the inverse square holds good in predicting output at extended SSDs.
  - ➤ The effective SSD for a given energy and field size may be determined by plotting $\sqrt{I_0/I_g}$ as a function of air gap g, as shown in Figure 14A.8.

  In the graph, I_0 is the dose at depth d_0 (e.g., depth of maximum dose), I_g the dose with gap g between the standard calibration SSD (nominal) and the extended treatment SSD (nominal), and $^*f$ the effective SSD.

  - ➤ The effective SSD varies with energy and field size. A table of effective SSDs as a function of energy and field size is needed to meet various clinical situations.

X-RAY CONTAMINATION

The x-ray contamination dose at the end of the electron range can be determined from the tail of the depth-dose curve by reading off the dose value at the point where the tail becomes straight (Figure 14A.3).

- The x-ray contamination dose in a patient is contributed by bremsstrahlung interactions of electrons with the scattering foils, chambers, collimator jaws, applicator, air, and the body tissues.

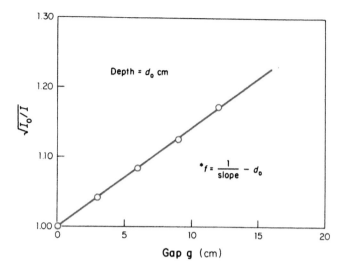

Figure 14A.8. Determination of effective source to surface distance. (From Khan FM, Sewchand W, Levitt SH. Effect of air space on depth dose in electron beam therapy. *Radiology.* 1978;126:249, with permission.)

- The biggest source of x-ray contamination is the scattering foil system.
- The x-ray contamination dose increases with increase in energy.
- In a modern linear accelerator, typical x-ray contamination dose to a patient ranges from approximately 0.5% to 1% in the energy range of 6 to 12 MeV; 1% to 2%, from 12 to 15 MeV; and 2% to 5%, from 15 to 20 MeV.
- For regular electron beam treatments, the dose contributed by the x-ray contamination is not of much concern. However, even the small amounts of x-ray contamination become critical in total skin electron therapy used for the treatment of mycosis fungoides.

LECTURE

14B

REFERENCE
Khan FM. *The Physics of Radiation Therapy*, 4th edition, 2009. Chapter 14 "Electron Beam Therapy"

Electron Beam Treatment Planning

 TOPIC OUTLINE

The following topics will be discussed in this lecture:

- Choice of energy and field size
- Corrections for surface contour and beam obliquity
- Corrections for tissue inhomogeneities
- Use of bolus
- Adjacent fields
- Field shaping
- Internal shielding
- Electron arc therapy
- Total skin electron therapy
- Treatment planning algorithms

CHOICE OF ENERGY AND FIELD SIZE

The choice of beam energy is dictated, in general, by the location and extent of the planning target volume (PTV).

- According to the ICRU Report 71 (2004), the electron energy should be selected so that the maximum of the depth curve ("peak dose") is located at (or close to) the center of PTV. This point should be selected as the *ICRU Reference Point* for target dose prescription and reporting.
- The choice of field size should be based on the adequacy of isodose coverage of the PTV.
- In the selection of energy and field size, it is important to ensure that the minimum dose to the PTV is adequate to sterilize the tumor and that the maximum dose does not exceed the tolerance of normal tissues within and around the PTV. These considerations not only depend on the total dose delivered but also on the dose-fractionation regimen used.

CORRECTIONS FOR SURFACE CONTOUR AND BEAM OBLIQUITY

An irregular or curved surface changes the depth dose distribution in a patient because of the air gaps and beam obliquity relative to the surface. Whereas the air gaps decrease the electron fluence incident on the surface, the beam obliquity affects the spatial distribution of scatter in the patient. The net result is an altered depth dose distribution.

- *Effect of beam obliquity*: The effect of beam obliquity on the central axis depth dose curve relative to a perpendicularly incident beam (0° angle of incidence) is shown in Figure 14B.1.

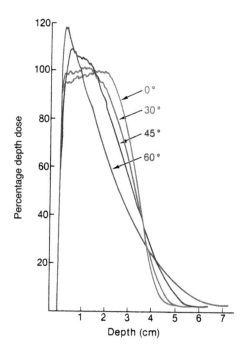

Figure 14B.1. Change in depth dose with the angle of obliquity for a 9-MeV electron beam. (From Ekstrand KE, Dixon RL. The problem of obliquely incident beams in electron beam treatment planning. *Med Phys.* 1982;9:276, with permission.)

- ➤ As seen in Figure 14B.1, beam obliquity for the same incident electron fluence (same source-to-surface distance [SSD]) gives rise to the following effects:

  - The magnitude of the maximum dose (peak dose) is increased.

  - The depth dose curve is shifted toward the surface. Consequently, the therapeutic range (e.g., d_{90}) of the beam is reduced.

  - Percent x-ray contamination is increased.

- *Effect of surface curvature*: If the beam is incident on a curved surface, the depth dose distribution along the ray lines is affected by both the increasing air gap and the increasing beam obliquity. This is seen in Figure 14B.2.

  - ➤ As seen in Figure 14B.2, the combined effect of increasing air gap and the increasing angle of obliquity results in the isodose curves becoming increasingly shallower laterally.

- *Effect of sudden change in contour*: Sharp surface irregularities produce localized hot and cold spots in the underlying medium due to changes in the spatial scatter distribution (Figure 14B.3).

  - ➤ Electrons are predominantly scattered outward by steep projections and inward by steep depressions in the contour. These can give rise to significantly large hot spots (along with the corresponding cold spot), as seen Figure 14B.3.

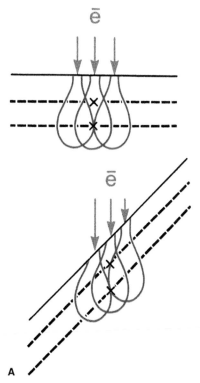

Figure 14B.2. A: A schematic illustration of how the relative orientation of pencil beams changes with the angle of obliquity. For a parallel beam, this effect would increase dose at the shallower points and decrease dose at the deeper points as the angle of obliquity is increased. (Redrawn from Ekstrand KE, Dixon RL. Obliquely incident electron beams. *Med Phys.* 1982;9:276.) (*continued*)

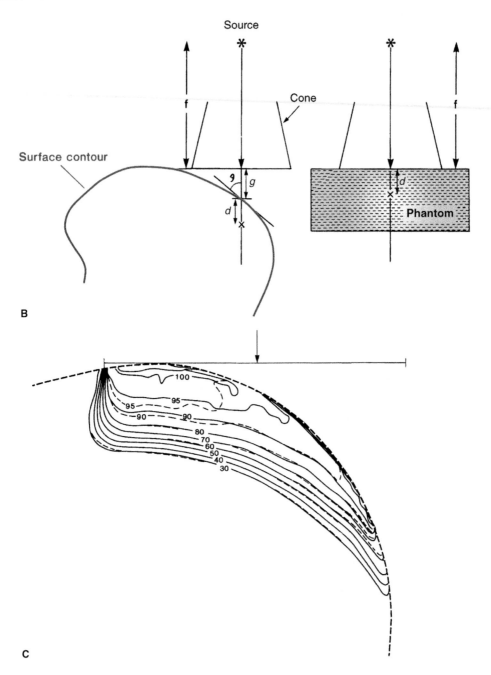

Figure 14B.2. (*Continued*) **B:** A diagrammatic representation of irradiation of a chest wall with sloping surface. The gap g and depth d for a point are measured along the fan line (the line joining the point to the effective source location). θ is the angle between the fan line and normal to the tangent to the sloping surface. The figure on the right represents the reference setup, with beam incident normal, with no air gaps between the cone end and the phantom. **C:** Comparison of measured (*solid lines*) and calculated (*dashed lines*) isodose distribution for a beam incident on a polystyrene cylindrical phantom. The measured distribution represents isodensity distribution obtained with a film sandwiched in the phantom according to the procedure outlined in 14.3B. The calculated distribution was obtained with a computer using a divergent pencil beam algorithm. Both distributions are normalized to the D_{max} in a reference setup in which the beam is incident normally on a flat phantom with no air gaps between the cone end and the phantom. 12-MeV electrons; field size 18×12 cm; effective source-to-surface distance = 70 cm.

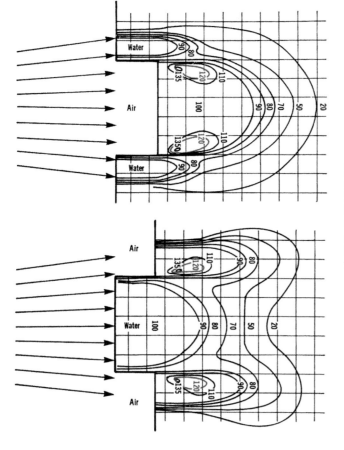

Figure 14B.3. Effect of sharp surface irregularities on electron beam isodose distributions. (From Dutreix J. Dosimetry. In: Gil G, Gayarre G, eds. *Symposium on High-energy Electrons.* Madrid: General Directorate of Health; 1970:113, with permission.)

➤ In practice, sharp contour irregularities may be smoothed out with an appropriately shaped bolus to reduce the hot spots.

➤ If a bolus is used to reduce beam penetration in a selected part of the field, its edges should be appropriately tapered to minimize the edge effect.

CORRECTIONS FOR TISSUE INHOMOGENEITIES

Electron beam depth dose distribution can be significantly altered in the presence of tissue inhomogeneities such as bone, lung, and air cavities.

• For a uniform slab of inhomogeneity that is larger than the field, the dose distribution may be corrected by using equivalent thickness based on electron density. The dose at a point is determined by calculating the effective depth, d_{eff}, along the ray line:

$$d_{eff} = d - z(1 - \rho_e)$$

where d is the actual depth from the surface, z the overlying thickness of inhomogeneity, and ρ_e the electron density (electrons/cm^3) of inhomogeneity relative to that of water.

• Approximate values of ρ_{en} for lung, soft bone (e.g., sternum), and hard bone are 0.25, 1.1, and 1.65, respectively.

• Small inhomogeneities (smaller than the field) present a more complex situation. The electron scatter from the inhomogeneity causes hot and cold spots behind the edges. The magnitude and the angle of scatter depend on the beam energy and the scattering power of the inhomogeneity. Figure 14B.4 shows an example.

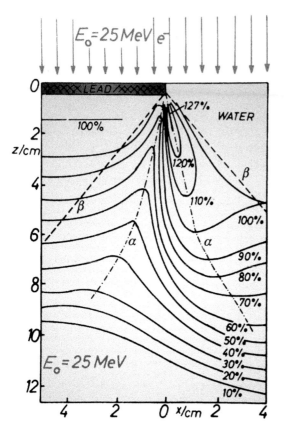

Figure 14B.4. Isodose distribution behind an edge of a thin lead slab in water. Angle α denotes the maxima of dose change and angle β of negligible change. (From Pohlit W, Manegold KH. Electron-beam dose distribution in inhomogeneous media. In: Kramer S, Suntharalingam N, Zinninger GF, eds. *High Energy Photons and Electrons.* New York: John Wiley; 1976:243, with permission.)

USE OF BOLUS

Bolus is often used in electron beam therapy to: (a) flatten out an irregular surface, (b) reduce the penetration (energy) of the electrons, and (c) build up the surface dose (buildup bolus).

- Ideally, the bolus material should be tissue equivalent in terms of stopping power and scattering power. Examples of nearly tissue-equivalent boluses: paraffin wax, polystyrene, solid water, Superstuff, and Superflab.

- If the bolus is approximately but not exactly tissue equivalent, a depth-scaling factor based on effective density may be used to correct the depth dose distribution.

- A plate of low atomic number material such as acrylic or polystyrene is sometimes used to reduce the energy of an electron beam. Such plates are known as *decelerators*.

- The bolus or a decelerator must be placed in close contact with the patient surface.

- A tissue-equivalent bolus or decelerator placed on the patient surface is considered part of the patient in determining depth dose distribution. Accordingly, the treatment SSD is set at the top surface of the bolus or decelerator.

ADJACENT FIELDS

When two adjacent electron fields are abutting on the surface, there is a danger of delivering excessively high doses in the overlap region at depth. On the other hand, separating the fields may seriously underdose superficial parts of the target volume.

- Because the tumors treated with electrons are mostly superficial, the electron fields are usually abutted on the surface and the resulting hot spots are taken into account in evaluating the treatment plan.

- Sometimes the abutting electron fields are tilted away from each other to avoid geometric overlap. The angle of tilt must be based on the uniformity of combined isodose distribution.

- The hot spots due to field abutment on the surface may or may not be acceptable, depending on their magnitude, extent, and location. Similar considerations apply to electron fields adjacent to x-ray fields.

- If an electron field is abutted at the surface with a parallel photon field (e.g., fields used in the treatment of some head and neck tumors), a hot spot develops on the side of the photon field (Figure 14B.5). This is caused by scattering of electrons from the electron field into the photon field.

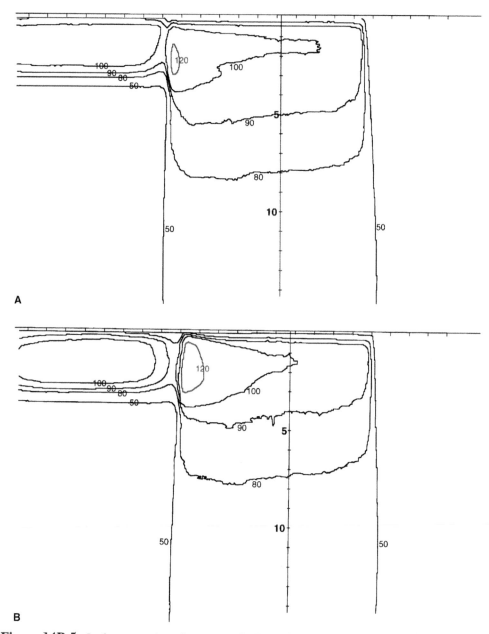

Figure 14B.5. Isodose curves in a plane perpendicular to the junction line between abutting photon and electron fields. 9-MeV electron beam; field size = 10 × 10 cm; 6-MV photon beam; SSD = 100 cm. **A:** Electron beam at standard source-to-surface distance (SSD) of 100 cm. **B:** Electron beam at extended SSD of 120 cm. (From Johnson JM, Khan FM. Dosimetric effects of abutting extended SSD electron fields with photons in the treatment of head and neck cancers. *Int J Radiat Oncol Biol Phys.* 1994;28:741–747, with permission.)

FIELD SHAPING

Lead (or Cerrobend) cutouts are often used to give shape to the treatment field and to protect the surrounding normal tissues or a critical organ. These cutouts are placed either directly on the skin surface (in the case of lead) or at the lower end of the treatment applicator (in the case of Cerrobend).

Figure 14B.6 shows a plot of minimum lead thickness required to stop electrons as a function of the most probable electron energy incident on lead.

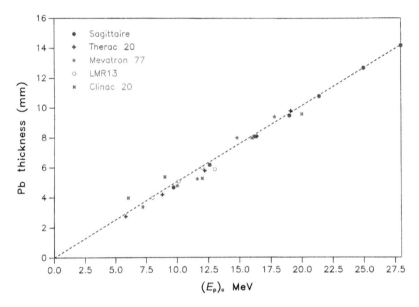

Figure 14B.6. A plot of published data for minimum lead thickness required to stop primary electrons as a function of electron energy incident on lead. (From Khan FM, Doppke K, Hogstrom KR, et al. Clinical electron-beam dosimetry. Report of AAPM Radiation Therapy Committee Task Group No. 25. *Med Phys.* 1991;18:73, with permission.)

- The data plotted in Figure 14B.6 have a slope of approximately 2 mm/MeV. That means that for blocking, the minimum thickness of lead required in mm is approximately given by the electron energy in MeV divided by 2.
- Field shaping, in general, affects output factor as well as depth dose distribution, depending on beam energy and the extent of field blocking.
- The output factor and the depth dose distribution at a point in the blocked field are not affected if the field radius drawn from the point of interest in any direction is larger than the minimum radius required for lateral scatter equilibrium.
- The minimum field radius, R_{eq}, in cm, required for lateral scatter equilibrium, is given by:

$$R_{eq} \cong 0.88\sqrt{(E_p)_0}$$

where $(E_p)_0$ is the most probable energy at the surface in MeV.

- If the blocked field radius in any direction is less than R_{eq}, the output factor and depth dose distribution would differ from those of the unblocked field. A special dosimetry is needed in that case to determine the output factor as well as the depth dose distribution.

INTERNAL SHIELDING

In some situations, such as the treatment of lip, buccal mucosa, and eyelid lesions, internal shielding is useful to protect the normal structures beyond the target volume.

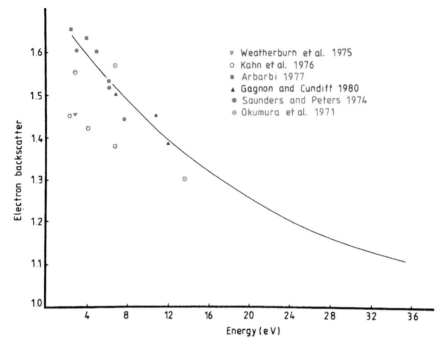

Figure 14B.7. Electron backscatter from lead as a function of mean electron energy at the interface. The solid line represents the best fit to the experimental data of Klevenhagen et al. (reprinted by permission from Benedetti GR, Dobry H, Traumann L. Computer programme for determination of isodose curves for electron energies from 5–42 MeV. *Electromedica (Siemens)*. 1971;39:5784).

- Lead shields, encased in low atomic material, may be used to reduce the transmitted dose to an acceptable value.
- The thickness of lead required (in mm) to block the electrons is approximately given by $E/2$, where E is the average energy in MeV of electrons incident on the lead shield.
- Electrons backscattered from lead increase the dose to tissues on the entrance side of the beam. This enhancement in dose at the tissue–lead interface can be quite substantial, for example, 70% to 30% in the range of 1 to 20 MeV (Figure 14B.7).
- To dissipate the effect of electron backscatter, a suitable thickness of low atomic number absorber such as bolus may be placed between the lead shield and the preceding tissue surface.
- Eyeshields are designed using the same principles to protect the lens as well as reduce the dose enhancement due to backscatter. Some commercially available eyeshields consist of tungsten shields coated with plastic and can be inserted under the eyelid like a contact lens. The thickness of tungsten should be sufficient to reduce the dose to the lens to an acceptably low value for the given treatment conditions.

ELECTRON ARC THERAPY

Electron arc technique is suitable for treating superficial tumors along curved surfaces.

- *Depth dose distribution:* Depth dose distribution in tissues treated with arc therapy is altered due to field motion.
  - ➤ The depth dose curve shifts slightly to the right, that is, the beam appears to penetrate deeper than for a stationary beam (Figure 14B.8).
  - ➤ The surface dose is reduced and the bremsstrahlung dose at the isocenter is increased.
  - ➤ The above-noted effects on dose distribution are caused by a phenomenon known as the *velocity effect:* a deeper point is exposed to the beam longer than a shallower point, resulting

in lower surface dose, apparent enhancement of beam penetration, and greater accumulation of x-ray dose at the isocenter.

- *Scanning field width:* A geometric field width of 4 to 8 cm at the isocenter is recommended for most clinical situations.

- *Location of isocenter:*

  ➤ The isocenter of beam rotation should be placed at a point approximately equidistant from the surface contour for all beam angles.

  ➤ The depth of isocenter must be greater than the maximum range of electrons so that there is no accumulation of electron dose at the isocenter.

- *Field shaping:* In electron arc therapy, additional collimation is required at the patient surface.

  ➤ Lead strips or cutouts may be placed at or close to the skin surface to define the arc as well as the field limits in the length direction (Figure 14B.9).

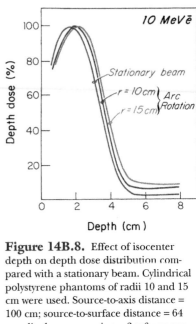

Figure 14B.8. Effect of isocenter depth on depth dose distribution compared with a stationary beam. Cylindrical polystyrene phantoms of radii 10 and 15 cm were used. Source-to-axis distance = 100 cm; source-to-surface distance = 64 cm; diaphragm opening = 3 × 6 cm; arc angle = 120°. (From Khan FM, Fullerton GD, Lee JM, et al. Physical aspects of electron-beam arc therapy. *Radiology.* 1977;124:497, with permission.)

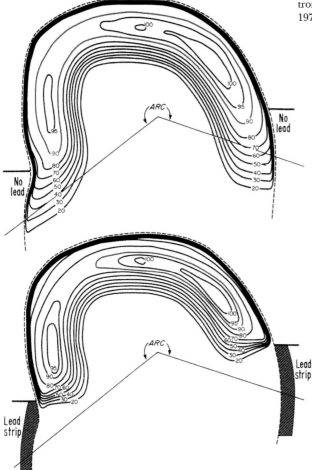

Figure 14B.9. Isodose distribution in arc rotation with and without lead strips at the ends of the arc, using a section of an Alderson Rando phantom closely simulating an actual patient cross section. Arc angle = 236°; average radius of curvature = 10 cm; beam energy = 10 MeV; lead strip thickness = 6 mm; field size at the surface = 4.2 × 8.5 cm. (From Khan FM, Fullerton GD, Lee JM, et al. Physical aspects of electron-beam arc therapy. *Radiology.* 1977;124:497, with permission.)

➤ Custom shielding (Cerrobend casts or lead cutouts molded on to the surface) may be used to define the treatment field and sharpen dose distribution at the field edges.

TOTAL SKIN ELECTRON THERAPY

Electrons in the energy range of 6 to 9 MeV may be used for treating superficial lesions covering large areas of the body, such as mycosis fungoides and other cutaneous lymphomas. Treatment techniques are designed to treat superficial skin lesions down to approximately 1 cm depth and without exceeding bone marrow tolerance. Several techniques have been devised to meet these goals:

a) *Translational technique*, in which a horizontal patient on a stretcher is translated relative to a vertical beam of electrons of sufficient width to cover the transverse dimensions of the patient;

b) *Large field technique*, in which a standing patient is treated at a large SSD with a combination of broad beams directed from different patient orientations;

c) *Rotational technique*, in which the patient, standing on a rotating platform, is treated with a large field at a large SSD.

• *Modified Stanford technique*: This technique is a version of the large field technique in which a standing patient is treated with six dual fields at a large SSD (~4 m). Each dual field (one up and one down) is directed at six patient orientations (anterior, posterior, and four obliques). An acrylic scatter plate ($\simeq$ 1 cm in thickness for a 9-MeV electron beam) may be placed in front of the patient to provide additional scatter to the electron beam. The treatment setup is illustrated in Figure 14B.10.

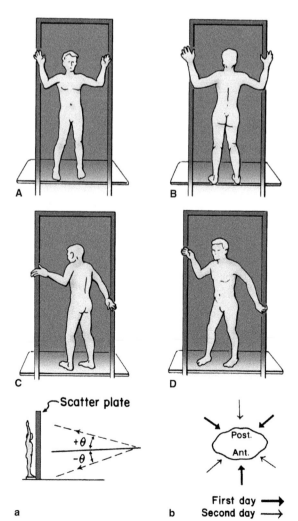

Figure 14B.10. Patient positions for the six-field Stanford technique. Patient is treated by two beams at each position, one beam directed 15° below horizontal and the other 15° above horizontal. (From Page V, Gardner A, Karzmark CJ. Patient dosimetry in the treatment of large superficial lesions. *Radiology.* 1970;94:635, with permission.)

➤ The objective of dual fields (one directed toward the head and the other toward the feet) is to avoid direct beam incidence on the bone marrow–bearing regions of the body (spine, ribs, and pelvis).

➤ The dual-field technique allows middle sections of the body to be treated with electrons scattered by air out of the main beam. Because the x-ray contamination is mostly forward directed along the beam central axes, the x-ray dose to the mid-section (outside the geometric field) is minimal.

➤ The angle of the dual fields relative to the horizontal direction is determined dosimetrically so that along the height of the patient, the composite dose profile is uniform within ±10% over a length of approximately 200 cm (Figure 14B.11).

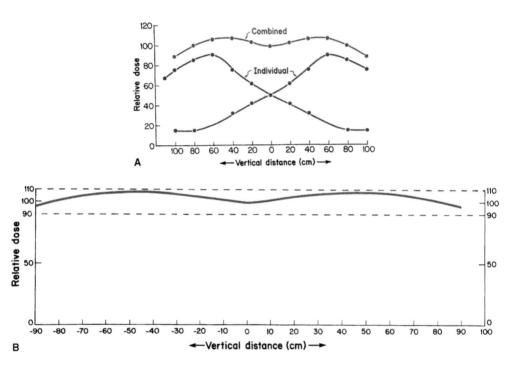

Figure 14B.11. Combining individual beam profiles to obtain a composite profile with ±10% dose variation in the vertical direction. **A:** Data for 9 MeV; source-to-surface distance = 410 cm; scatter plate-to-phantom distance = 20 cm; individual profile beam angle = 12° relative to horizontal axis. A dual field angle $\theta = \pm 11°$ is obtained by combining the profiles as shown. **B:** Confirmatory beam profile for the dual field using $\theta \pm 11°$. (From Khan FM. Total skin electron therapy: technique and dosimetry. In: Purdy JA, ed. *Advances in Radiation Oncology Physics.* AAPM Monograph No. 19. New York: American Institute of Physics; 1990:466, with permission.)

➤ The dose uniformity in the transverse direction should be within ±10% (Figure 14B.12).

➤ The composite depth dose distribution for the six dual-field techniques may be determined by film dosimetry in a cylindrical polystyrene phantom placed at the treatment SSD. Figure 14B.13 gives the results of such a measurement.

TREATMENT PLANNING ALGORITHMS

Pencil beam algorithms based on multiple scattering theories are most commonly used for electron beam treatment planning. These theories assume small-angle multiple scattering approximation in which an elementary pencil beam penetrating a scattering medium is very nearly Gaussian in its lateral spread at all depths.

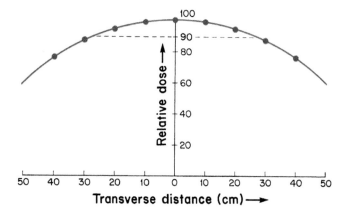

Figure 14B.12. Transverse dose profile showing width of the profile within ±90% dose relative to central axis. (From Khan FM. Total skin electron therapy: technique and dosimetry. In: Purdy JA, ed. *Advances in Radiation Oncology Physics.* AAPM Monograph No. 19. New York: American Institute of Physics; 1990:466, with permission.)

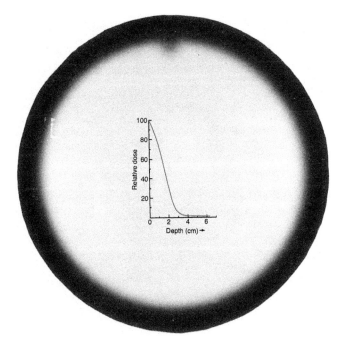

Figure 14B.13. Composite depth dose distribution for six dual fields obtained with a dosimetry film sandwiched in a cylindrical polystyrene phantom exposed under treatment conditions. Irradiation conditions are given in Figure 14.46. (From Khan FM. Total skin electron therapy: technique and dosimetry. In: Purdy JA, ed. *Advances in Radiation Oncology Physics.* AAPM Monograph No. 19. New York: American Institute of Physics; 1990:466.)

- The dose distribution in a pencil electron beam incident on a uniform phantom looks like a teardrop or onion (Figure 14B.14).

- The pencil beam is characterized by two components: a) Its central axis depth dose distribution; and b) its lateral distribution.

- The central axis depth dose for the pencil beam is represented by a mathematical function that is normalized to the depth dose distribution for a broad field.

- The lateral spread is represented by σ, the root mean square radial displacement of electrons as a result of multiple Coulomb scattering.

- Eyges (1948) predicted σ theoretically by extending the small-angle multiple scattering theory of Fermi to slab geometry of any composition. Considering $\sigma_x(z)$ in the x–z plane,

$$\sigma_x^2(z) = \frac{1}{2} \int \left(\frac{\theta^2}{\rho l}(z') \right) \rho(z')\,(z - z')^2\,dz'$$

where $\theta^2/\rho l$ is the mass angular scattering power and ρ is the density of the slab phantom.

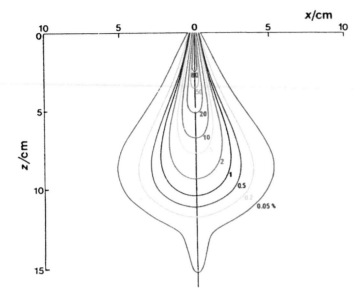

Figure 14B.14. Pencil beam dose distribution measured with a narrow beam of 22 MeV energy incident on a water phantom. (From International Commission on Radiation Units and Measurements. *Radiation Dosimetry: Electron Beams with Energies between 1 and 50 MeV.* Report 35. Bethesda, MD: International Commission on Radiation Units and Measurements; 1984:36, with permission.)

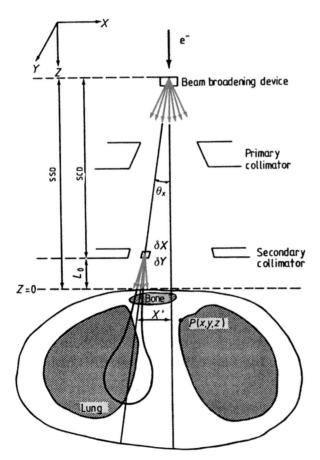

Figure 14B.15. Schematic representation of the Hogstrom algorithm for electron beam treatment planning. (From Hogstrom KR, Mills MD, Almond PR. Electron beam dose calculation. *Phys Med Biol.* 1981;26:445, with permission.)

- The spread parameter σ increases with depth until a maximum spread is achieved. Beyond this depth there is a precipitous loss of electrons as their larger lateral excursion causes them to run out of energy.

- The total dose distribution in a field of any size and shape can be calculated by summing dose contributions to a point by all the pencil beams. Mathematically,

$$D_{(x,y,z)} = \iint d_{\mathrm{p}}(x - x', y - y', z)\, dx'\, dy'$$

where $d_{\mathrm{p}}(x, y, z)$ is the dose contributed to point (x, y, z) by a pencil beam whose central axis passes through (x', y', z).

- Practical implementation of the above algorithm was carried out by Hogstrom et al. (1981) and was subsequently adopted by several commercial treatment-planning systems. Figure 14B.15 shows a schematic representation.

- The pencil beam σ in the Hogstrom algorithm is calculated by the Fermi-Eyges equation. By correlating electron linear collision stopping power and linear angular scattering power relative to that of water with CT numbers, effective depth and σ are calculated for inhomogeneous media. Thus, the method allows pixel-by-pixel calculation of heterogeneity correction.

REVIEW QUESTIONS • Chapter 14

In multiple choice questions, more than one option may be correct.

1. Absorbed dose to tissue from clinical electron beams is predominantly due to which type of interaction?

   a) Inelastic collisions with nuclei
   b) Inelastic collisions with electrons
   c) Elastic collisions with nuclei
   d) Elastic collisions with electrons

2. Electrons in the clinical range of energies lose energy in water approximately at the rate of:

   a) 0.5 MeV/cm
   b) 1.0 MeV/cm
   c) 2.0 MeV/cm
   d) 3.0 MeV/cm

3. The energy of clinical electron beams is specified as the:

   a) Maximum energy at the surface
   b) Minimum energy at the surface
   c) The most probable energy at the surface
   d) The half-value layer in water

4. The practical range (R_p) of a broad electron beam in water is 6 cm. Its most probable energy in MeV at the surface is approximately:

   a) 6
   b) 9
   c) 12
   d) 15

5. The depth of 50% dose (R_{50}) for a broad beam of electrons is 3.8 cm. Its average energy in MeV at the surface is approximately:

   a) 6
   b) 9
   c) 12
   d) 15

6. Which of the following detectors require corrections in measuring percentage depth dose in electron beams?

   a) Ion chamber
   b) Film
   c) Unshielded diode
   d) TLD chips
   e) All of the above

7. For a lateral electron neck field, the minimum depth to the spinal cord is 5 cm. What is the maximum electron energy in the list below whose practical range is less than the cord depth?

   a) 6
   b) 9
   c) 12
   d) 16

8. The higher the energy of an electron beam:

   a) The greater is the percentage surface dose
   b) The greater is the bremsstrahlung dose to the patient
   c) The sharper is the dose fall-off beyond the 90% depth dose
   d) Greater is the electron backscatter from lead

9. The minimum thickness of lead required to block a 15 MeV electron beam is approximately:
   a) 2 mm
   b) 5 mm
   c) 8 mm
   d) 11 mm

10. Virtual SSD for electron beams:
    a) Corresponds to the target-to-surface distance
    b) Corresponds to the scattering foil-to-surface distance
    c) Gives an accurate fit to inverse square law for beam intensity as a function of distance for all energies and field sizes
    d) Relates to beam divergence

11. An electron beam incident obliquely with respect to the surface (for the same SSD) tends to:
    a) Increase the magnitude of peak dose
    b) Decrease the depth of peak dose
    c) Decrease the depth of 90% dose
    d) Increase the percentage surface dose

12. If an electron field abuts a parallel photon field at the surface:
    a) A hot spot is expected in the photon field
    b) A hot spot is expected in the electron field
    c) A hot spot is expected in both the fields
    d) A cold spot is expected in both the fields

13. According to the ICRU Report 71:
    a) The target dose should be prescribed at the 80% dose level
    b) The peak dose should occur somewhere in the middle of PTV
    c) The beam energy should be selected so that the deepest part of the tumor receives 80% depth dose
    d) The ICRU reference point for dose reporting should be at the isodose surface that just covers the PTV

14. In electron arc therapy:
    a) The depth dose curve is shifted deeper than for the stationary beam
    b) The surface dose is higher than for the stationary beam
    c) The x-ray dose at the isocenter is higher than in the stationary beam
    d) The depth dose curve remains the same as for the stationary beam

BRACHYTHERAPY

Low-Dose-Rate Brachytherapy: Rules of Implantation and Dose Specification

 TOPIC OUTLINE

The following topics will be discussed in this lecture:

➤ Brachytherapy sources
➤ Calibration of brachytherapy sources
➤ Calculation of dose distribution
➤ Rules of implantation
➤ Dose specification and recording

BRACHYTHERAPY SOURCES

In the early days, brachytherapy was carried out mostly with radium (needles and tubes) or radon (seeds). Currently, only the artificially produced radioisotopes are used. These include: ^{137}Cs, ^{192}Ir, ^{198}Au, ^{125}I, and ^{103}Pd.

- *Cesium-137*: ^{137}Cs tubes are used mostly for low-dose-rate (LDR) intracavitary brachytherapy such as in the treatment of uterine cervix.

  ➤ Average γ-ray energy ~0.66 MeV

  ➤ Half-life ~30 years

  ➤ HVL ~5.5 mm lead

- *Iridium-192*: ^{192}Ir sources are fabricated in several different forms, depending on their use. The most commonly used forms:

  ➤ ^{192}Ir seeds contained in nylon ribbons for interstitial implantation;

  ➤ High-intensity iridium source, welded at the end of a flexible cable, for high-dose-rate (HDR) brachytherapy.

    • Average photon energy of 0.4 MeV

    • Half-life ~74 days

    • HVL ~2.5 mm lead

- *Gold-198*: [198]Au seeds have been used mostly in eye plaques for treating intraocular tumors such as choroidal melanoma. Currently ^{125}I seeds are most commonly used for eye plaques.
  - ➤ Average γ-ray energy ~0.4 MeV
  - ➤ Half-life ~2.7 days
  - ➤ HVL ~2.5 mm lead
- *Iodine-125*: [125]I seeds are used for permanent implants such as in the treatment of early-stage prostate cancer.
  - ➤ Average photon energy ~28 keV
  - ➤ Half-life ~59 days
  - ➤ HVL ~0.025 mm lead
- *Palladium-103*: [103]Pd seeds have the same clinical application as that of ^{125}I seeds.
  - ➤ Average photon energy ~21 keV
  - ➤ Half-life ~17 days
  - ➤ HVL ~0.01 mm lead

CALIBRATION OF BRACHYTHERAPY SOURCES

- *Specification of source strength*: The American Association of Physicists in Medicine (AAPM) recommends the quantity *air kerma strength* for the specification of brachytherapy sources.
  - ➤ The air kerma strength is defined as the air kerma rate (μGy/h) at a specified distance (usually 1 m) from the source center along the perpendicular bisector.
  - ➤ The units for air kerma strength are $\mu Gym^2\ h^{-1}$.
  - ➤ The air kerma strength is related to exposure rate by the following equation:

$$S_k = \dot{X}_l \left(\frac{\overline{W}}{e} \right) l^2$$

  Where S_k is the air kerma strength at a specified distance l, $\dot{X}_l$ the exposure rate at l, and $\dfrac{\overline{W}}{e}$ the average energy absorbed per unit charge of ionization in air.

  - ➤ The air kerma strength is determined from exposure rate that may be measured by using an ion chamber, for example, a large-volume ion chamber in open-air geometry, a "reentrant"-type well chamber or a dose calibrator supplied with a suitable standard source.
  - ➤ Calibration of brachytherapy sources should be directly traceable to the National Institute of Standards and Technology (NIST) or an Accredited Dosimetry Calibration Laboratory (ADCL).
  - ➤ Traceability means that the sources should be calibrated by direct comparison with a NIST- or ADCL-calibrated source of the same kind, that is, the same radionuclide with the same encapsulation, size, and shape.
  - ➤ If a well-type ionization chamber is used, it should bear a calibration factor determined with a NIST- or ADCL-calibrated source of the same kind.

CALCULATION OF DOSE DISTRIBUTION

Traditionally, the dose distribution around a brachytherapy source has been calculated using the Sievert integral. The method consists of dividing the line source into small elementary sources and applying inverse square law and filtration corrections to each. Since the introduction of sources of complex design such as ^{125}I and [103]Pd, the Sievert integral method has given way to Monte Carlo calculations and/or direct measurements to determine the dose distributions. To translate these results into treatment planning systems, a more modular approach is used (AAPM TG-43) in which the effects of several physical factors on dose rate distribution are considered separately.

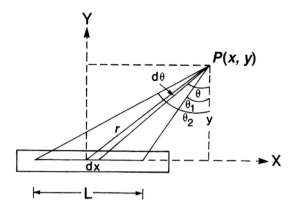

Figure 15.1. Diagram illustrating geometric relationships used in calculation of exposure at point *P*, from a linear source.

- *TG-43 formalism*: This calculation model involves the following functions:

  Referring to Figure 15.1,

  ➤ *Dose rate constant* for the source, Λ, defined as the dose rate per unit air kerma strength at 1 cm along the transverse axis of the source.

  ➤ Air kerma strength, S_K, at 1 cm

  ➤ *Geometry factor*, $G(r, \theta)$, that accounts for the geometric falloff of the photon fluence with distance from the source and depends on the distribution of radioactive material.

  ➤ *Radial dose function*, $g(r)$, that accounts for radial dependence of photon absorption and scatter in the medium along the transverse axis

  ➤ *Anisotropy factor*, $F(r, \theta)$, that accounts for the angular dependence of photon absorption and scatter in the encapsulation and the medium.

    - The dose rate, $\dot{D}(r, \theta)$, at point *P* with polar coordinates (r, θ) in a medium (e.g., water) from the center of a source of air kerma strength S_K can be expressed as:

$$\dot{D}(r,\theta) = \Lambda S_K \frac{G(r,\theta)}{G(1, \pi/2)} F(r,\theta)\, g(r)$$

    - The dose rate constant, Λ, depends on the type of source, its construction, and its encapsulation.

    - For a point source, $G(r, \theta) = 1/r^2$ (inverse square law) and $F(r, \theta)$ is replaced by a distance-dependent anisotropy function, $\phi_{an}(r)$.

RULES OF IMPLANTATION AND DOSE SPECIFICATION (INTERSTITIAL)

- *General principles*: The sources of predetermined strength are implanted in a predetermined geometric pattern to achieve the following goals:

  a) Desired dose distribution:

    - Adequate dose coverage of clinical target volume (CTV)

    - Minimum dose to normal tissues and organs at risk

  b) Desired dose rate:

    - High therapeutic ratio*

- *Dose distribution (uniform or nonuniform?)*:

  In brachytherapy, the importance of dose uniformity is debatable. EXAMPLE:

  ➤ Paterson-Parker (P-P) system specifies uniform distribution of source activity to attain "uniform dose" (within ±10% in the specified plane of treatment).

---

*Therapeutic ratio = [damage to tumor cells]/[damage to normal calls] for the same dose.

➤ Quimby, Paris, and computer* systems specify uniform source activity that inevitably results in nonuniform dose in the specified plane (higher dose in the center than in the periphery).

- *Source spacing*:
  - ➤ Linear source activity variable in P-P but constant in other implant systems
  - ➤ Constant source spacing for a given implant
  - ➤ Sources to be implanted 1 cm apart for small size implants
  - ➤ Larger spacing (up to 1.5 cm) recommended for larger size implants in the Paris and computer systems
  - ➤ Crossing needles recommended, if possible, in the P-P and Quimby systems
  - ➤ Longer sources used instead in the Paris and computer systems to provide adequate dose coverage of the CTV

- *Dose specification*: "Stated" or prescribed dose should be:
  - ➤ In accordance with the implant system rules, to the exclusion of the others
  - ➤ Based on published clinical data for best outcome

EXAMPLES:

- *Paterson-Parker*:
  - ➤ *Planar implants*: Stated dose to be 10% higher than the minimum dose in a parallel plane 0.5 cm away;
  - ➤ *Volume implants*: Stated dose to be 10% higher than the minimum dose within the implanted volume.

- *Quimby*:
  - ➤ *Planar implants*: Stated dose to be the maximum dose in the plane of treatment (e.g., 0.5 cm away);
  - ➤ *Volume implant*: Stated dose to be the minimum dose within the implanted volume.

- *Paris*:
  - ➤ Stated dose to be the value of the reference isodose surface or 85% of the basal dose (Figure 15.2).

- *Computer*:
  - ➤ Stated dose to be the value of the isodose surface that just covers the implant boundary (which should correspond to the CTV boundary) (Figure 15.3).

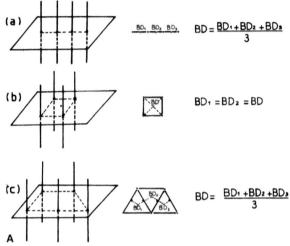

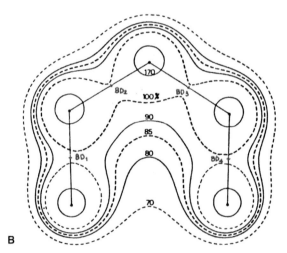

Figure 15.2. Determination of basal dose (BD) in implants using the Paris system. **A:** Line sources implanted in patterns of (a) single plane, (b) squares, and (c) triangles. **B:** Isodose curves in central plane of a volume implant using the Paris system. The isodose values are normalized to the average basal dose, which is given by $1/4(BD_1 + BD_2 + BD_3 + BD_4)$. (From Dutreix A, Marinello G. In: Pierquin B, Wilson JF, Chassagne D, eds. *Modern Brachytherapy*. New York: Masson; 1987, with permission).

*Computer system is modified Paris system, used at the University of Minnesota.

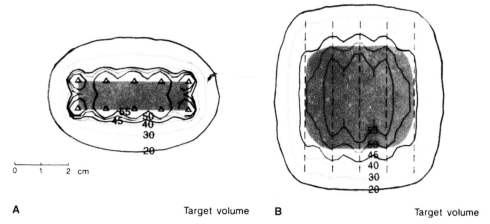

A   Target volume   **B**   Target volume

Figure 15.3. Isodose curves for a volume implant using two parallel planes containing five ^{192}Ir line sources per plane. **A:** Central cross-sectional plane. **B:** Longitudinal plane through middle of implant. Prescription dose is specified on the 45-cGy/h isodose curve, which just encloses the implant in the central cross-sectional plane. (From Khan FM. Brachytherapy: rules of implantation and dose specification. In: Levitt SH, Khan FM, Potish RA, eds. *Technological Basis of Radiation Therapy.* Philadelphia, PA: Lea & Febiger; 1992:113, with permission).

- *Comparative summary*: Rules of implantation and dose specification for various interstitial implant systems are summarized in Table 15.1.

RULES OF IMPLANTATION AND DOSE SPECIFICATION (INTRACAVITARY)

- *Source loading*:
  - ➤ *Uterine cervix*: ^{137}Cs tubes of specific strengths are loaded into specific applicators (e.g., Fletcher-Suit) (Figure 15.4).
  - ➤ *Uterine corpus*: sources of specific strength loaded into Heyman capsules.

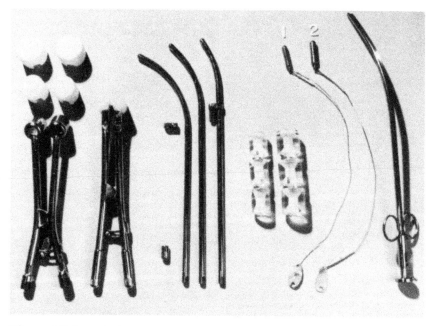

Figure 15.4. A Fletcher-Suite applicator set. (From Fletcher GH. *Textbook of Radiotherapy.* 2nd ed. Philadelphia, PA: Lea & Febiger; 1973:620, with permission).

TABLE 15.1	Rules of Interstitial Implant Systems			
Characteristic	*Paterson-Parker*	*Quimby*	*Paris*	*Computer[a]*
Linear strength	Variable (full intensity, 0.66 mg-Ra/cm; half-intensity, 0.33 mg-Ra/cm)	Constant (full intensity, 1 mg-Ra/cm; half-intensity, 0.5 mg-Ra/cm)	Constant (0.6–1.8 mg-Ra eq/cm)	Constant (0.2–0.4 mg-Ra eq/cm)
Source distribution	Planar implants: Area <25 cm², 2/3 Ra in periphery; area 25–100 cm², 1/2 Ra in periphery. Area >100 cm², 1/3 Ra in periphery	Uniform	Uniform	Uniform
	Volume implants Cylinder: belt, four parts; core, two parts; each end, one part Sphere: shell, six parts; core, two parts Cube: each side, one part; core, two parts	Uniform distribution of sources throughout the volume	Line sources arranged in parallel planes	Line sources arranged in parallel planes or cylindrical volumes
Line source spacing	Constant approximately 1 cm apart from each other or from crossing ends	Same as Paterson-Parker	Constant, but selected according to implant dimensions— larger spacing used in large volumes; 8-mm minimum to 15-mm maximum separation	Constant, 1–1.5 cm, depending on size of implant (larger spacing for larger-size implants)
Crossing needles	Crossing needles required to enhance dose at implant ends	Same as Paterson-Parker	Crossing needles not used; active length 30%–40% longer than target length	Crossing needles not required; active length of sources 30%–40% longer than target length

[a]The computer system used at the University of Minnesota Hospital.
From Khan FM. Brachytherapy: rules of implantation and dose specification. In: Levitt SH, Khan FM, Potish RA, eds. *Technological Basis of Radiation Therapy*. Philadelphia, PA: Lea & Febiger; 1992:113, with permission.

- *Dose specification (ca. cervix, using tandem, and ovoids)*:
  - ➤ *The Manchester system*: The dose prescription and implant duration are based on evaluating dose rates at:
    - Point A
    - Point B
    - Bladder point
    - Rectum point

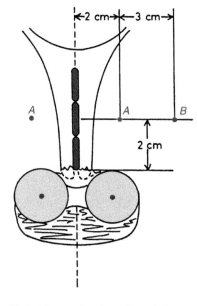

Figure 15.5. Original definition of points *A* and *B*, according to the Manchester system. (From Meredith WJ. *Radium Dosage: The Manchester System*. Edinburgh: Livingstone; 1967, with permission).

- Definitions of points A and B, according to the Manchester system, are illustrated in Figure 15.5.

- The total dose is prescribed at point A.

- The maximum dose to bladder and rectum should be, as far as possible, less than the dose to point A (e.g., 80% or less of the dose to point A).

➤ *Limitations of point A:*

a) It relates to the position of the sources and not to a specific anatomic structure;

b) Dose to point A is very sensitive to the position of the ovoid sources relative to the tandem sources, which should not be the determining factor in deciding on implant duration;

c) Depending on the size of the cervix, point A may lie inside or outside the tumor. Thus, the dose prescription at point A could risk underdosage of large cervical cancers or overdosage of small ones (Figure 15.6).

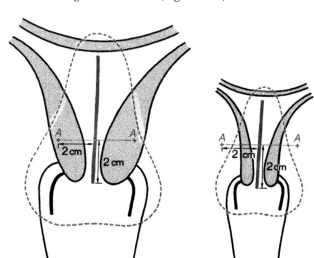

Figure 15.6. Variation of point *A* relative to anatomy. **A:** Point *A* inside large cervix, resulting in underdosage. **B:** Point *A* outside small cervix, resulting in overdosage. (From Pierquin B, Wilson JF, Chassagne D, eds. *Modern Brachytherapy*. New York: Masson; 1987, with permission).

A **B**

➤ *The ICRU system:*

The dose is prescribed as the value of an isodose surface that just surrounds the target volume. Figure 15.7 illustrates the concept of target volume.

A. ONLY INTRACAVITARY TREATMENT

B. COMBINED INTRACAVITARY AND EXTERNAL BEAM THERAPY

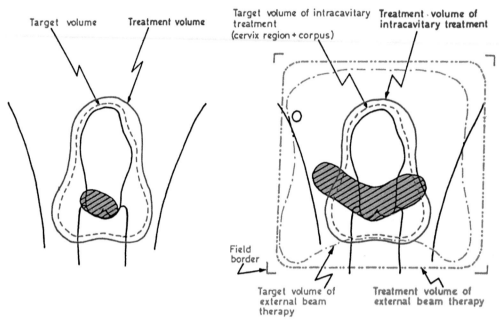

Figure 15.7. Definition of target and treatment volumes for brachytherapy and external beam treatment. (From International Commission on Radiation Units and Measurements [ICRU]. *Dose and Volume Specification for Reporting Intracavitary Therapy in Gynecology.* ICRU Report No. 38. Bethesda, MD: International Commission on Radiation Units and Measurements; 1985, with permission).

- Table 15.2 summarizes the ICRU system of dose specification, which includes recording of various treatment parameters:

  - *Description of the technique.* Minimum information should include the applicator type, source type and loading, and orthogonal radiographs of the application.

  - *Total reference air kerma.* By this parameter is meant the total air kerma strength of sources times the implant duration.

TABLE 15.2	Data Needed for Reporting Intracavitary Therapy in Gynecology

Description of the technique
Total reference air kerma
Description of the reference volume
    Dose level if not 60 Gy
    Dimensions of reference volume (height, width, thickness)
Absorbed dose at reference points
    Bladder reference point
    Rectal reference point
    Lymphatic trapezoid
    Pelvic wall reference point
Time–dose pattern

From International Commission on Radiation Units and Measurements (ICRU). *Dose and Volume Specification for Reporting Intracavitary Therapy in Gynecology.* ICRU Report No. 38. Bethesda, MD: International Commission on Radiation Units and Measurements; 1985.

- *Reference volume.* The reference volume is the volume of the isodose surface that just surrounds the target volume. The reference volume is approximated by $(d_h \times d_w \times d_t)$ cm^3, as seen in Figure 15.8.

Plane a

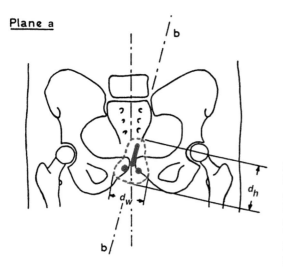

Plane b

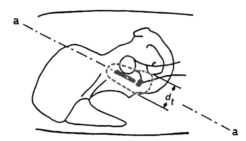

Figure 15.8. Determination of the reference isodose surface dimensions. d_w, width; d_h, height; d_t, thickness. (From International Commission on Radiation Units and Measurements [ICRU]. *Dose and Volume Specification for Reporting Intracavitary Therapy in Gynecology.* ICRU Report No. 38. Bethesda, MD: International Commission on Radiation Units and Measurements; 1985, with permission).

- *Prescription dose.* The prescription isodose value of 60 Gy includes the dose contribution from the external beam.
- *Bladder point.* The bladder point is localized by using a Foley catheter, with the balloon filled with a contrast material (Figure 15.9).

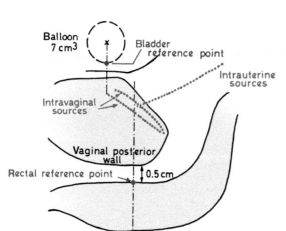

Figure 15.9. Localization of bladder and rectum points. (From International Commission on Radiation Units and Measurements [ICRU]. *Dose and Volume Specification for Reporting Intracavitary Therapy in Gynecology.* ICRU Report No. 38. Bethesda, MD: International Commission on Radiation Units and Measurements; 1985, with permission).

- *Rectal point.* On the lateral radiograph, the rectal point is located on a line drawn from the middle of the ovoid sources, 5 mm behind the posterior vaginal wall (Figure 15.9).

- *Lymphatic trapezoid of Fletcher.* These points correspond to the para-aortic and iliac nodes and are shown in Figure 15.10.

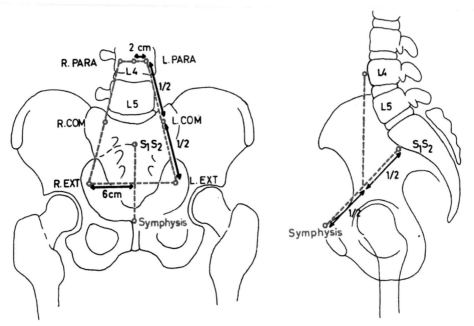

Figure 15.10. Determination of reference points corresponding to the lymphatic trapezoid of Fletcher. (From International Commission on Radiation Units and Measurements [ICRU]. *Dose and Volume Specification for Reporting Intracavitary Therapy in Gynecology.* ICRU Report No. 38. Bethesda, MD: International Commission on Radiation Units and Measurements; 1985, with permission).

- *Pelvic wall points.* These points are identified from the A/P and lateral radiographs, as shown in Figure 15.11.

- *Time dose pattern.* The duration and time sequence of the implant relative to the external beam treatment should be recorded.

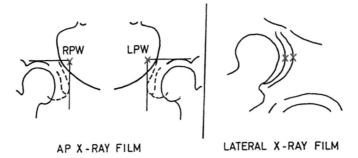

AP X-RAY FILM   LATERAL X-RAY FILM

Figure 15.11. Definition of pelvic wall points, LPW (left pelvic wall) and RPW (right pelvic wall). **Left:** Anteroposterior (AP) view. **Right:** Lateral view. (From International Commission on Radiation Units and Measurements [ICRU]. *Dose and Volume Specification for Reporting Intracavitary Therapy in Gynecology.* ICRU Report No. 38. Bethesda, MD: International Commission on Radiation Units and Measurements; 1985, with permission).

REVIEW QUESTIONS • Chapter 15

In multiple choice questions, more than one option may be correct.

1. A ^{137}Cs source is replaced in a remote LDR afterloader system after 10 years of service. If the initial source strength of both the old and the new sources is 60 mCi, what is the percentage reduction in treatment time that would occur for the same implant after the replacement?

    a) 0 (no change in treatment time)
    b) 5
    c) 12
    d) 21
    e) 26

2. Which of the following brachytherapy radioisotopes has the greatest HVL?

    a) ^{60}Co (average energy 1.25 MeV)
    b) ^{226}Ra (average energy 0.83 MeV)
    c) ^{137}Cs (average energy 0.66 MeV)
    d) ^{198}Au (average energy 0.41 MeV)
    e) ^{125}I (average energy 0.028 MeV)

3. Which of the following is/are a traceable calibration(s)?

    a) Calibration of a source using an ADCL-calibrated well chamber
    b) Calibration of a source at NIST or an ADCL
    c) Intercomparison of a source with a NIST- or ADCL-calibrated source of the same kind
    d) Intercomparison with a ^{137}Cs source

4. Which of the following most significantly effects brachytherapy dose distributions?

    a) Inverse square law
    b) Absorption within tissue
    c) Scatter within tissue
    d) Tissue heterogeneities
    e) Use of point or line source model

5. Which of the following sources exhibit dose reductions of ~1% per centimeter from attenuation and scatter within the first few cm?

    a) ^{137}Cs
    b) ^{125}I
    c) ^{198}Au
    d) ^{192}Ir
    e) All of the above

6. What is the initial dose rate of a permanent ^{125}I prostate seed implant designed to deliver a prescription dose of 144 Gy?

    a) 0.07 cGy/hr
    b) 0.5 cGy/hr
    c) 7 cGy/hr
    d) 50 cGy/hr
    e) 5 Gy/hr

7. Isodose curves around a linear brachytherapy source show dips near the ends because:

    a) The linear activity of the source is less near the ends.
    b) Radiation suffers greater attenuation due to oblique filtration.
    c) β-Particles are mixed with γ-rays.
    d) Measurement close to the source ends cause artifacts.

8. The Paterson-Parker system of interstitial implants is designed to:
   a) Give uniform distribution of source activity within the implanted area.
   b) Give dose uniformity of ±10% to the target area in the plane of implant.
   c) Give dose uniformity of ±10% to the target area in parallel planes at 0.5 cm from the implanted plane.
   d) Higher dose at the center and less dose to the periphery of implant.

9. The Quimby system of interstitial implants is designed to:
   a) Give uniform distribution of source activity within the implanted area.
   b) Give dose uniformity of ±10% to the target area in the plane of implant.
   c) Give dose uniformity of ±10% to the target area in parallel planes at 0.5 cm from the implanted plane.
   d) Give dose uniformity equivalent to that of Paterson-Parker but with equal intensity sources.

10. In the Paris system of interstitial implants:
    a) Crossing needles are required to adequately cover the target area.
    b) Spacing between ^{192}Ir wires or ribbons should not exceed 1 cm.
    c) There is higher dose at the center and less dose at the periphery of implant.
    d) Dose is specified by the 85% value of the basal dose.

11. The ICRU system of dose specification for GYN intracavitary implants:
    a) Specifies dose prescription at point A
    b) Requires the recording of dose at point B
    c) Requires the recording of doses at the bladder and rectal points
    d) Requires the recording of doses at points on the Trapezoid of Fletcher

16

RADIATION PROTECTION

REFERENCE

Khan FM. *The Physics of Radiation Therapy*, 4th edition, 2009. Chapter 16 "Radiation Protection"

Radiation Protection and Shielding Design

 TOPIC OUTLINE

The following topics will be discussed in this lecture:

➤ Dose equivalent
➤ Effective dose equivalent
➤ Background radiation
➤ Low-level radiation effects
➤ Effective dose-equivalent limits
➤ Shielding design for radiation installations
➤ Protection against brachytherapy sources
➤ Radiation protection surveys
➤ Radiation monitoring instruments
➤ Personnel monitoring
➤ NRC regulations

DOSE EQUIVALENT

The dosimetric quantity relevant to radiation protection is the dose equivalent (H). It is defined as:

$$H = D \cdot Q$$

where D is the absorbed dose and Q the quality factor for the radiation.

- The Q-factor in radiation protection is a conservative value based on a range of relative biological effectiveness related to linear energy transfer (LET) of the radiation. EXAMPLE: The recommended Q-factors are:

  ➤ X-rays, γ-rays, electrons   1
  ➤ Thermal neutrons   5
  ➤ Fast neutrons, heavy particles   20

- The SI unit for dose equivalent is sievert (Sv).

$$1\,\text{Sv} = 1\,\text{J/kg}$$

The older unit of dose equivalent is rem.

$$1\,\text{rem} = 10^{-2}\,\text{Sv}$$

EFFECTIVE DOSE EQUIVALENT

The effective dose equivalent (H_E) is defined as "the sum of the weighted dose equivalents for irradiated tissues or organs". Mathematically:

$$H_E = \sum W_T H_T$$

where W_T is the weighting factor of tissue T and H_T is the mean dose equivalent received by tissue T.

- The weighting factor represents the proportionate stochastic risk (e.g., cancer induction) of tissue when the body is irradiated uniformly. They are derived from *risk coefficients* (i.e., risk per unit dose equivalent) for various body tissues.

BACKGROUND RADIATION

The background radiation is contributed principally by three sources: terrestrial radiation, cosmic radiation, and radiation from radioactive elements in our bodies.

- The terrestrial radiation varies over the earth because of differences in the amount of naturally occurring elements in the earth's surface.
- Cosmic radiation levels change with elevation.
- The internal irradiation arises mainly from ^{40}K in our body, which emits β- and γ-rays and decays with a half-life of 1.3×10^9 years.

- The total effective dose equivalent for a member of the population in the United States from various sources of natural background radiation is approximately 3.0 mSv/year (300 mrem/year).

LOW-LEVEL RADIATION EFFECTS

The harmful effects of radiation may be classified into two general categories: *stochastic* effects and *nonstochastic* effects. The National Council on Radiation Protection and Measurements (NCRP) defines these effects as:

- A stochastic effect is one in which "the probability of occurrence increases with increasing absorbed dose but the severity in affected individuals does not depend on the magnitude of the absorbed dose." EXAMPLE: the development of a radiation-induced cancer or genetic effects.

- A nonstochastic effect is one "which increases in severity with increasing absorbed dose in affected individuals, owing to damage to increasing number of cells and tissues." EXAMPLES: radiation-induced organ atrophy, fibrosis, lens opacification, blood changes, and decrease in sperm count.

- Whereas no threshold dose can be predicted for stochastic effects, it is possible to set threshold limits for nonstochastic effects that are significant or seriously health impairing.

- For the purpose of radiation protection, a cautious assumption is made that "the dose–risk relationship is strictly proportional (linear) without threshold, throughout the range of dose equivalent and dose equivalent rates of importance in routine radiation protection."

- According to the linear threshold model for stochastic effects, the lifetime risk is given by:

Lifetime risk = Risk coefficient × Dose equivalent

EFFECTIVE DOSE-EQUIVALENT LIMITS

NCRP recommendations on exposure limits of radiation workers are based on the following criteria:

   a) At low radiation levels, the nonstochastic effects should be essentially avoided;

   b) The predicted risk for stochastic effects should not be greater than the average risk of accidental death among workers in "safe" industries;

   c) ALARA principle should be followed, for which the risks are kept *as low as reasonably achievable*, taking into account social and economic factors.

- The "safe" industries are defined as those having an associated annual fatality accident rate of 1 or less per 10,000 workers, that is, an average annual risk of 10^{-4}.

- The NCRP (Reports 91 and 116) has recommended exposure limits for radiation workers and the general population (Table 16.5 in the Textbook). These limits do not include exposure received from medical procedures or the natural background.

- Radiation workers are limited to an annual effective dose equivalent of 50 mSv (5 rem) and the general public is not to exceed one-tenth of this value: 5 mSv (0.5 rem) for infrequent exposure and 1 mSv (0.1 rem) for continuous or frequent exposure.

- Students under the age of 18 who may be exposed to radiation as a result of their educational or training activities should not receive more than 1 mSv (0.1 rem) per year.

- The pregnant woman who is a radiation worker can be considered as an occupationally exposed individual, but the fetus cannot. The total dose equivalent limit to an embryo-fetus is 5 mSv (0.5 rem), with the added recommendation that exposure to the fetus should not exceed 0.5 mSv (0.05 rem) in any month.

SHIELDING DESIGN FOR RADIATION INSTALLATIONS

Radiation protection guidelines for the design of structural shielding for radiation installations are discussed in the NCRP Reports 102 and 151.

- Protective barriers are designed to ensure that the dose equivalent received by any individual does not exceed the applicable maximum permissible value.

- The areas surrounding the room are designated as *controlled* or *noncontrolled*, depending on whether the exposure of persons in the area is under the supervision of a radiation protection supervisor.

- Protection is required against three types of radiation: the primary radiation, the scattered radiation, and the leakage radiation through the source housing. A barrier sufficient to attenuate the useful beam to the required degree is called the *primary barrier*. The required barrier against stray radiation (leakage and scatter) is called the *secondary barrier*. These barriers are illustrated in Figure 16.1.

- The calculation of barrier thicknesses involves the following factors:

  ➤ *Workload (W)*: For megavoltage machines, the workload is usually stated in terms of weekly dose delivered at 1 m from the source. This can be estimated by multiplying the number of patients treated per week with the dose delivered per patient at 1 m. W is expressed in Gy/week at 1 m.

  ➤ *Use factor (U)*: Fraction of the operating time during which the radiation under consideration is directed toward a particular barrier.

  ➤ *Occupancy factor (T)*: Fraction of the operating time during which the area of interest is occupied by the individual.

  ➤ *Distance (d)*: Distance in meters from the radiation source to the area to be protected. Inverse-square law is assumed for both the primary and stray radiation.

  ➤ *Maximum permissible dose equivalent (P)*: The maximum dose per week allowed in a given area outside the treatment room. For structural shielding, *P* is

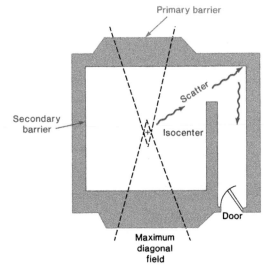

Figure 16.1. Schematic diagram of a megavoltage x-ray therapy installation (drawing not to scale). Radiation scatter from patient can reach the door, as shown.

taken as 0.1 mSv/week for controlled areas and 0.02 mSv/week for noncontrolled areas. (Note: These *P* values are recommended by the NCRP Report 151.)

- *Primary barrier*: If *B* is the transmission factor for the barrier to reduce the primary beam dose to the maximum permissible dose *P* in the area of interest, then the required transmission factor *B* is given by:

$$B = \frac{P \cdot d^2}{WUT}$$

- *Secondary barrier for scattered radiation*: The required barrier transmission factor B_s is given by:

$$B_s = \frac{P}{\alpha WT} \cdot \frac{400}{F} \cdot d^2 \cdot d'^2$$

where α is the fractional scatter at 1 m from the scatterer, for beam area of 400 cm^2 incident at the scatterer, *d* the distance from source to the scatterer, *d'* the distance from the scatterer to the area of interest, and *F* the area of the beam incident at the scatterer in cm^2.

> - For megavoltage beams, α is usually assumed to be 0.1% for 90° scatter.
> - For megavoltage beams, the maximum energy of the 90° scattered photons is 511 keV.
> - At smaller scattering angles the scattered beam has greater energy or penetrating power. In addition, a greater fraction of the incident beam is scattered at smaller angles.
> - The use factor for the secondary barrier is considered unity.

- *Secondary barrier for leakage radiation*: The transmission factor B_L for the leakage barrier is given by:

$$B_L = \frac{P \cdot d^2}{0.001\, WT} \quad [\text{Therapy above 500 kVp}]$$

where the factor 0.001 is the allowed leakage fraction (0.1% of the primary beam) from the source housing.

> - The quality of leakage radiation is approximately the same as that of the primary beam.
> - For megavoltage therapy installations, the leakage barrier usually far exceeds that required for the scattered radiation, because the leakage radiation is more penetrating than the scattered radiation.

- *Door shielding*

   Unless a maze entranceway is provided, the door must provide shielding equivalent to the wall surrounding the door. A maze arrangement, on the other hand, drastically reduces the shielding requirements for the door.

> - The function of the maze is to prevent direct incidence of radiation at the door.
> - If the inner wall of the maze is sufficiently thick against leakage radiation, the door is exposed mainly to the multiply scattered radiation of significantly reduced intensity and energy.
> - In a properly designed maze, the required shielding in the door turns out to be less than 6 mm of lead in most cases.
> - In the case of x-ray beams of energy >10 MV, the barriers as well as the door must provide adequate shielding against contaminant neutrons.
> - With a long maze (>5 m), the door receives reduced neutron fluence. A few inches of a hydrogenous material such as polyethylene may be added to the door to thermalize the neutrons and reduce the neutron dose further.

- *Shielding against neutrons*

   High-energy x-ray beams (e.g., >10 MV) are contaminated with neutrons. These are produced by high-energy photons and electrons incident on the various materials of target, flattening filter, collimators, and other shielding components.

> - The cross sections for (e, n) reactions are smaller by a factor of about 10 than those for (γ,n) reactions. Because of this, the neutron production during electron beam therapy mode is quite small compared with that during the x-ray mode.

➤ In the 15 to 25 MV x-ray therapy modes, the neutron dose equivalent along central axis is approximately 0.5% of the x-ray dose and falls off to approximately 0.1% outside the field.

➤ The energy spectrum of emitted neutrons within the x-ray beam is similar to the uranium fission spectrum, showing a broad maximum in the range of 1 MeV.

➤ The neutron energy is considerably degraded after multiple scattering from walls, roof, and floor, and consequently, the proportion of the fast neutron (>0.1 MeV) reaching the inside of the maze is usually small.

➤ Concrete barriers designed for x-ray shielding are sufficient for protection against neutrons. However, the door must be protected against neutrons that diffuse into the maze and reach the door.

PROTECTION AGAINST BRACHYTHERAPY SOURCES

This subject has been dealt with in detail in NCRP Report 40.

• *Storage*: The storage room typically has the following:

➤ Lead-lined safes with lead-filled drawers.

➤ A shielded area for source preparation.

➤ A sink for cleaning source applicators. The sink should be provided with a filter or trap to prevent loss of any source.

➤ The storage area should be ventilated by a direct filtered exhaust to the outdoors. This precaution is taken so that if a source ruptures, the radionuclide is not drawn into the general ventilation system of the building.

➤ The door to the radioisotope facility must be kept secure under lock and key.

• *Source preparation*: A source preparation bench should be provided close to the safe. Many facilities are equipped with a protective "L-block," made up of lead with a leaded-glass viewing window.

➤ Brachytherapy sources must never be touched with the hands. Suitably long forceps should be used to provide as much distance as practical between a source and the operator.

➤ The operator must be aware of the effectiveness of *time*, *distance*, and *shielding* in radiation protection. Exposures of individuals can be greatly reduced if: a) the time spent in the vicinity of the sources is minimized; b) the distance from the sources is maximized; and c) there is a protective barrier or shield between the source and the operator, whenever possible.

• *Source transportation*: The sources can be transported in lead containers or leaded carts. The thickness of lead required will depend on the type of source and the amount of radioactive material to be transported.

• *Leak testing*: Leak testing of sources is usually specified by the United States Nuclear Regulatory Commission (USNRC) or state regulations.

➤ A source is considered to be leaking if a presence of 0.005 μCi or more of removable contamination is measured.

➤ A leaking source should be returned to a suitable agency that is authorized for the disposal of radioactive materials.

RADIATION PROTECTION SURVEYS

After the installation of radiation equipment, a qualified expert must carry out a radiation protection survey of the installation. The survey includes:

- Equipment survey to check equipment specifications and interlocks related to radiation safety.

- Area survey to check environmental safety.

• The leakage radiation through the source housing should be measured with an ionization chamber of appropriate volume or sensitivity (e.g., survey meter). These measurements should be made in selected directions in which leakage is expected to be the highest.

- The leakage radiation dose rate from the head of the machine in any direction at a distance of 1 m from the source must not exceed 0.1% of the primary beam dose rate at 1 m.
- The environmental safety will be considered acceptable if no person is likely to receive more than the applicable dose equivalent limit, considering the actual operating conditions, including workload, use factor, occupancy factor, and attenuation and scattering of the useful beam by the patient.

RADIATION MONITORING INSTRUMENTS

In measuring low levels of radiation as in protection surveys, the instrument must be sensitive enough to measure such low levels. The detectors most often used for this purpose are the ionization chambers and Geiger counters.

- *Ion chamber survey meter:* An ionization chamber used for low-level x-ray measurements (of the order of milliroentgens/hour) has a large volume (~600 ml) to obtain high sensitivity (Figure 16.2).

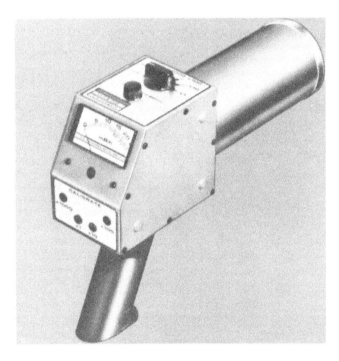

Figure 16.2. A Cutie Pie survey meter. (Courtesy of the Victoreen Instrument Division, Cleveland, OH.)

- ➤ Radiation survey around a linear accelerator installation should be made by a calibrated ion chamber survey meter.
- ➤ The survey meter is usually calibrated for exposure in a γ-ray beam from a cesium or a radium brachytherapy source using open-air measurement geometry and a large distance (in which the exposure can be predicted as a function of distance from the source by inverse square law).
- *Geiger-Müller counter:* The G-M tube is much more sensitive than the ionization chamber. For example, the Geiger counter can detect individual photons or individual particles that cannot be observed in an ionization chamber.
  - ➤ G-M counter is primarily used for detecting or counting radiation rather than measuring exposure or dose.
  - ➤ Although a Geiger counter is useful for preliminary surveys, ionization chamber survey meters are recommended for quantitative measurement of radiation exposures.
- *Neutron meters:*
  - ➤ Neutron measurements in or near the primary x-ray beam can be made with passive detectors such as activation detectors, without being adversely affected by pulsed radiation. An activation

detector can be used either as a bare threshold detector (e.g., phosphorus detector) or inside a moderator (e.g., gold foil surrounded by polyethylene).

➤ Outside the treatment room, it is a common practice to use two detectors that respond predominantly to one or the other radiation—x-rays or neutrons. For example, a Cutie Pie survey meter (large-volume ion chamber) may be used to measure x-rays without being affected by the presence of neutrons. Neutrons may be measured by a rem meter (e.g., BF_3 counter), without being affected by x-rays. Figure 16.3 shows one of the commercially available neutron survey meters.

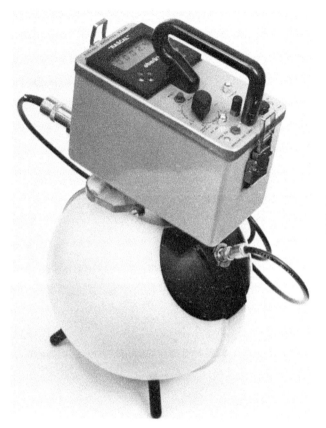

Figure 16.3. A portable neutron rem counter, "Rascal." (Courtesy of Eberline, Santa Fe, NM.)

➤ The rem meter shown in Figure 16.3 is a BF_3 proportional counter surrounded by a cadmium-loaded polyethylene sphere to moderate the neutrons. The response of the meter is displayed in terms of neutron count rate and millirem/hour.

➤ The neutron survey meter is calibrated using a Pu-Be neutron source that has been calibrated by the National Institute of Standards and Technology (NIST).

PERSONNEL MONITORING

Personnel monitoring must be used in controlled areas for occupationally exposed individuals.

• Cumulative radiation monitoring is mostly performed with film badges, although thermoluminescent dosimetry badges are also used in some cases.

• Because the badge is mostly used to monitor whole body exposure, it should be worn on the chest or abdomen.

• Special badges, in addition, may be worn to measure exposure to specific parts of the body (e.g., hands) if higher exposures are expected during a particular procedure.

• Radiation monitoring during a particular procedure may also be performed with pocket dosimeters. These instruments are useful where exposure needs to be monitored more frequently than possible with the regular film badges.

NRC REGULATIONS

The USNRC controls the use of radioactive materials in this country.

- The USNRC has an agreement with a number of states, called the *agreement states*, that allows these states to enforce the NRC regulations.

- The NRC regulations that govern the medical use of radioactive materials are contained in the Code of Federal Regulations 10 CFR Part 35. They are revised from time to time. A licensee must abide by the most current regulations in force.

REVIEW QUESTIONS • Chapter 16

✔ **TEST YOURSELF**

Review questions for this chapter are provided online.

In multiple choice questions, more than one option may be correct.

1. Naturally occurring sources of radiation include:

   a) Cosmic radiation
   b) Medical imaging
   c) Terrestrial radiation
   d) Internal radiation
   e) All of the above

2. Which of the following is best described as a stochastic event?

   a) Skin erythema
   b) Epilation (hair loss)
   c) Lens opacification
   d) Tissue necrosis
   e) None of the above

3. When dealing with brachytherapy sources, which of the following should be kept at a minimum to reduce exposure?

   a) Time spent in the vicinity of the sources
   b) Distance between the operator and the source material
   c) Shielding between the operator and the source material
   d) All of the above

4. Which of the following detectors may be used to determine the adequacy of a primary barrier?

   a) Ionization chamber survey meter
   b) Geiger-Müller counter
   c) Farmer-type ionization chamber
   d) Scintillation detector
   e) BF_3 proportional counter

5. Assuming risk coefficient of 10^{-2} Sv^{-1} for radiation protection purposes, what is the risk for members of the general public if they are exposed to the annual effective dose-equivalent limit for infrequent exposure: [Consult Table 16.5 in the Textbook.]

   a) 5×10^{-4}
   b) 1×10^{-4}
   c) 5×10^{-5}
   d) 1×10^{-5}

6. A linac vault is designed to treat 30 patients per 8 hour day, 5 days a week. The primary barrier on one of the walls protects a clerical office. The distance from the *isocenter to the office* (i.e., 0.3 m beyond the end of the primary barrier) is 7 m. If the shielding design goal is 0.02 mSv/week, how many tenth-value layers (TVLs) are needed in the primary barrier, assuming an average treatment dose of 3 Gy/patient?

   a) 4.24
   b) 4.76
   c) 4.94
   d) 5.06
   e) 5.55

7. In the above problem, how many inches of concrete (density = 2.35 g/cm^3) are required for the barrier? [Use barrier transmission curves in Figure 16.2 of the Textbook.]

    a) 54
    b) 63
    c) 70
    d) 78
    e) 85

8. Suppose the construction of the vault and the linac installation are complete as specified in problem 6. What would be the expected instantaneous dose rate in μGy/hour in the office when the beam is directed at the barrier with a maximum field size and a dose rate of 2 Gy/minute?

    a) 5
    b) 14
    c) 21
    d) 28

9. In the above problem, what would be the transmitted dose equivalent in mSv/week in the office, assuming the same workload and use factor as in problem 6?

    a) 0.01
    b) 0.02
    c) 0.03
    d) 0.05

10. A 6-MV linear accelerator is planned to be installed to deliver up to 200 treatments per week. The thickness of concrete (density 2.35 g/cm^3) required for a wall separating the treatment room and an office of a nonradiation worker ($P = 0.02$ mSv/week) is approximately: [Assume average dose/treatment of 300 cGy at isocenter at 1 m, isocenter-to-wall distance of 3 m, and the wall being perpendicular to the axis of rotation of the unit. Use barrier transmission curves in Figure 16.2 of the Textbook.]

    a) 32 inches
    b) 47 inches
    c) 52 inches
    d) 60 inches

11. In the above problem, the thickness of concrete required to adequately shield the office against *scattered radiation only* would be approximately: [Assume 40 × 40 cm^2 field size at the patient.]:

    a) 10 inches
    b) 14 inches
    c) 22 inches
    d) 27 inches

12. In designing structural shielding for a 10-MV linear accelerator vault, the beam quality is taken as:

    a) 10 MV for the primary beam
    b) 10 MV for the leakage radiation
    c) 3.3 MeV for the scattered radiation at all angles
    d) 0.511 MeV for scattered radiation at 90°

13. A calibrated rem meter (moderated BF$_3$ proportional counter) is used to measure radiation outside the door of a 20 MV linac room. The radiation quantity thus measured represents primarily:

    a) The dose equivalent from x-rays
    b) The dose equivalent from neutrons
    c) The dose equivalent from x-rays and neutrons
    d) The dose equivalent from x-rays, neutrons, and β-particles, if present.

14. According to the U.S. Nuclear Regulatory Commission (USNRC) regulations, each medical institution licensee shall establish a radiation safety committee to oversee the use of byproduct material. The committee *must* include:

    a) The department head
    b) The authorized user
    c) The radiation safety officer (RSO)
    d) A medical physicist
    e) A representative of management who is neither the RSO nor an authorized user
    f) A nurse

15. According to the NRC, the term "medical event" applies to a treatment administration with byproduct material in which:

    a) The total dose delivered differs from the prescribed dose by 20% or more.
    b) The fractionated dose delivered differs from the prescribed dose, for a single fraction, by 30% or more.
    c) The dose is delivered to the wrong patient.
    d) The dose to an organ exceeds 0.05 Sv from a leaking sealed source.

16. A licensee may release a patient with radiopharmaceutical material only if it is ensured that:

    a) The activity remaining in the patient is less than 0.005 μCi.
    b) The dose rate at 1 foot from the patient is less than 5 mrem/h.
    c) The activity remaining in the patient is less than 30 μCi.
    d) The dose rate at 1 m from the patient is less than 2 mrem/h.
    e) The dose rate at 1 m from the patient is less than 5 mrem/h.

QUALITY ASSURANCE

REFERENCE

Khan FM. *The Physics of Radiation Therapy*, 4th edition, 2009. Chapter 17 "Quality Assurance"

Quality Assurance and Maintenance

 TOPIC OUTLINE

The following topics will be discussed in this lecture:

➤ Program goals
➤ Equipment QA: acceptance testing, commissioning, and periodic checks
  • Linear accelerator
  • Brachytherapy
  • Simulator
  • Treatment planning system

PROGRAM GOALS

A quality assurance (QA) program in radiation oncology is essentially a set of policies and procedures to maintain the quality of patient care. The American College of Radiology ("*Blue Book*" [1991]) specifies the following general goals:

1. The QA program should provide objective, systematic monitoring of the quality and appropriateness of patient care. Such a program is essential for all activities in Radiation Oncology.

2. The QA program should be related to structure, process, and outcome, all of which can be measured.

   - *Structure* includes the staffing, equipment, and facility.

   - *Process* covers the pre- and post-treatment evaluations and the actual treatment application.

   - *Outcome* is documented by the frequency of accomplishing stated objectives, usually tumor control, and by the frequency and seriousness of treatment-induced sequelae.

3. The QA program should be comprehensive—it should include administrative, clinical, physical, and technical aspects of radiation oncology.

4. The QA program should involve teamwork among administrators, radiation oncologists, nurses, medical physicists, dosimetrists, and therapists.

5. For a QA program to be effective, all the staff involved with the radiation oncology service must be well coordinated and committed to QA.

EQUIPMENT QA: ACCEPTANCE TESTING, COMMISSIONING, AND PERIODIC CHECKS

ACCEPTANCE TESTING

Whereas installation of major equipment is carried out by the vendor personnel, the acceptance testing and commissioning are the responsibility of the institution's physicist.

- **Linear Accelerator**: The vendor, together with the physicist, first performs all the tests in accordance with the company's procedure manual. Any deviations or additions stipulated in the bid specifications are then addressed to complete the acceptance testing process. The following checks are performed as part of the acceptance testing:

  ➤ *Radiation Survey*: As soon as the installation has reached a stage at which a radiation beam can be generated, the physicist performs a *preliminary radiation survey* of the treatment facility (discussed in Chapter 16).

    - The survey is evaluated to ensure that during the testing of the machine the exposure levels outside the room will not exceed permissible limits.

    - After completion of the installation, a formal radiation protection survey is carried out, including the measurement of head leakage; area survey, and tests of interlocks, warning lights, and emergency switches.

    - The survey is evaluated for conditions that are expected to exist in the clinical use of the machine, for example, workload, use factors, and occupancy factors.

  ➤ *Jaw Symmetry*: Each pair of collimator jaws moves symmetrically with respect to the central axis of the beam. The jaw symmetry may be checked mechanically with a machinist's dial indicator. The symmetry error should not exceed 1 mm.

  ➤ *Coincidence of Collimator Axis, Light Beam Axis, and Cross-hair*: As the collimator is rotated through 180°, the intersection of the light field diagonals and the cross-hair images should remain coincident within acceptable tolerance (within 2-mm diameter).

  ➤ *Coincidence of Light Field and Radiation Field*: This check may be performed using film. The alignment between the light beam and the x-ray beam should be within ± 2 mm.

  ➤ *Mechanical Isocenter*: Mechanical isocenter is the intersection point of the axis of rotation of the collimator and the axis of rotation of the gantry.

    - For an acceptable alignment, the isocenter should stay within a 2-mm-diameter circle when the collimator is rotated through its full range of rotation.

    - The isocenter should stay within 2-mm-diameter circle when the gantry is rotated.

  ➤ *Radiation Isocenter*: The radiation isocenter is the center of rotation of the beam central axis when the gantry is rotated. This point in space can be determined with a ready-pack film. The procedure consists of closing down one set of jaws and obtaining slit images as the gantry is rotated through a series of different angles. The image pattern thus obtained is known as the *star pattern*, as shown in Figure 17.1.

    The alignment of the radiation isocenter with the axes of the collimator, gantry, and table rotation should be within a 2-mm-diameter sphere.

  ➤ *Multileaf Collimator (MLC)*: The following tests are recommended by the AAPM TG-50 (AAPM Report No. 72 [2001]):

    - *Projected leaf width at isocenter*: The projected leaf width at the isocenter is specified by the vendor. It can be verified radiographically.

    - *Calibration of leaf positions*: Accuracy of leaf positions can be checked radiographically. Misalignment of any leaf with its neighbor would be visible on the film.

    - *Leaf travel*: Maximum specified ranges of leaves travel should be checked in both directions.

    - *Leaf speed*: Individual leaves should move smoothly and continuously over the entire range of their travel. The maximum specified speed should be verified.

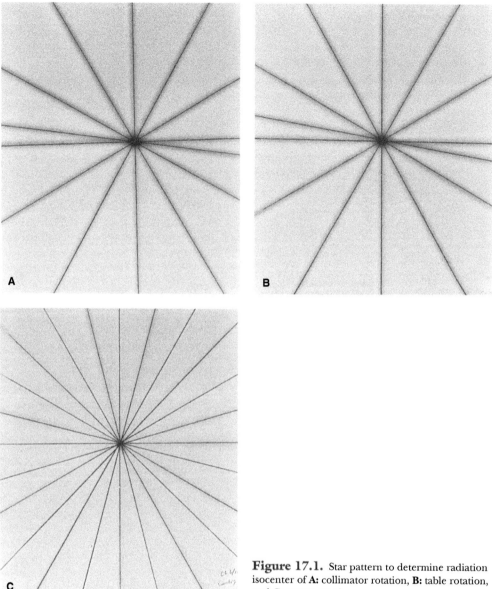

Figure 17.1. Star pattern to determine radiation isocenter of **A:** collimator rotation, **B:** table rotation, and **C:** gantry rotation.

- *Transmission*: Transmission of radiation through leaves, interleaves, and the leaves and jaws combined should be measured and checked against manufacturer's specifications. The measurements may be performed with a dosimetry film or an ion chamber.

- *Leakage*: Leakage of radiation between leaf faces in the closed position should be measured. These measurements should be checked against values specified by the manufacturer.

- *Field shaping*: Accuracy of field shaping software to create irregularly shaped fields with MLC should be checked as specified by the vendor. A series of typical irregular field shapes should be digitized and compared with MLC-generated fields optically and radiographically.

➤ *X-ray Beam Performance*:

- *Energy*: The acceptance criterion for energy is usually specified in terms of depth-dose variance from the published data for a 10 × 10 cm field size, 100 cm SSD, and 10 cm depth. A difference of ≤2% in the depth dose or ionization ratio is acceptable.

- *Field flatness*: Field flatness for photon beams may be defined as the transverse variation of dose relative to the central axis over the central 80% of the field size at 10 cm depth in a plane perpendicular to the central axis (Figure 17.2). A dose variation of ± 3% relative to the central axis value is considered acceptable.

- *Field symmetry*: The cross-beam profiles obtained for flatness also can be used for symmetry. The dose profile should not differ more than 2% at any pair of points located symmetrically on opposite sides of the central axis.

➤ *Electron Beam Performance*:

- *Energy*: The most probable energy at the surface, $(E_p)_o$, is determined from the practical range, R_p, obtained from a depth–dose curve for a broad beam (e.g., 20 × 20 cm^2 field). The energy thus measured should be within approximately ±0.5 MeV of the nominal energy shown on the accelerator control panel.

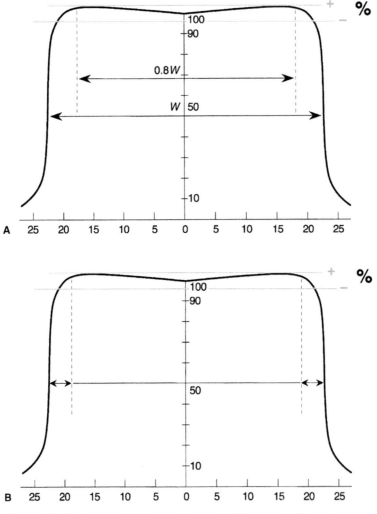

Figure 17.2. Alternate definitions of photon field flatness. **A:** Flatness is measured within a region bounded by 80% of the field width (*W*). **B:** Flatness is measured within a region bounded by lines drawn a certain distance (e.g., 2 cm) inside from the field edges. Depth of measurement is specified at 10 cm.

- *Flatness*: The AAPM (TG-25 Report) recommends that the flatness of an electron beam be specified in a reference plane perpendicular to the central axis, at the depth of the 95% isodose beyond the depth of dose maximum. The variation in dose relative to the dose at central axis should not exceed ±5% (optimally to be within ±3%) over an area confined within lines 2 cm inside the geometric edge of fields equal to or larger than 10 × 10 cm.

- *Field symmetry*: For the above conditions, the cross-beam profile in the reference plane should not differ more than 2% at any pair of points located symmetrically on opposite sides of the central axis.

➤ *Monitor Chambers*: Linearity of monitor chambers should be checked as a function of dose rate and for special operating conditions such as total body irradiation, total skin irradiation, and arc rotation.

- *Wedge filters*: Wedge isodose distribution for a 10 × 10 cm field may be used to check wedge angle. The measured wedge angles should be within ±2° of the values specified.

➤ *Miscellaneous Checks*:

- Isocenter shift with couch motion up and down should not exceed ±2 mm.
- Optical distance indicators should be accurate within ±2 mm.
- Field size indicators should be accurate within ±2 mm.
- Gantry angle and collimator angles should be accurate within 1°.
- Laser lights should be aligned with the isocenter within ±2 mm.
- Tabletop sag with lateral or longitudinal travel under a distributed weight (similar to patient) of 180 lb should not exceed 2 mm.
- The tennis racket insert for the couch should not sag more than 0.5 cm under the above-stated conditions.
- Other ancillary devices provided with the accelerator should be checked in accordance with the vendor's specifications or as specified in the purchase contract.

- **Simulator**: Acceptance testing of a simulator may be divided into two parts:
  a) Checking of the geometric and spatial accuracies. This part is similar to the acceptance testing of a linear accelerator.
  b) Performance evaluation of the x-ray generator and the associated imaging system. This part deals with the simulator performance like a diagnostic x-ray and fluoroscopic unit.

  Table 17.5 of the Textbook gives the list of acceptance tests and tolerances recommended by the British Institute of Radiology.

- **Brachytherapy—Manual Afterloaders**: The following procedures are recommended to evaluate intracavitary sources and manual afterloading applicators.

  ➤ *Source Identity*: Source dimensions may be checked by physical measurement or by radiography. The serial number and color-coding can be checked by visual inspection (behind the leaded glass window).

  ➤ *Source Uniformity and Symmetry*: An autoradiograph of a brachytherapy source reveals distribution of activity as well as active length.

  ➤ *Source Calibration*: A well-ionization chamber (e.g., a dose calibrator) with a standard source of the same kind may be used for these calibration checks. Differences should not exceed ±5% from the vendor-stated values.

  ➤ *Applicator Evaluation*: The internal structure of applicators may be examined by orthogonal radiographs using a 4- or 6-MV x-ray beam.

- **Brachytherapy—Remote Afterloaders**: Acceptance procedures for remote afterloading equipment may be broadly divided into:

  ➤ Operational testing of the afterloading unit
  ➤ radiation safety check of the facility

➤ checking of source calibration and transport

➤ checking of treatment planning software

Acceptance testing procedures for remote afterloaders are listed in Table 17.6 of the Textbook.

COMMISSIONING

Most equipment is ready for clinical use after acceptance testing. However, some equipment requires additional data before it can be used in conjunction with patient treatments. For example, a linear accelerator cannot be used for patient treatments until it has been calibrated and all the beam data and necessary parameters for treatment planning have been obtained.

- **Linear Accelerator**: Table 17.7 of the Textbook gives a list of typical data that are required for commissioning a linear accelerator. Commissioning is complete only after the beam data have been input into the treatment-planning computer and the computer-generated dose distributions have been checked.

- **Treatment Planning System**: Acceptance testing and commissioning of a treatment-planning computer system include both hardware and software. The tests include (but not limited to):

  ➤ Checking the accuracy and linearity of input digitizers, output plotters, and printers.

  ➤ Checking the accuracy of beam modeling and dose distributions for a selected set of treatment conditions against measured distributions or manual calculations.

  ➤ Algorithm verification—its accuracy, precision, limitations, and special features.

Extensive QA guidelines and recommendations for 3D treatment planning systems may be found in the AAPM TG-53 Report.

PERIODIC CHECKS

A periodic QA program is designed to maintain the system within its acceptable performance standards.

- **Linear Accelerator**: The periodic QA for linear accelerators recommended by the AAPM (AAPM TG-40 Report) is summarized in Tables 17.8 and 17.9 of the Textbook.

- **^{60}Co unit**: QA of ^{60}Co teletherapy should be similar to that of a linear accelerator except that some aspects of the QA are mandated by the Nuclear Regulatory Commission (NRC) or the state (if an Agreement State). Table 17.10 of the Textbook contains the NRC requirements as well as recommendations by the AAPM TG-40.

- **Radiographic simulator**: Geometric accuracy of a radiographic simulator must be comparable with that of the linear accelerator. The periodic QA program for simulators as recommended in AAPM TG-40 Report is summarized in Table 17.11 of the Textbook.

- **CT simulator**: QA program for a CT simulator is detailed by the AAPM Task Group No. 66. Periodic tests are recommended daily, monthly, and annually. These tests are summarized in Tables 17.12A and 17.12B of the Textbook.

REVIEW QUESTIONS • Chapter 17

✔ TEST YOURSELF

Review questions for this chapter are provided online.

In multiple choice questions, more than one option may be correct.

1. According to the AAPM TG-40 recommendations, the x-ray output constancy check should be performed:
   a) Daily
   b) Twice a week
   c) Once a week
   d) Once a month

2. According to the AAPM TG-40, the tolerance for x-ray or electron output constancy check with a field instrument using temperature and pressure correction is specified at plus or minus:
   a) 1%
   b) 2%
   c) 3%
   d) 4%
   e) 5%

3. According to the AAPM TG-40, the tolerance for the light/radiation field alignment is specified at plus or minus:
   a) 1 mm
   b) 2 mm
   c) 3 mm
   d) 4 mm
   e) 5 mm

4. According to the AAPM TG-40, the tolerance for rotation isocenter is specified at:
   a) 2-mm diameter for collimator
   b) 2-mm diameter for gantry
   c) 1-mm diameter for radiation beam central axis
   d) 5-mm diameter for couch

5. According to the AAPM TG-50, the tolerance for the field generated by the MLC versus the simulator film or DRR is specified at plus or minus:
   a) 1 mm
   b) 2 mm
   c) 3 mm
   d) 4 mm
   e) 5 mm

6. Which of the following statements regarding dosimetric accuracy is/are correct:
   a) Evidence points to the need for dosimetric accuracy of approximately 3% in the target dose delivered.
   b) Overall treatment beam calibration accuracy is estimated to be approximately 1%.
   c) An ion chamber calibrated with a ^{60}Co exposure calibration factor from an ADCL has a cumulative uncertainty of approximately 1.5%.
   d) None of the above is correct

7. Which of the following tests are recommended for remote afterloading brachytherapy units?
   a) Timer accuracy and end-time effects
   b) Monthly radiation survey around the radiation facility
   c) Proper functionality of radiation detectors
   d) Verify door will not open while source is out.

8. For HDR remote afterloaders:
   a) Source leak test is not necessary since the source is automatically retracted in the device safe.
   b) Source positional accuracy test should be performed monthly.
   c) The tolerance of the source positional accuracy test is ±1 mm.
   d) Cylindrical ion chambers in free-air geometry can be used to perform source strength calibration.
   e) Calibration of the HDR source strength should be performed monthly.

9. Which of the following tolerance(s) is recommended by the BIR for treatment simulators?
   a) Accuracy of 0° position for rotation of gantry should be ±1°.
   b) Maximum displacement of the x-ray beam axis from the radiation isocenter should be within 2 mm.
   c) Average luminance at the normal treatment distance should meet or exceed 40 lux.
   d) Maximum difference between numerical field indication and dimensions of the x-ray field should be less than 1.0 mm.

10. According to the AAPM Report 83 (TG #66) on CT simulator QA:
    a) CT number accuracy for water should be checked daily.
    b) Tolerance for CT number accuracy for water is specified at 0 ± 5 HU.
    c) Spatial resolution should be checked monthly per manufacturer specifications.
    d) Electron density to CT number conversion should be checked annually.

18

TOTAL BODY IRRADIATION

REFERENCE

Khan FM. *The Physics of Radiation Therapy*, 4th edition, 2009. Chapter 18 "Total Body Irradiation"

Total Body Irradiation: Techniques and Dosimetry

 TOPIC OUTLINE

The following topics will be discussed in this lecture:
- ➤ Role of total body irradiation
- ➤ Techniques
- ➤ Dosimetry
- ➤ Compensators
- ➤ In vivo patient dosimetry

ROLE OF TOTAL BODY IRRADIATION

The role of total body irradiation (TBI) is to destroy the recipient's bone marrow and tumor cells, and to immunosuppress the patient sufficiently to avoid rejection of the donor bone marrow transplant.

- TBI with megavoltage photon beams is most commonly used as **part of the conditioning regimen for bone marrow transplantation**, which is used in the treatment of (for example):
  - ➤ Leukemia
  - ➤ Aplastic anemia
  - ➤ Lymphoma
  - ➤ Multiple myeloma
  - ➤ Autoimmune diseases
  - ➤ Inborn errors of metabolism
- Although chemotherapy alone can be used as a conditioning regimen, addition of TBI is considered beneficial for certain diseases and clinical conditions because:
  - a) TBI allows the delivery of almost homogeneous dose (within 10%) to the entire body including "sanctuary areas" where chemotherapy may not be effective;
  - b) Selected parts of the body (e.g., lungs, kidneys, and head) can be partially or fully shielded, if desired.

TECHNIQUES

The choice of a particular technique depends on the available equipment, photon beam energy, maximum possible field size, treatment distance, dose rate, patient dimensions, and the need to shield selectively certain body structures.

- An anteroposterior (AP/PA) technique generally provides a better dose uniformity along the longitudinal body axis but the patient positioning, other than standing upright, may pose problems.
- Bilateral TBI (treating from left and right) can be more comfortable to the patient if seated or laying down supine on a TBI couch, but presents greater variation in body thickness along the path of the beam.
- Compensators are usually required to achieve dose uniformity along the body axis to within ±10%, although extremities and some noncritical structures may exceed this specification.

  ➤ *Beam energy:* The choice of photon beam energy is dictated by the patient thickness, its variation along the axis of the patient, and the specification of dose homogeneity. Figure 18.1 shows that the ratio of the maximum dose to the midline dose is a function of energy and patient thickness when parallel-opposed beams are used.

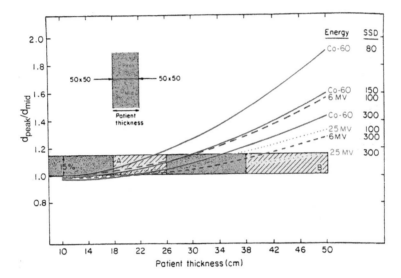

Figure 18.1. A plot of the ratio of dose at d_{max} (d_{peak}) to that at the midplane (d_{mid}) as a function of patient thickness for a number of beam energies. The shaded region represents a 15% spread in the ratio. Regions A and B represent the range of adult patient thickness in the anteroposterior and lateral directions, respectively. SSD, source-to-surface distance in centimeters. (From American Association of Physicists in Medicine. *The Physical Aspects of Total and Half Body Photon Irradiation.* AAPM Report No. 17. Colchester, VT: AIDC; 1986, with permission.)

➤ *Initial dose buildup:*
- Dose buildup data obtained at normal source-to-surface distance (e.g., 100 cm) do not apply accurately at TBI distances (e.g., 400 cm) because of the longer distance and the intervening air.
- Most TBI protocols do not require skin sparing.
- A bolus or a beam spoiler may be used to build up the surface dose to at least 90% of the prescribed TBI dose. A large spoiler screen of 1- to 2-cm thick acrylic is sufficient to meet these requirements, provided the screen is placed as close as possible to the patient surface.

- *Patient support/positioning devices:* Patient support and positioning devices are designed to implement a given treatment technique. Important criteria include patient comfort, stability, and reproducibility of setup and treatment geometry that allows accurate calculation and delivery of dose in accordance with the TBI protocol.

Total body irradiation bilateral fields

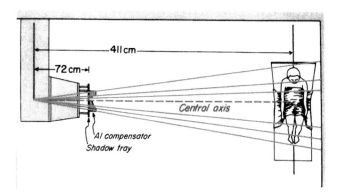

Figure 18.2. Schematic diagram illustrating patient setup geometry for the bilateral total body irradiation technique. (From Khan FM, Williamson JF, Sewchand W, et al. Basic data for dosage calculation and compensation. *Int J Radiat Oncol Biol Phys.* 1980;6:745–751, with permission.)

- *Bilateral TBI technique*: This technique involves bilateral fields (left and right lateral opposing fields) with the patient seated on a couch in a semi-fetal position (Figure 18.2).

  ➤ Lateral body thickness varies considerably along the patient axis. Therefore, compensators are needed for head and neck, lungs, and legs to achieve dose uniformity within approximately ±10% along the sagittal axis of the body.

  ➤ Dose prescription is specified by the relevant protocol and, for the bilateral technique, is usually at the midpoint of the body cross section at the level of umbilicus. *The reference thickness for compensation is the lateral diameter of the body at the level of umbilicus.*

- *AP/PA TBI technique*: The patient is irradiated AP/PA by parallel-opposed fields while positioned in a standing upright position at the TBI distance (Figure 18.3).

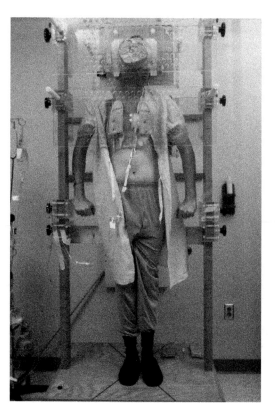

Figure 18.3. Patient in the standing total body irradiation (TBI) position with the head turned sideways for shielding of the brain. A five half-value-layer Cerrobend block is mounted on an acrylic plate attached to the TBI stand. (From Dusenbery KE, Gerbi BJ. Total body irradiation in conditioning regimens for bone marrow transplantation. In: Levitt SH, Khan FM, Potish RA, et al., eds. *Technological Basis of Radiation Therapy.* Philadelphia, PA: Lippincott Williams & Wilkins; 1999:499–518, with permission).

➤ The standing AP/PA technique allows shielding of certain critical organs (e.g., lungs and brain) from excessive photon dose and boosting the dose to superficial tissues in the shadow of the blocks with electrons to makeup for the deficit. The protocol does not require compensators.

➤ The AP/PA technique can also be adopted for treating small children in the reclining position (Figure 18.4).

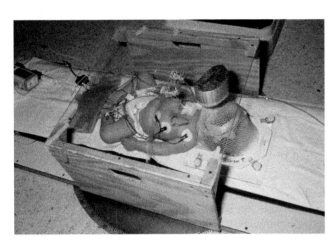

Figure 18.4. Pediatric patient in the reclining total body irradiation position on the floor. The legs are placed in the "frog-legged" position to cover the entire patient in the radiation field with adequate margins. Brain-sparing shielding block is placed on top of an acrylic tray to shadow the central part of the skull with the head turned sideways.

DOSIMETRY

Dosimetric data for the calculation of dose per monitor unit (MU) may be acquired in a phantom directly at the TBI distance or derived from the data obtained under standard conditions (at isocenter). The latter must be checked for accuracy at the TBI distance.

• *Dose/MU calculation formalism*: The formalisms used for regular isocentric techniques (discussed in Chapter 10) may be used also for TBI. The basic equation to calculate dose per monitor unit at the point of prescription using the TMR formalism is:

$$D/MU = k \cdot TMR(d, r_e) \cdot S_c(r_c) \cdot S_p(r_e) \cdot (f/f')^2 \cdot OAR_d \cdot \text{TF}$$

where

D/MU is the dose per monitor unit to be delivered at the prescription point;

k is the calibration dose/MU at the reference depth of maximum dose;

TMR is the tissue–maximum ratio at depth d for the patient-equivalent field size (r_e) at the point of prescription;

S_c is the collimator scatter factor for the field size projected at isocenter (r_c);

S_p is the phantom scatter factor for the patient-equivalent field size (r_e);

f is the source-to-calibration point distance;

f' is the source-to-patient axis distance at the prescription point;

OAR_d is the off-axis ratio at depth d;

TF is the transmission factor for the block tray, beam spoiler, or any other absorber placed between the machine diaphragm and the patient.

COMPENSATORS

The thickness of compensator required along a ray line depends on the tissue deficit relative to the reference depth at the dose prescription point, material of the compensator (e.g., its density), distance of the compensator from the point of dose compensation, depth of the point of dose compensation, field size, and beam energy (see Chapter 12). A TBI compensator may be designed using the thickness ratio method or the effective attenuation coefficient method.

- *Thickness ratio method:* The thickness of a compensator, t_c, at any point in the field is given by:

$$t_c = \text{TD} \cdot (\tau/\rho_c)$$

where

TD is the tissue deficit relative to the reference depth at the prescription point;

τ is the thickness ratio (the ratio of the required tissue-equivalent compensator thickness along a ray line to the tissue deficit along the same line); ρ_c is the density of compensator relative to water.

- ➤ The thickness ratio τ depends on several variables, for example, depth of the point of dose compensation, the amount of tissue deficit, the distance of compensator from the point of dose compensation, field size, and beam energy.
- ➤ It has been shown that a single value of 0.7 for τ gives a compensation accuracy of approximately ±5% for all beam energies and TBI conditions.

- *Effective attenuation coefficient method:* In this method, the thickness of a compensator, t_c, at any point in the field may be calculated from the following equations:

$$I/I_0 = [T(A_R, d_R)/T(A, d)] \cdot \text{OAR}_d$$
$$= \exp(-\mu_{\text{eff}} t_c)$$

where

I and I_0 are doses at the point of compensation with and without the compensator, respectively;

$T(A_R, d_R)$ and $T(A, d)$ are tissue–phantom ratios or TMRs for the reference body cross section and the section to be compensated, respectively;

A_R and A are equivalent fields at the midline depths d_R and d, for the reference body cross section and the section to be compensated, respectively;

OAR_d is off–axis ratio at the point of compensation relative to the prescription point;

μ_{eff} is the effective linear attenuation coefficient for the compensator measured at the TBI distance.

IN VIVO PATIENT DOSIMETRY

After a particular TBI technique has been commissioned for clinical use, it is recommended that an in vivo dosimetry check be performed on the first 20 or so patients.

- In vivo dosimetry check may be performed using thermoluminescent dosimeters (TLD) or diodes placed on the patient's surface at strategic locations. The dosimeters should be surrounded by suitable buildup bolus.

- The measured doses should be compared with the expected doses at the surface under the dose buildup condition.

- An agreement of ±5% between the calculated and measured doses is considered acceptable.

REVIEW QUESTIONS • Chapter 18

In multiple choice questions, more than one option may be correct.

1. Which of the following statement(s) is/are true about TBI treatments:

   a) Dosimetry is designed to give a uniform dose along the midplane of the patient within ±5%.
   b) Dosimetry is designed to give a superficial dose of >90% of the prescribed dose.
   c) TBI is used in the treatment of leukemia, aplastic anemia, lymphoma, multiple myeloma, autoimmune diseases, and inborn errors of metabolism.
   d) A beam spoiler is used to lower the average energy of the beam.
   e) High-Z eye shields are employed to protect the lens from opacification.

Questions 2 to 4 refer to a 10-MV TBI procedures with the patient midplane positioned 4 m from the source. For all problems, assume the patient-effective field size is 30×30 cm^2, $S_c(r_c = 40) = 1.04$, $S_p(r_p = 30) = 1.03$, TF = 0.90, and use the 10-MV TMR Table A.11.2 in the textbook where appropriate. The machine is calibrated to give 1 cGy/MU under normalization conditions (10×10 cm^2, $d = d_m$, 100 cm SAD).

2. A patient to be treated with a bilateral TBI technique has a lateral thickness at the umbilicus (i.e., prescription point) of 32 cm. If the protocol calls for a midplane dose rate of 5 to 10 cGy/min, what accelerator dose rate should be selected for this treatment?

   a) 100 MU/min
   b) 200 MU/min
   c) 300 MU/min
   d) 400 MU/min
   e) 500 MU/min

3. For the inverse square law, photon scatter from the flattening filter causes the effective source position to be shifted slightly toward the isocenter. For most conventional treatments (i.e., to points near the isocenter), this effect is small and can be ignored. If the effective source position is 98 cm from the isocenter, what is the dosimetric error from neglecting this effect in problem 2?

   a) <0.5%
   b) 1%
   c) 3%
   d) 5%
   e) 10%

4. A patient is treated with an AP/PA technique using the same machine and using partial-thickness Cerrobend blocks ($\mu_{eff} = 0.3$ cm^{-1}) to reduce the lung dose to 50% of the prescribed dose. Neglecting OAR$_d$, if the patient's thicknesses at the umbilicus and chest are 26 and 32 cm, respectively, compute the lung block thickness for an AP/PA lung thickness of 24 cm. Use the Ratio of TMR technique to account for the lung heterogeneity, assuming a relative electron density of 0.25.

   a) 1.3 cm
   b) 2.5 cm
   c) 2.8 cm
   d) 3.5 cm
   e) 3.7 cm

5. For the bilateral TBI technique:

   a) Compensators are necessary only for the head and extremities.
   b) The arms should shadow the lungs to provide dose compensation for lungs.
   c) Additional electron treatments are necessary to the lung for boost.
   d) The reference thickness for compensation is the lateral diameter of the body at umbilicus, including the thickness of the arms.

6. A patient is to be treated using bilateral TBI technique. The reference thickness for dose prescription (at the umbilicus) is 30 cm. The lateral thickness of neck is 10 cm. What should be the thickness of an aluminum compensator for the neck?

   [Given: 10-MV x-rays, SAD = 100 cm, source-to-compensator distance = 50 cm, source-to-patient axis distance = 400 cm, field size at isocenter = 40 × 40 cm², equivalent field size at the dose prescription point = 30 × 30 cm², equivalent field size at the midpoint of neck = 20 × 20 cm², and the effective linear attenuation coefficient for the aluminum compensator is = 0.0923 cm⁻¹.]

   a) 1.5 cm
   b) 2.0 cm
   c) 2.5 cm
   d) 3.0 cm

7. In problem 6, if the compensator is constructed with a thickness ratio (τ) of 0.7, what would be the thickness of the aluminum compensator?

   a) 1.6 cm
   b) 2.1 cm
   c) 2.6 cm
   d) 3.2 cm

8. What is the percentage error in dose at the midpoint of neck in using the compensator designed in problem 7, assuming the compensator designed in problem 6 to be correct?

   a) 1
   b) 2
   c) 3
   d) 4

9. In problem 6, what would be the thickness of aluminum compensator if the attenuation coefficient for aluminum given in Table A-7 (Appendix) of the Textbook is used instead of the effective attenuation coefficient? [Hint: The effective energy of a 10-MV x-ray beam is ~3 MeV.]

   a) 1.4 cm
   b) 1.9 cm
   c) 2.4 cm
   d) 2.9 cm

10. What is the percentage error in dose at the midpoint of neck in using the compensator designed in problem 9, assuming the compensator designed in 6 to be correct?

   a) 1
   b) 2
   c) 3
   d) 4

THREE-DIMENSIONAL CONFORMAL RADIATION THERAPY

LECTURE

19

REFERENCE
Khan FM. *The Physics of Radiation Therapy*, 4th edition, 2009. Chapter 19 "Three-Dimensional Conformal Radiation Therapy"

3D Conformal Radiotherapy: Dosimetry and Treatment Planning

 TOPIC OUTLINE

The following topics will be discussed in this lecture:

➤ Definition
➤ Dose calculation algorithms
➤ Treatment planning process
➤ Delivery of 3D CRT and verification

DEFINITION

By three-dimensional conformal radiotherapy (3D CRT), we mean radiation therapy that is based on 3D anatomic information, uses 3D dose distributions, and designs and delivers treatment plans that conform as closely as possible to the planned target volume in terms of adequate dose to the tumor and minimum possible dose to normal tissue.

DOSE CALCULATION ALGORITHMS

Broadly, the dose calculation algorithms fall into three categories: (a) correction based, (b) model based, and (c) Monte Carlo. These are discussed in Lecture 12B. Their application and limitations relative to 3D CRT are outlined below:

• *Correction-based algorithms*: These algorithms are semi-empirical. They are based primarily on measured data (e.g., percentage depth doses and cross-beam profiles) obtained in a cubic water phantom. Corrections are applied to the measured data to calculate dose distributions in a patient.

  ➤ Examples of correction-based computer algorithms include Clarkson integration using scatter–air ratios, delta volume, and dose spread array.

  ➤ Limitations of the correction-based algorithms include their inability to calculate dose accurately in all treatment situations, for example, treatments where electronic equilibrium may not exist such as those involving initial buildup region, lung irradiation with high-energy beams, or very small fields as in stereotactic radiotherapy.

287

- *Model based algorithms*: Unlike correction-based algorithms, the model-based algorithms do not involve reconstructing measured data before correcting it for the given patient situation. The treatment situation is modeled from first principles.

  ➤ Examples of model-based algorithms include pencil beam convolution, convolution/super-position of dose kernels, and Monte Carlo.

  ➤ Model-based algorithms are capable of calculating dose in 3D geometries including most situations of electronic disequilibrium. Consequently, these methods are more accurate in calculating dose distribution in the buildup region, lung, and in small fields.

  ➤ None of the algorithms, except Monte Carlo, are sufficiently accurate at tissue interfaces.

TREATMENT PLANNING PROCESS

The treatment planning process for the 3D CRT involves the following steps:

- *Imaging data acquisition*: Anatomic images of high quality are required to accurately delineate target volumes and normal structures. Modern imaging modalities include computed tomography (CT), magnetic resonance imaging, ultrasound, single photon emission tomography, and positron emission tomography. These are discussed in Lecture 12A.

  ➤ Although CT is the most commonly used procedure for treatment planning, other modalities offer special advantages in imaging certain types of tumors and locations.

- *Image registration*: The term *registration* as applied to images is a process of correlating different image data sets to identify corresponding structures or regions.

  ➤ Computer programs are now available that allow *image fusion*, for example, mapping of structures seen in study A onto the images seen in study B.

  ➤ Various registration techniques include point-to-point fitting, interactively superimposing images in the two data sets, and surface or topography matching. An example of image fusion of a CT and magnetic resonance imaging study is shown in Figure 19.1.

- *Image segmentation*: The term *image segmentation* in treatment planning refers to slice-by-slice delineation of anatomic regions of interest, for example, external contours, target volumes, critical normal structures, and anatomic landmarks. Figure 19.2 shows an example of a segmented image for prostate treatment planning.

  ➤ The segmented regions can be rendered in different colors and can be viewed in *beam's eye view* (BEV) configuration or in other planes using *digitally reconstructed radiographs*.

  ➤ Segmentation is also essential for calculating *dose–volume histograms* (DVHs) for the selected regions of interest.

- *Beam aperture design*: Designing beam aperture is aided by the BEV capability of the 3D treatment-planning system. Figure 19.3 shows examples of BEV of beam apertures and dose distributions in transverse, sagittal, and coronal planes.

- *Field multiplicity*: Combination of multileaf collimators and independent jaws provides almost unlimited capability of designing multiple fields of any shape. Targets and critical structures can be viewed in the BEV configuration individually for each field.

- *Plan optimization*: Traditionally, treatment plans can be optimized iteratively by using multiple fields, beam modifiers (e.g., wedges and compensators, etc.), beam weights, and appropriate beam directions.

- *Plan evaluation*: Criteria for an optimal plan include both the biologic and the physical aspects of radiation oncology.

  ➤ *Biologic criteria*: To achieve quantitative biologic end points, models have been developed involving biologic indices such as *tumor control probability* (TCP) and *normal tissue complication probability* (NTCP).

    • *TCP and NTCP*: Although clinical data required to validate TCP and NTCP models are scarce, the concepts are important in plan evaluation.

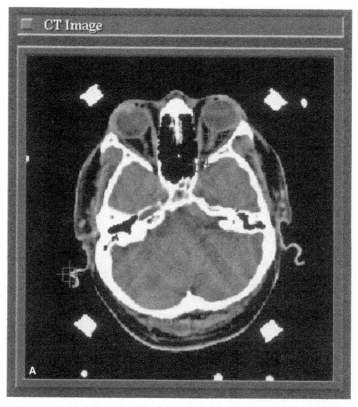

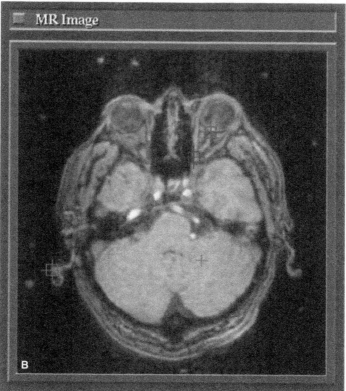

Figure 19.1. An example of fusion between **A:** computed tomography (CT) and **B:** magnetic resonance (MR) images. Three points of correlation were selected for fusion. (*continued*)

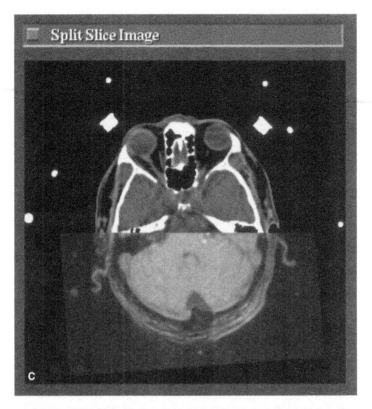

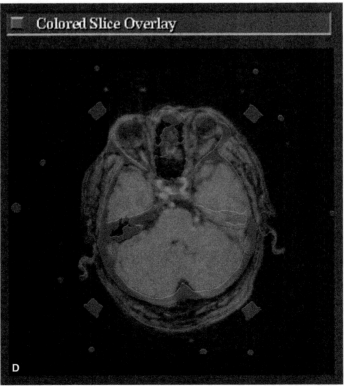

Figure 19.1. (*Continued*) **C:** Split slice image shows correlation at the interface of two images. **D:** Fused image shows slice overlay with CT as red and MR as green.

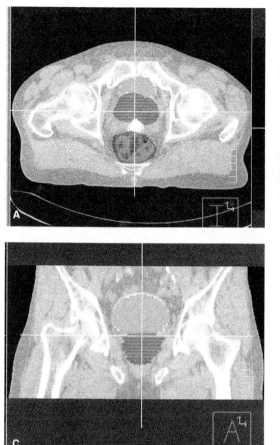
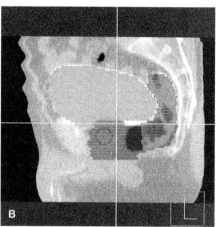

Figure 19.2. Image segmentation for prostate treatment planning. Prostate gland, bladder, and rectum are delineated in different colors. Segmented structures are shown in **A:** transverse, **B:** lateral, and **C:** coronal planes.

Currently most evaluations are carried out on the basis of physical end points, namely, dose distribution within the specified target volumes and dose to *critical organs or organs at risk.*

➤ *Physical criteria:* Tools for the physical aspects of plan evaluation are:
- Isodose curves and surfaces: Dose distributions of competing plans are evaluated by viewing isodose curves in individual slices, orthogonal planes (e.g., transverse, sagittal, and coronal), or 3D isodose surfaces.

➤ The dose distribution is usually normalized to be 100% at the point of dose prescription. This point should be the *International Commission on Radiation Units and Measurements (ICRU) Reference Point* (ICRU Reports 50 and 62), located at the center (or central parts) of the *planning target volume* (PTV).

- *Dose–volume histograms*: The DVH is a tool for evaluating a given plan or comparing competing plans.

DVH may be represented in two forms: the cumulative and the differential.

1. The *cumulative (or integral)* DVH is a plot of the volume of a given structure receiving a certain dose or higher as a function of dose. This is the most common method to display dose to structures in a 3D CRT treatment plan.

2. The *differential* DVH is a plot of volume receiving a dose within a specified dose interval (or dose bin) as a function of dose. The differential form of DVH shows the extent of dose variation within a given structure.

Figure 19.4 shows a 3D CRT plan of glioblastoma with isodose curves and DVHs.

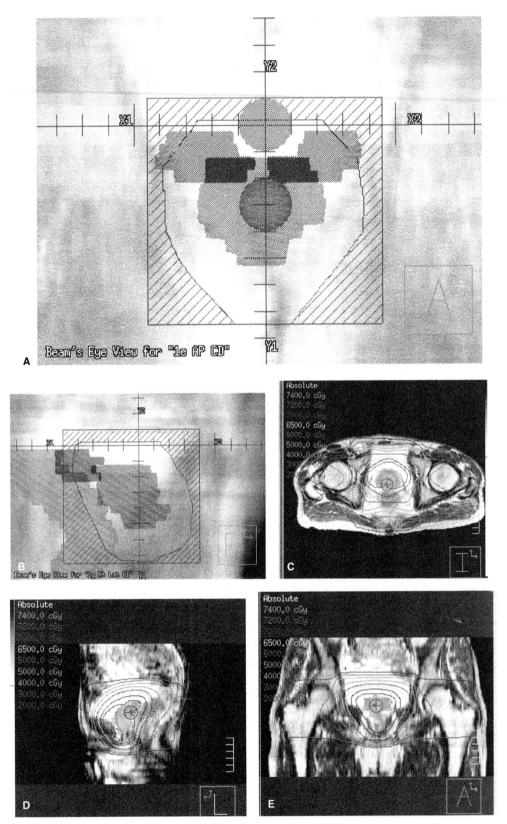

Figure 19.3. **A:** Beam's eye view of anterior-posterior and **B:** left-right lateral fields used in the treatment of prostate gland. Composite (initial plus boost) isodose curves for a four-field plan are displayed in **C:** transverse, **D:** sagittal, and **E:** coronal planes.

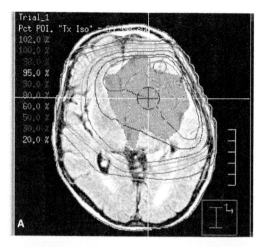

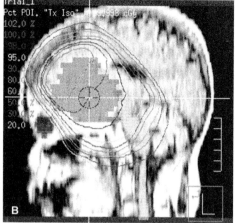

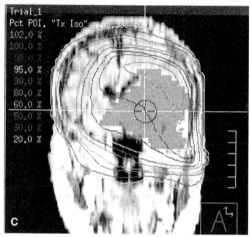

Figure 19.4. A three-dimensional plan for the treatment of glioblastoma is displayed. Isodose curves in **A:** transverse, **B:** lateral, and **C:** coronal planes are used to evaluate the plan. (*continued*)

DELIVERY OF 3D CRT AND VERIFICATION

Implementation of a 3D plan requires spatial registration of the treatment plan with the patient's anatomical landmarks or fiducial markers and the treatment machine. This may be accomplished by comparing the digitally reconstructed radiographs with images obtained by one or more of the following techniques:

- Port films
- Electronic portal imaging device images
- In-room CT scans
- Kilovoltage cone-beam CT
- Megavoltage cone-beam CT
- Helical tomotherapy scans

The above techniques are discussed in Lectures 12 and 25.

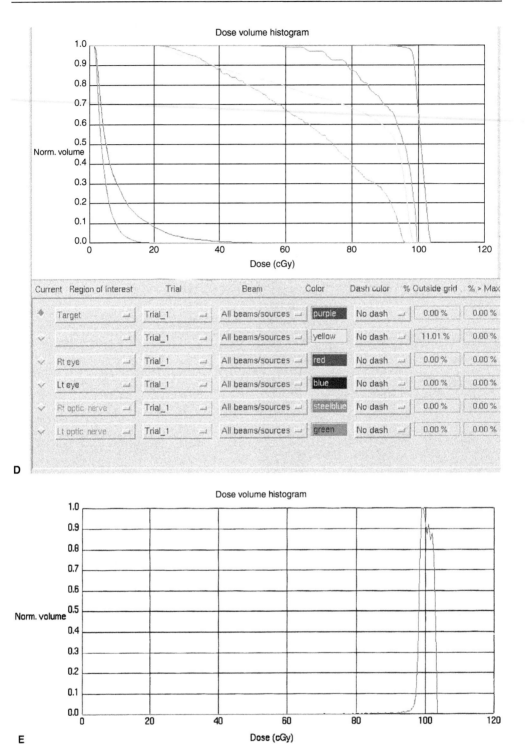

Figure 19.4. (*Continued*) **D:** Cumulative dose–volume histogram (DVH) is also useful in the evaluation process. **E:** Differential DVH shown here for the tumor only is more of an academic interest.

REVIEW QUESTIONS • Chapter 19

✔ **TEST YOURSELF**

Review questions for this chapter are provided online.

In multiple choice questions, more than one option may be correct.

1. In 3D CRT, using multiple photon beams, the ICRU reference point for dose prescription is selected to be:

   a) The point of maximum dose in the PTV
   b) The point of minimum dose in the PTV
   c) The point in the center (or central parts) of the PTV
   d) The point at the isodose level that just covers the PTV

2. The term image registration applies to a process of:

   a) Identifying anatomical landmarks and external fiducials
   b) Correlating CT numbers with electron density of tissues
   c) Correlating patient position with side lasers or infrared surface markers
   d) Comparing and fusing images from one study to those from another

3. Image segmentation refers to:

   a) Dividing the image into segments of high spatial resolution
   b) Adjusting grid size to compute dose distribution in greater detail
   c) Software function that divides the image into subimages for positioning beamlets of different weights for iterative optimization of treatment plan
   d) Slice-by-slice delineation of targets and organs at risk

4. Cumulative DVH is a plot of volume of a given structure receiving:

   a) A certain dose or higher as a function of dose
   b) A certain dose or lower as a function of dose
   c) A certain dose on the average as a function of dose
   d) A certain dose over the volume interval as a function of dose

5. Differential DVH is a plot of volume of a given structure receiving:

   a) A dose higher than the corresponding dose on the abscissa
   b) A dose lower than the corresponding dose on the abscissa
   c) A certain dose within a specified dose interval as a function of dose
   d) Receiving a certain dose most frequently as a function of dose

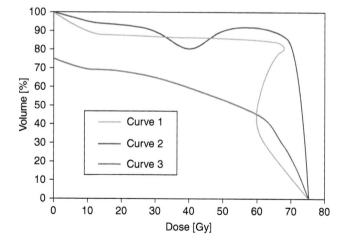

6. Which of the three curves shown above are possible cumulative DVHs:

   a) Curve 3
   b) Curves 2 and 3
   c) Curves 1 and 2
   d) None of the curves
   e) All of the curves

7. Which of the following is/are required to obtain an accurate DVH of a region of interest (ROI):

   a) The CT data set must include entire volume of the ROI
   b) Treatment fields must encompass entire volume of the ROI
   c) At least one treatment field must intersect a portion of the ROI
   d) The dose grid must include the entire ROI volume.
   e) The CT slice spacing must be 2 mm or less.

8. A conformal arc is defined as an arc treatment where the MLC conforms to the shape of the PTV at each gantry angle. What advantage(s) might this treatment have over a conventional 3D CRT?

   a) Reduced volume of normal tissue irradiated
   b) Reduce volume of normal tissue irradiated to high dose levels (e.g., >80% Rx)
   c) Reduced treatment time
   d) Avoidance of radiation passing through critical structures
   e) Optimized beam weighting with gantry angle.

9. 3D volume information allows the use of noncoplanar beam geometries. What advantage(s) might this treatment have over traditional axial coplanar beam geometry?

   a) Reduced volume of normal tissue irradiated
   b) Less CT scan data required for planning
   c) More options to avoid critical structure irradiation
   d) Reduced treatment time

INTENSITY-MODULATED RADIATION THERAPY

REFERENCE
Khan FM. *The Physics of Radiation Therapy,* 4th edition, 2009. Chapter 20 "Intensity-Modulated Radiation Therapy"

IMRT: Commissioning, Treatment Planning, and Delivery

 TOPIC OUTLINE

The following topics will be discussed in this lecture:
➤ Definition and principle
➤ Plan optimization
➤ IMRT delivery
➤ IMRT commissioning
➤ Dosimetry checks
➤ Quality assurance
➤ Dose calculation algorithms
➤ Clinical applications

DEFINITION AND PRINCIPLE

The term intensity-modulated radiation therapy (IMRT) refers to a radiation therapy technique in which nonuniform fluences are delivered to the patient from different directions to optimize the composite dose distribution.

- The treatment criteria for plan optimization are specified by the planner and the optimal fluence profiles for a given set of beam directions are determined through "inverse planning."

- The inverse planning software divides each field into "beamlets" and adjusts their weights or intensities to satisfy predefined dose distribution criteria for the composite plan.

- The optimally modulated fluences are converted into multileaf collimator (MLC) leaf sequence files, which are electronically transmitted to the linear accelerator equipped with the required software and hardware to deliver the intensity-modulated beams (IMBs) as calculated.

PLAN OPTIMIZATION

A number of algorithms have been devised to calculate optimum intensity profiles for IMRT beams. These methods, which are based on inverse planning, can be divided into two broad categories:

1. *Analytic methods*: These involve mathematical techniques in which the desired dose distribution is inverted by using a back projection algorithm. EXAMPLE: If one assumes that the dose

distribution is the result of convolutions of a point-dose kernel and kernel density, then the reverse is also possible, namely, by deconvolving a dose kernel from the desired dose distribution, one can obtain kernel density or fluence distribution in the patient. These fluences can then be projected onto the beam geometry to create incident beam intensity profiles.

2. *Iterative methods*: These involve optimization techniques in which beamlet weights for a given number of beams are iteratively adjusted to minimize the value of a cost function, which quantitatively represents deviation from the desired goal.

➤ The cost function may be a least square function, for example, a quadratic function representing the cost as the root mean squared difference between the desired dose to a volume or structure and the realized dose.

➤ The optimization algorithm attempts to minimize the overall cost at each iteration until the desired goal (close to a predefined dose distribution) is achieved.

➤ An optimization process, called *simulated annealing* has been devised that allows the system to accept some higher costs in pursuit of a global minimum. As the optimization process proceeds, the acceptance probability decreases exponentially until an optimal solution is achieved. The process is analogous to a skier descending from a hilltop to the lowest point in a valley.

IMRT DELIVERY

Many classes of intensity-modulated systems have been devised. These include compensators, wedges, transmission blocks, dynamic jaws, moving bar, MLCs, tomotherapy collimators, and scanned elementary beams of variable intensity. Of these, the computer-controlled MLC is the most commonly used device for delivering IMBs.

• *MLC as intensity modulator*: A computer-controlled MLC is not only useful in shaping beam apertures for conventional radiotherapy, it can also be programmed to deliver IMRT. This has been done in three ways:

➤ *Multisegmented static fields delivery (or Segmented-MLC IMRT)*: This method of IMRT delivery is commonly known as "step-and-shoot" or "stop-and-shoot."

• The patient is treated by multiple fields and each field is subdivided into a set of subfields irradiated with uniform beam intensity levels.

• The subfields are created by the MLC and delivered in a stack arrangement one at a time in sequence without operator intervention. The accelerator is turned off while the leaves move to create the next subfield. The composite of dose increments delivered to each subfield creates the IMB as planned by the treatment planning system.

• The advantage of step-and-shoot method is the ease of implementation from the engineering and safety points of view.

• A possible disadvantage is the instability of some accelerators when the beam is switched "off" (to reset the leaves) and "on" within a fraction of a second.

• Figure 20.1 is an example of intensity-modulated fluence profile generated by the step-and-shoot method and compared with calculated and measured dose.

➤ *Dynamic fields delivery (or DMLC IMRT)*: The method has been commonly called by several names: the "sliding window," "leaf-chasing," "camera-shutter," and "sweeping variable gap."

• In this technique the corresponding (opposing) leaves sweep simultaneously and unidirectionally, each with a potentially different velocity as a function of time.

• The period for which the aperture between leaves remains open (dwell time) allows the delivery of variable intensity to different points in the field.

• The DMLC algorithm for the sliding window is based on the following principles:

- If the spatial gradient of the intensity profile is positive (increasing fluence), the leading leaf should move at the maximum speed and the trailing leaf should provide the required intensity modulation.

- If the gradient is negative (decreasing fluence), the trailing leaf should move at the maximum speed and the leading leaf should provide the required intensity modulation.

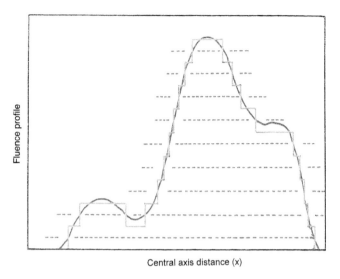

Figure 20.1. Generation of one-dimensional intensity modulation profile. All left leaf settings occur at positions where the fluence is increasing and all right leaf settings occur where the fluence is decreasing. (From Web S. *The Physics of Conformal Radiotherapy*. Bristol, UK: Institute of Physics Publishing; 1997:131, with permission.)

Central axis distance (x)

➤ *Intensity-modulated arc therapy*: The intensity-modulated arc therapy technique combines the dynamic motion of the MLC with arc rotation of the accelerator gantry.

  • During IMAT, the MLC moves dynamically to shape each subfield while the gantry is rotating and the beam is on all the time.

  • Each arc is programmed to deliver one subfield at each gantry angle.

  • The superimposition of subfields (through multiple arcs) creates the intensity modulation of fields at each beam angle.

➤ *Tomotherapy*: Tomotherapy is an IMRT technique in which the patient is treated slice by slice by IMBs in a manner analogous to computed tomography (CT) imaging. A special collimator is designed to generate the IMBs as the gantry rotates around the longitudinal axis of the patient.

➤ *Helical tomotherapy*: This is a method of IMRT delivery in which the linac head and gantry rotate while the patient is translated through the doughnut-shaped aperture in a manner analogous to a helical CT scanner.

  • In the helical tomotherapy, the problem of interslice matchlines is minimized because of the continuous helical motion of the beam around the longitudinal axis of the patient.

  • The tomotherapy unit also provides megavoltage CT scanning for image-guided radiation therapy.

  • Schematic diagrams of the tomotherapy unit and its operation are shown in Figure 20.2A and B. Figure 20.2C shows a photograph of a commercial tomotherapy unit.

IMRT COMMISSIONING

The clinical implementation of IMRT requires careful testing of its component systems: the IMRT treatment-planning system and the IMB delivery system. Details of the commissioning procedures are provided in the American Association of Physicists in Medicine Report 27 (2003). The following tests represent a few selected examples.

  • *Mechanical testing of DMLC*: To assure accurate delivery of IMBs, it is essential that the speed, acceleration, and position of leaves are controlled precisely and accurately as planned.

    ➤ *Test 1—stability of leaf speed*: Individual pairs of opposed leaves should be tested for stability of their speed. This can be accomplished by measuring dose profiles generated by different leaf pairs that are made to move at different speeds (Figure 20.3). Any fluctuations should indicate instability of leaf motion.

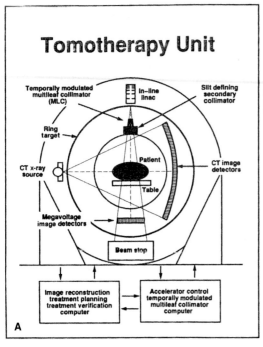

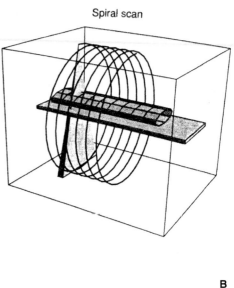

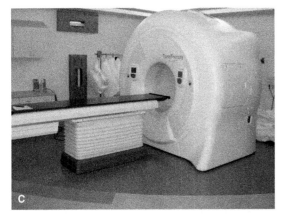

Figure 20.2. **A**, **B:** Schematic diagram of the tomotherapy unit. (From Mackie TR, Holmes T, Swerdloff S, et al. Tomotherapy: a new concept for the delivery of conformal radiotherapy using dynamic collimation. *Med Phys.* 1993;20:1709–1719, with permission.) **C:** Photograph of tomotherapy unit (Tomotherapy Inc., Madison, WI, USA) at the University of Minnesota.

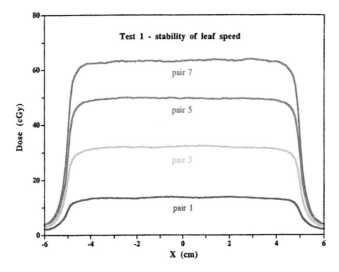

Figure 20.3. Dose profiles obtained with test 1 to check the stability of leaf speed. (From Chui CS, Spirou S, LoSasso T. Testing of dynamic multileaf collimation. *Med Phys.* 1996;23:635–641, with permission.)

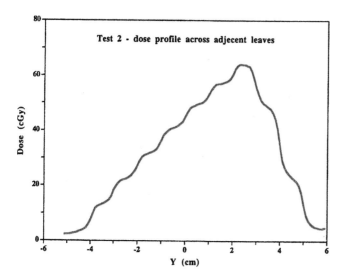

Figure 20.4. Dose profile resulting from test 2 to check dose profile between adjacent leaves. The exposed film is scanned across the leaves in the direction perpendicular to the leaf motion. Because of the spread of secondary electrons and scattered photons, there is no flat dose region within the width of the leaves. (From Chui CS, Spirou S, LoSasso T. Testing of dynamic multileaf collimation. *Med Phys.* 1996;23:635–641, with permission.)

➤ *Test 2—dose profiles across adjacent leaves*: The film obtained with test 1 described above may be scanned in the direction perpendicular to leaf motion (Figure 20.4). In this test one should look for any irregularity in the expected dose profile pattern in the direction perpendicular to the path of leaf motion.

➤ *Test 3—leaf acceleration and deceleration*: Discontinuities in planned intensity profiles could possibly occur as a result of acceleration or deceleration of leaves due to inertia. The extent of any such problem may be determined by repeating test 1 and intentionally interrupting the beam several times (Figure 20.5).

➤ *Test 4—positional accuracy of leaves*: To test the positional accuracy of leaves, the left and right leaves of an opposed pair are made to travel at the same speed but with a time lag between them. Each leaf is instructed to stop at the same position for a fixed duration of beam-on time and then continues its motion as before. Different pairs are instructed to stop at different positions. The uniformity of dose profiles in this case will indicate accurate leaf positioning (Figure 20.6).

➤ *Test 5—overall mechanical check*: The leaves are driven in fixed steps (e.g., 2 cm) with 1-mm-wide gaps created at the stop positions. This will give rise to a pattern of straight dark lines on an irradiated film as shown in Figure 20.7. The test is also known as the Picket Fence test.

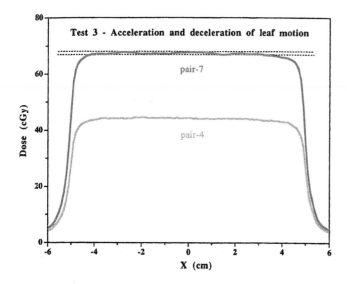

Figure 20.5. Dose profiles resulting from leaf acceleration and deceleration (test 3). A dose variation of ±1% is shown by dotted lines. (From Chui CS, Spirou S, LoSasso T. Testing of dynamic multileaf collimation. *Med Phys.* 1996;23:635–641, with permission.)

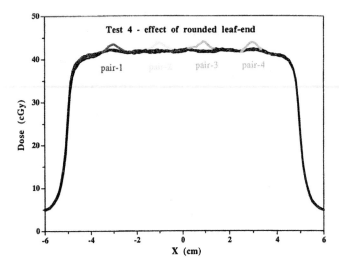

Figure 20.6. Dose profile resulting from test 4 to check positional accuracy and the effect of rounded leaf end. A hot spot of approximately 5% in dose is seen in all profiles. (From Chui CS, Spirou S, LoSasso T. Testing of dynamic multileaf collimation. *Med Phys.* 1996;23:635–641, with permission.)

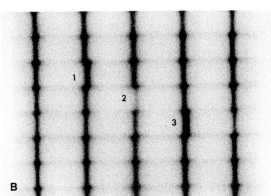

Figure 20.7. Routine mechanical check (test 5). All 26 pairs produce dark lines on film at equally placed positions. If there is a positional error in any leaf, the location or width of the dark lines would differ from the other pairs. **A:** Normal condition with no discernible positional error. **B:** Shift of dark lines caused by an intentional error of 1 mm introduced in three leaf pairs. (From Chui CS, Spirou S, LoSasso T. Testing of dynamic multileaf collimation. *Med Phys.* 1996;23:635–641, with permission.)

DOSIMETRY CHECKS

A series of dosimetric checks have been recommended as part of IMRT commissioning and quality assurance. The following examples pertain to the "sliding window" technique and include measurements of MLC transmission, transmission through leaf ends, head scatter, and dose distribution in selected intensity-modulated fields.

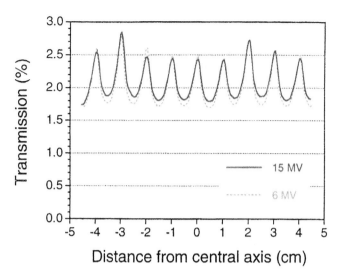

Figure 20.8. The midleaf and interleaf transmission measured with film at isocenter. Transmission is the ratio of dose with the multileaf collimator blocked to that with the field open. Field size = 10×10 cm^2 and depth = 15 cm. (From LoSasso T, Chui CS, Ling CC. Physical and dosimetric aspects of a multileaf collimation system used in the dynamic mode for implementing intensity-modulated radiotherapy. *Med Phys.* 1998;25:1919–1927, with permission.)

- *MLC transmission*: Transmission through the MLC may be determined by measuring dose per monitor unit (MU) in a phantom with the MLC closed and dividing it by dose per MU measured with the MLC open. Figure 20.8 shows the results obtained for a Varian MLC.

- *Head scatter*: A comparative influence of head scatter, MLC transmission, and the rounded edge transmission on target dose versus leaf gap for a dynamic field delivery is shown in Figure 20.9. It is seen that the overall effect of the head scatter as a percentage of the target dose is minimal for this technique. As part of the commissioning procedure, these data should be measured and accounted for in the treatment-planning system.

- *Treatment verification*: The following checks may be used to verify relative dose distribution as well as absolute dose delivered by DMLC for selected fields and treatment plans:

  ➤ *Sliding aperture field*: Using a film placed perpendicular to central axis and at a suitable depth in a phantom (e.g., 10 cm), dose distribution for a 10×10 cm^2 field generated by a sliding MLC aperture (e.g., 5-mm wide) may be compared with a 10×10 cm^2 static field. Absolute dose may also be verified by film dosimetry or by an ion chamber in a water phantom.

  ➤ *Individual field dose distribution*: Individual IMRT fields generated by the treatment planning system may be verified by film dosimetry in a cubic phantom at a suitable depth. These comparisons may also be made using multidetector arrays. Commercial systems are available, which allow side-by-side comparison of calculated compared to measured dose distributions.

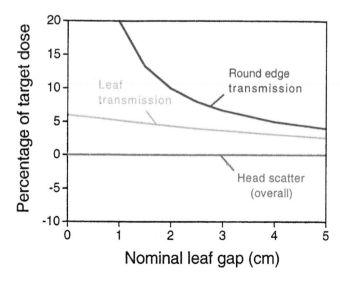

Figure 20.9. Relative contribution of multileaf collimator transmission through midleaf, rounded edge, and overall head scatter. (From LoSasso T, Chui CS, Ling CC. Physical and dosimetric aspects of a multileaf collimation system used in the dynamic mode for implementing intensity modulated radiotherapy. *Med Phys.* 1998;25:1919–1927, with permission.)

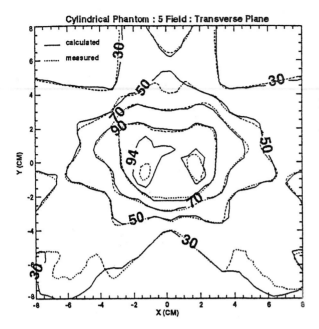

Figure 20.10. Comparison of calculated and measured dose distribution with corrections for multileaf collimator transmission and head scatter. (From LoSasso T, Chui CS, Ling CC. Physical and dosimetric aspects of a multileaf collimation system used in the dynamic mode for implementing intensity modulated radiotherapy. *Med Phys.* 1998;25:1919–1927, with permission.)

➤ *Multiple field plan*: An IMRT plan of a particular patient may be set up on a cylindrical or a cubic phantom to compare the calculated compared to measured distribution. Figure 20.10 is an example of such a comparison.

QUALITY ASSURANCE

A few of the periodic quality assurance tests are listed in Table 20.1. More detailed discussion of various tests and procedures is provided in the American Association of Physicists in Medicine Report 82 (2003).

DOSE CALCULATION ALGORITHMS

Dose calculation algorithms for IMRT are basically the same as those for standard 3D treatment planning (see Chapter 19) except for the dynamic features of multileaf collimation. In-air fluence

TABLE 20.1	IMRT Quality Assurance Program[a]	
Frequency	Procedure	Tolerance
Before first treatment	Individual field verification, plan verification	3% (point dose), other per clinical significance
Daily	Dose to a test point in each IMRT field	3%
Weekly	Static field vs. sliding window field dose distribution as a function of gantry and collimator angles	3% in dose delivery
Annually	All commissioning procedures: stability of leaf speed, leaf acceleration and deceleration, multileaf collimator transmission, leaf positional accuracy, static field vs. sliding window field as a function of gantry and collimator angles, standard plan verification	3% in dose delivery, other per clinical significance

IMRT, intensity-modulated radiation therapy.
[a]As an example for a "sliding window" IMRT program.

distribution is first calculated based on the time (or MUs) a point is exposed to in the open part of the MLC window and the time it is shielded by the leaves. Corrections are applied to take into account leaf edge penumbra, interleaf transmission, and head scatter as a function of MLC aperture and jaw position.

- *In-air fluence distribution*: The algorithm reconstructs the fluence distribution by integrating an output function, which is dependent on whether the point is in the open portion of the field or under the MLC, for example:

$$\Psi(x, y) = \int I_{air}(x,y,t) \cdot T(x,y,t)\, dt$$

where $\Psi(x, y)$ is the photon energy fluence in air at a point (x, y) and $I_{air}(x, y, t)$ the beam intensity or energy fluence rate at time t; $T(x, y, t)$ the leaf transmission factor at any time t, being unity when the point is in the open portion of the field and a transmission fraction when under a jaw or leaf.

- *Depth dose distribution*: Once the photon energy fluence distribution incident on the patient has been calculated, any of the methods discussed in Chapter 19 may be used to compute depth dose distribution. The most commonly used methods are the pencil beam and the convolution/superposition. Monte Carlo techniques are also under development but are considered futuristic at this time because of their limitation on computation speed.

- *Monitor unit calculations*: A manual calculation of monitor units for IMRT is difficult, if not impossible. Reliance is usually made on the treatment planning system to calculate monitor units, following the same algorithm as used in the calculation of dose distribution. The user, however, is encouraged to develop or acquire an independent MU calculation system.

CLINICAL APPLICATIONS

IMRT can be used for any treatment for which external beam radiation therapy is an appropriate choice, *except* where intrafractional motion of the target is large, such as in lung tumors. The basic difference between conventional radiotherapy (including 3D CRT) and IMRT is that the latter provides an extra degree of freedom, that is, intensity modulation, in achieving dose conformity. Especially targets of concave shape surrounding sensitive structures can be treated conformally with steep dose gradients outside the target boundaries—a task that is almost impossible to accomplish with conventional techniques. Figure 20.11 is an example of such a target.

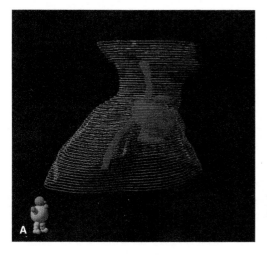
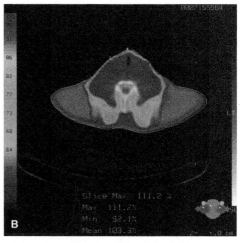

Figure 20.11. **A:** A concave-shaped target of a thyroid tumor in close vicinity of spinal cord and **B:** the intensity-modulated radiation therapy–generated isodose plan in a transverse slice.

REVIEW QUESTIONS • Chapter 20

✔ **TEST YOURSELF**

Review questions for this chapter are provided online.

In multiple choice questions, more than one option may be correct.

1. The intensity-modulated radiation therapy (IMRT) with photons is a radiation therapy technique in which:
   a) Photon energy is modulated to adjust beam penetration across the field.
   b) Photon fluence is modulated to obtain the desired dose distribution.
   c) Photon energy fluence is modulated to obtain the desired dose distribution.
   d) Dose rate in the patient is modulated to obtain the desired dose distribution.

2. In IMRT, the relative contribution to the target dose from collimator transmission scatter is greatest for:
   a) Leaf transmission
   b) Round edge transmission
   c) X-ray jaws
   d) Overall head scatter

3. The typical average value of leakage dose from the multileaf collimator (MLC) relative to the primary dose is approximately:
   a) 0.1%
   b) 1%
   c) 2%
   d) 5%

4. Compared to the four-field box technique, the total number of monitor units (MU) required for an IMRT plan using four fields is:
   a) Approximately the same
   b) Substantially less
   c) Substantially greater
   d) Greater or less depending on the target depth and field sizes

5. In generating an intensity-modulated profile in minimum time with the dynamic MLC:
   a) The opposing pair of leaves should move with equal but variable speed.
   b) The leading leaf should move at the maximum speed and the trailing leaf should provide the required intensity modulation, if the gradient of the intensity profile is positive (increasing fluence).
   c) The trailing leaf should move at the maximum speed and the leading leaf should provide the required intensity modulation, if the spatial gradient of the intensity profile is negative (decreasing fluence).
   d) The two leaves should move with equal and maximum speed, if the spatial gradient of the intensity profile is zero.

6. If majority of the patients are to be treated with IMRT instead of conventional radiotherapy, the structural shielding should be greater for the:
   a) Primary barrier
   b) Barrier for scattered radiation
   c) Barrier for leakage radiation
   d) Secondary barrier

7. The difference between an IMRT and 3-D CRT delivery typically includes:
   a) Non-uniform (modulated) beam intensities
   b) Patient-specific beam-shaping
   c) Inverse planning for dose optimization
   d) Dosimetric or biological objectives with relative weights
   e) Significantly more complex dose calculation algorithm

8. IMRT Delivery techniques include:

   a) Intensity modulated arc therapy
   b) Conformal arc therapy
   c) Helical tomotherapy
   d) Dynamic MLC delivery (DMLC)
   e) Segmental MLC delivery (SMLC)

9. The term "step-and-shoot" is sometimes used to describe which IMRT delivery technique?

   a) Helical tomotherapy
   b) Serial tomotherapy
   c) IMAT
   d) Segmental MLC—IMRT
   e) Dynamic MLC—IMRT

10. For a "step-and-shoot" IMRT treatment delivery, an MLC controller system introduces a 50 millisecond delay between the monitor chamber signal reaching a control point and beam termination. If the initial segment of a field is set to receive 2 MU, what percent error does this delay introduce for this segment if the linac's output is set to 600 MU/min?

    a) <1
    b) 5
    c) 10
    d) 25
    e) 250

11. Which MLC test(s) are unique to dynamic MLC delivery?

    a) Linac performance for small MU delivery.
    b) Leaf positional accuracy
    c) Inter- and intra-leaf leakage
    d) Tongue- and groove effect
    e) Leaf speed accuracy

12. The contribution of MLC leakage to the total dose from an IMRT field:

    a) Is the largest component of the dose
    b) Increases with increase in leaf speed
    c) Increases with increase in leaf gap width
    d) May be neglected in the final dose calculation
    e) None of the above.

STEREOTACTIC RADIATION THERAPY

REFERENCE
Khan FM. *The Physics of Radiation Therapy*, 4th edition, 2009. Chapter 21 "Stereotactic Radiation Therapy"

LECTURE

21

Stereotactic Radiotherapy and Radiosurgery

 TOPIC OUTLINE

The following topics will be discussed in this lecture:

➤ Definition and principle
➤ Stereotactic radiosurgery techniques
➤ Dosimetry
➤ Dose calculation algorithms
➤ Quality assurance
➤ Clinical applications

DEFINITION AND PRINCIPLE

Stereotactic radiation therapy (SRT) is an external beam radiation therapy procedure that uses a combination of stereotactic apparatus and multiple noncoplanar beams directed at a small but well-defined tumor.

- When SRT is applied to a tumor in the brain or spine using a single fraction, it is called *stereotactic radiosurgery* (SRS). If it is applied to tumors outside the brain or spine, it is called *stereotactic body radiation therapy* (SBRT).

- In SRS, the accuracy of beam delivery is strictly controlled by a specially designed stereotactic apparatus (e.g., head frame) that immobilizes the patient during treatment and is used through all steps of the process: imaging, target localization, head immobilization, and treatment setup.

- In SBRT, the accuracy is aided by appropriate patient immobilization and image-guided radiation therapy procedures during treatment.

- The acceptable mechanical accuracy in terms of the radiation isocenter displacement from the specified target center is ±1.0 mm.

- Currently there are three types of radiation modalities used in SRT: ^{60}Co γ-rays, megavoltage x-rays, and heavy charged particles.

- Dose fractionation in SRT may involve a single fraction or hyperfractionated treatments, usually between three and five.

STEREOTACTIC RADIOSURGERY TECHNIQUES

Two SRS techniques are described below: linac-based x-ray knife (or x-knife), and gamma knife.

- *X-ray knife*: This technique consists of using multiple noncoplanar arcs of circular or dynamically shaped x-ray beams converging on to the machine isocenter, which is stereotactically placed at the center of imaged target volume. Figure 21.1 shows a schematic of patient treatment setup.

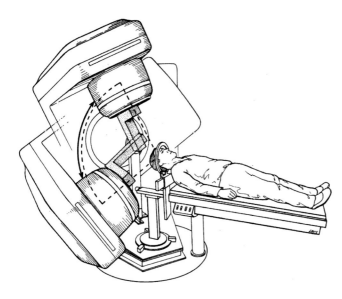

Figure 21.1. Schematic of patient treatment setup showing gantry positions and independent support stand subgantry to maintain isocenter accuracy independent of the linac isocenter accuracy. (From Friedman WA, Bova FJ. The University of Florida radiosurgery systems. *Surg Neurol.* 1989;32:334, with permission.)

- ➤ *Shaping of dose distribution*: Dose distribution can be shaped to fit the target volume conformally by manipulating several parameters, such as:
  - Selectively blocking parts of a circular field
  - Shaping the beams-eye-aperture dynamically with a miniature multileaf collimator
  - Changing arc angles and beam weights
  - Using more than one isocenter
  - Combining stationary beams with arcing beams
- ➤ *Stereotactic frame*: The stereotactic frame for SRS refers to an apparatus that can be attached to the patient's skull as well as to the couch or pedestal for head positioning and immobilization.
  - The frame immobilizes the patient's head and provides coordinates that relate the center of imaged target to the isocenter of treatment.
  - Several frames have been developed for SRS. EXAMPLES: Leksell, Riechert-Mundinger, Todd-Wells, and Brown-Robert-Wells (BRW). Figure 21.2 shows a BRW frame.
  - A special relocatable head ring, called the Gill-Thomas-Cosman, has been designed for fractionated SRT. It uses a bite block system, headrest bracket, and Velcro straps attached to the BRW frame (Figure 21.3).
- ➤ *Beam collimation*: SRS is normally used for small lesions requiring much smaller fields than those for conventional radiation therapy.
  - To reduce geometric penumbra, a tertiary collimation system is used to bring the collimator diaphragm closer to the surface. This may be accomplished in two ways: 1) mounting long cones of different diameters (e.g., 5–50 mm) below the x-ray jaws; 2) installing a miniature multileaf collimator (e.g., micro-multileaf collimator by BrainLab), which can dynamically shape the field to cover the target conformally during arc rotation.

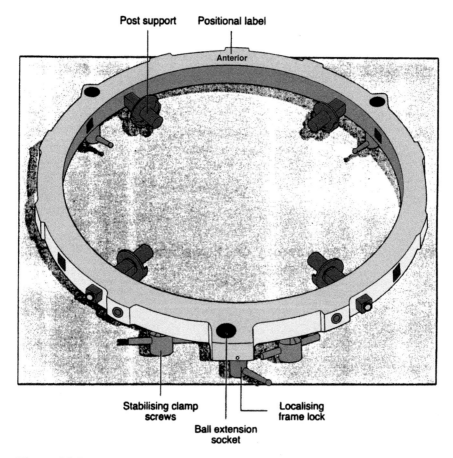

Post support   Positional label

Anterior

Stabilising clamp
screws

Ball extension
socket

Localising
frame lock

Figure 21.2. Schematic drawing of Brown-Robert-Wells frame. (From Cho KH, Gerbi BJ, Hall WA. Stereotactic radiosurgery and radiotherapy. In: Levitt SH, Khan FM, Potish RA, et al., eds. *Technological Basis of Radiation Therapy*. Philadelphia, PA: Lippincott Williams & Wilkins; 1999:147–172, with permission.)

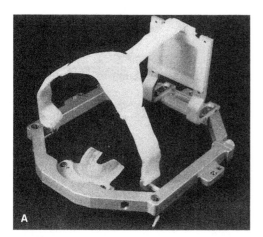
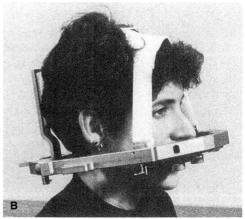

Figure 21.3. **A:** The Gill-Thomas-Cosman (GTC) relocatable head ring with bite block and Velcro straps. **B:** The GTC head ring worn by the patient. (From Cho KH, Gerbi BJ, Hall WA. Stereotactic radiosurgery and radiotherapy. In: Levitt SH, Khan FM, Potish RA, et al., eds. *Technological Basis of Radiation Therapy*. Philadelphia, PA: Lippincott Williams & Wilkins; 1999:147–172, with permission.)

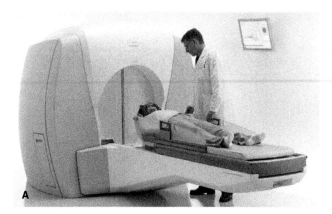
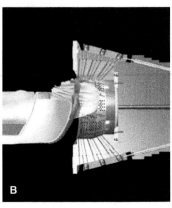

Figure 21.4. Leksell Gamma Knife Perfexion. **A:** Picture of Perfexion unit; **B:** Illustration of the Perfexion collimating system. Courtesy of Elekta Medical Systems. [http://www.elekta.com/healthcare_international_leksell_gamma_knife_perfexion.php]

- *Gamma knife*: The gamma knife delivers radiation to a target lesion in the brain by simultaneous irradiation with a large number of isocentric γ-ray beams. The most recent model of gamma knife unit is the Perfexion, by Elekta Oncology Systems, which is described below (Figure 21.4).

  ➤ In Perfexion, the γ-ray beams can be delivered by any number of 192 ^{60}Co sources, housed in a cylindrical configuration in five rings.

  ➤ The beams are collimated by a single 12-cm-thick tungsten collimator ring array that is subdivided into eight movable sectors, each holding 24 sources.

  ➤ There are three collimator sizes available: 4-, 8-, and 16-mm diameter.

  ➤ A sector containing 24 sources can be moved automatically to a collimator set with any one of the above sizes or to an off position in which all the sources are blocked.

  ➤ The source-to-focus distance for each ring varies from 37.4 to 43.3 cm.

  ➤ The patient is set up in the treatment position by a patient positioning system (PPS) that moves the whole patient (instead of just the patient's head as in the previous models) into preselected *X, Y, Z* stereotactic coordinates.

  ➤ The PPS requires a patient frame adapter that attaches to the standard stereotactic Leksell G frame worn by the patient. The frame adapter is docked directly to the PPS.

  ➤ The patient's head can be locked into one of three possible orientations, called *gamma angles*: 70° (chin up), 90° (chin horizontal), and 110° (chin down).

  ➤ Treatment target in the brain is localized with the Leksell's stereotactic frame attached to the patient's skull and by performing imaging studies, such as computed tomography (CT), magnetic resonance imaging, or angiography.

  ➤ The Perfexion gamma knife allows treatment of one or more tumors in the brain in a single session. It has the potential to treat lesions in the orbits, paranasal sinuses, and cervical spine.

DOSIMETRY

Typically there are three quantities of interest in SRS dosimetry: central axis depth dose distribution (percentage depth dose or tissue-maximum ratios), cross-beam profiles (off-axis ratios), and output factors ($S_{c,p}$ or dose/MU) for various field sizes.

- Depth dose distribution in small fields such as used in SRT should be measured with detectors of size as small as possible compared to the field size.

- For the measurement of central axis depth dose, an essential criterion is that the sensitive volume of the detector should lie within uniform electron fluence generated by photons (e.g., within ±0.5%).

- For a crossbeam profile measurement, the detector size is again important because of the steep dose gradients at the field edges. The dosimeter, in such a case, must have high spatial resolution to measure field penumbra accurately, which is critically important in SRS.

- Several different types of detector systems have been used in SRS dosimetry: ion chambers, film, thermoluminescent dosimeters, and diodes.

- There are advantages and disadvantages to each of the above detector systems. For example:
  - Ion chamber is the most precise and the least energy-dependent system but usually has a size limitation.
  - Film has the best spatial resolution but shows energy dependence and a greater dosimetric uncertainty (e.g., ±3%).
  - Thermoluminescent dosimeters show little energy dependence and can have a small size in the form of chips but suffer from about the same degree of dosimetric uncertainty as the film.
  - Diodes have small size but show energy dependence as well as possible directional dependence.

  Thus the choice of any detector system for SRS dosimetry depends on its size, the quantity to be measured, and the measurement conditions.

DOSE CALCULATION ALGORITHMS

In principle, any of the dose calculation algorithms discussed in Chapters 10 and 19 can be adopted for SRT dose calculations. However, the model-based algorithms (e.g., pencil beam convolution, kernel-based convolution/superposition, and Monte Carlo) are more accurate for heterogeneous tissues that might be encountered (e.g., in SBRT involving lung).

- One of the simplest methods of beam modeling in SRS is based on tissue–maximum ratios, off-axis ratios, exponential attenuation, output factors, and inverse-square law. The beam data are acquired specifically for the beam energy and circular fields, used in SRS, as discussed previously.

- The patient surface contour geometry is defined three dimensionally by CT scans. The multiple arc geometries are simulated by stationary beams separated by angles of 5° to 10°.

- The calculation grid spacing should be small (e.g., 2 × 2 mm) to minimize uncertainty in the calculated dose obtained through interpolation.

QUALITY ASSURANCE

The American Association of Physicists in Medicine (AAPM) TG-40, Report 54, and Report 101 are pertinent quality assurance (QA) protocols. These protocols should provide guidelines for an institution to design its QA program for SRT and SBRT. QA involves both the clinical and physical aspects of SRT. The physics part of the QA may be divided into two categories: treatment QA and routine QA.

- *Treatment QA*: Major components of treatment QA consist of checking:
  - ➤ Stereotactic frame accuracy including phantom base, CT/magnetic resonance imaging/angiographic localizer, pedestal, or couch mount.
  - ➤ Imaging data transfer, treatment plan parameters, target position, and monitor unit calculations.
  - ➤ Frame alignment with gantry and couch eccentricity, congruence of target point with radiation isocenter, collimator setting, cone diameter, couch position, patient immobilization, and safety locks.
  - ➤ Treatment console programming of beam energy, monitor units, arc angles, etc.

- *Routine QA*: A routine QA program is designed to check the hardware/software performance of SRS equipment on a scheduled frequency basis.
  - ➤ For the linear accelerator, the relevant QA protocol is the AAPM TG-40.
  - ➤ For the SRS, the routine QA schedule is recommended by the AAPM Report No. 54.

➤ For SRBT, the recommended QA is given in AAPM Report No. 101.

➤ A QA program for the gamma knife must be compliant with the state or Nuclear Regulatory Commission (NRC) regulations. An example program is published in the AAPM Report No. 54.

CLINICAL APPLICATIONS

- *Stereotactic radiosurgery*: SRS may be used, if indicated, to treat small well-localized tumors of the brain and spine. For example:
  - Arteriovenous malformations (treatment plan shown in Figure 21.5)
  - Meningiomas
  - Acoustic neuromas
  - Gliomas
  - Brain metastases
  - Cavernous angiomas
  - Pituitary adenomas (treatment plan shown in Figure 21.6)
  - Meningiomas
  - Oligodendrogliomas

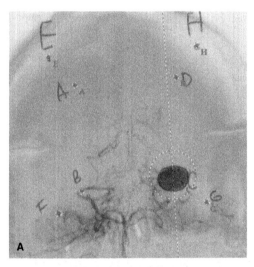

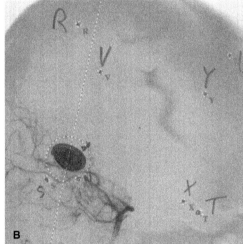

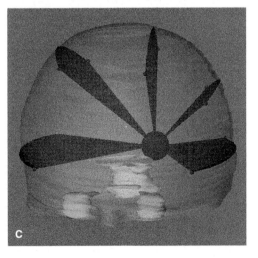

Figure 21.5. An example of stereotactic radiosurgery treatment of arteriovenous malformation. **A:** Anterior angiographic view of nidus. **B:** Lateral view of nidus. **C:** Beam arrangement using five noncoplanar arcs. Isodose surfaces (*color wash*) corresponding to 90% of the maximum dose are shown in the anterior view (**A**) and the lateral view (**B**).

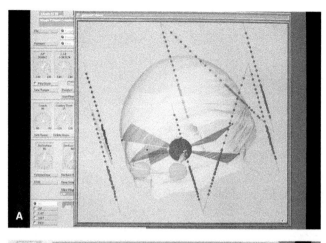

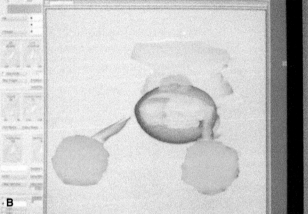

Figure 21.6. Fractional stereotactic radiation therapy of pituitary adenoma. **A:** Beam arrangement with five noncoplanar arcs. **B:** Prescription isodose surface covering the planning treatment volume.

- Certain functional brain disorders (e.g., trigeminal neuralgia)
- Spinal tumors

• *Stereotactic body radiation therapy*: SBRT is used to treat small localized tumors that lie outside the brain and spine. These techniques are frameless, that is, they do not use rigid stereotactic frames to immobilize the body. Instead, the tumor is localized through image guidance systems such as ExacTrac/Novalis Body System, CyberKnife, and helical tomotherapy.

➤ SBRT has been applied to the tumors in the lung, liver, pancreas, kidney, spine, and prostate.

REVIEW QUESTIONS • Chapter 21

✔ **TEST YOURSELF**

Review questions for this chapter are provided online.

In multiple choice questions, more than one option may be correct.

1. In stereotactic radiosurgery (SRS):
   a) All beams are coplanar.
   b) All beams are equally weighted.
   c) All beams are directed at the same point in the target volume.
   d) Geometric accuracy of isocenter localization of ±1 mm is acceptable.

2. For measuring central axis depth dose distribution in small fields such as used in SRS, which detector(s) may require corrections as a function of depth?
   a) Ion chamber
   b) TLD
   c) Diode
   d) Film

3. In a test CT phantom, the errors in individual coordinates of an imbedded target were measured to be 0.3 mm (AP), 0.2 mm (lat), and 0.5 mm (vert). The overall localization error for the CT image is approximately:
   a) 0.3 mm
   b) 0.6 mm
   c) 1.0 mm
   d) 1.5 mm

4. Beam collimation in the linac-based SRS may be provided by long cones mounted below the x-ray jaws. This tertiary collimation is provided *primarily* to:
   a) Assure accuracy of beam alignment
   b) Improve field flatness by side scatter from the cone walls
   c) Reduce transmission penumbra
   d) Reduce geometric penumbra

5. Stereotactic body radiation therapy (SBRT):
   a) Uses a custom-designed stereotactic frame with accuracy comparable to SRS
   b) Delivers higher doses in fewer fractions than the conventional 3D CRT
   c) Delivers a more uniform dose to PTV than possible with 3D CRT
   d) Needs less monitor units to deliver the same dose than with IMRT

6. Which disease(s)/disease site(s) is/are treated with SRS:
   a) Maxillary sinus
   b) Meningioma
   c) Rhabdomyosarcoma
   d) Acoustic neuroma
   e) Pituitary adenoma

7. Which of the following modalities are used to treat SRS/SRT:
   a) Protons
   b) HDR brachytherapy
   c) Neutrons
   d) γ-Ray photons
   e) High-energy electrons

8. SRS treatment plans are characterized by steep dose gradients, for example, >50%/cm, at the target periphery. What is the corresponding dosimetric uncertainty in this region if the spatial accuracy of the treatment delivery is ±1 mm?

   a) <0.5%
   b) 1%
   c) 2%
   d) >5%
   e) >50%

9. Acceptable detectors for the measurement of small field (i.e., <5 mm) output factors used in SRS include:

   a) Farmer-type ion chambers
   b) Diodes
   c) Film
   d) Fricke dosimetry
   e) Parallel plate ion chambers

10. Which measurements are typically made to commission a SRS/SRT program?

   a) TPR versus cone/field size
   b) Transmission factors
   c) OAR versus cone/field size
   d) Output factors versus cone/field size
   e) All of the above

11. The Elekta Gamma Knife:

   a) Uses a couple of hundred ^{60}Co sources aimed at a single focal point
   b) Delivers a 6-MV photon beam
   c) Uses a rotating source system to equally distribute the dose distribution
   d) Is slightly less accurate than a linac-based SRS system
   e) Was the first SRS system used in the world

HIGH-DOSE-RATE BRACHYTHERAPY

REFERENCE

Khan FM. *The Physics of Radiation Therapy*, 4th edition, 2009. Chapter 22 "High-Dose-Rate Brachytherapy"

High-Dose-Rate Brachytherapy: Dosimetry and Treatment Planning

 TOPIC OUTLINE

The following topics will be discussed in this lecture:

➤ High-dose-rate unit
➤ High-dose-rate applicators
➤ Facility design
➤ Licensing requirements
➤ HDR Source calibration
➤ Treatment planning
➤ Clinical applications
➤ Quality assurance

DEFINITION

The International Commission on Radiation Units and Measurements (Report 38) classifies high-dose-rate (HDR) brachytherapy as 20 cGy/minute or higher at the prescription point. In comparison, the prescription dose rate in low-dose-rate (LDR) brachytherapy ranges between 0.5 and 2 cGy/minute, depending on the implant.

HIGH-DOSE-RATE UNIT

Most HDR units contain a single source of ^{192}Ir of high activity (~10 Ci or 370 GBq). The dimensions of the source vary between 0.3 and 0.6 mm in diameter and 3.5 and 10 mm in length, depending on the HDR model. The ^{192}Ir source is welded to the end of a flexible drive cable. The cable with the source attached at the end is also called *source wire*. The HDR unit is equipped with several channels and an indexer system to direct the source to each channel. Channels are provided on a rotating turret in which any channel can be aligned with the source wire path. Applicators or catheters implanted in the patient are connected to the channels by catheters called *transfer tubes* or *transfer guides*. The positioning of the source at the programmed dwell positions in the applicators is accomplished in precise increments by the stepper motors. Figure 22.1 shows an HDR unit (Varian) as an example.

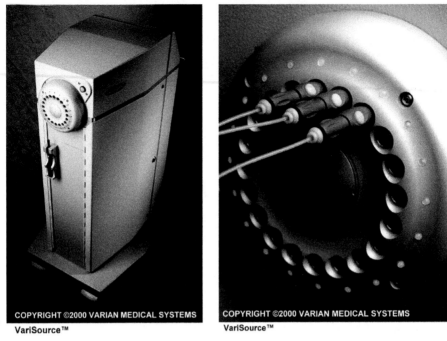

Figure 22.1. **A:** Picture of Varian high-dose-rate unit (VariSource). **B:** Channels on a rotating turret showing transfer guides inserted into the channels. (Courtesy of Varian Associates, Palo Alto, CA, USA).

- The positioning accuracy of the source is approximately ±1 mm.
- The dose control precision is provided by a 0.1-second dwell time resolution.
- In compliance with the Nuclear Regulatory Commission (NRC) regulations, the leakage radiation levels outside the unit do not exceed 1 mR/hour (0.01 mSv/hour) at a distance of 10 cm from the nearest accessible surface surrounding the safe with the source in the shielded position.

HIGH-DOSE-RATE APPLICATORS

Brachytherapy applicators used for LDR implants can also be used for HDR. For example, some of the most commonly used applicators, for various HDR applications, are the following:

- *Fletcher-Suit or Fletcher-Suit-Delclos*: These applicators are used for the treatment of gynecological malignancies of the uterus, cervix, and pelvic side walls.
- *Vaginal cylinder*: These are acrylic cylinders having various diameters and axially drilled holes to accommodate a stainless steel tandem. The applicator is suitable for treating tumors in the vaginal wall.
- *Rectal applicator*: Acrylic cylinders of different diameters are designed to treat superficial tumors of the rectum. Selective shielding is incorporated to spare normal tissue.
- *Intraluminal catheter*: Suitable diameter catheters of various lengths are available for treating intraluminal disease such as endobronchial carcinoma.
- *Nasopharyngeal applicators*: These applicators are used for treating nasopharyngeal tumors with HDR. The applicator set includes tracheal tube, catheter, and a nasopharyngeal connector.
- *Interstitial implants*: Hollow, stainless steel needles are implanted into the tumor following standard brachytherapy rules of implant (see Chapter 15) and closed ended catheters are inserted to accommodate the HDR source wire. EXAMPLES: prostate, breast, and some head and neck tumors.
- *Breast brachytherapy applicators*: Single or multiple-catheter-designed applicators placed postoperatively in lumpectomy cavities for partial breast irradiation. Devices may be surrounded by a saline-filled balloon.

FACILITY DESIGN

- *Room shielding*: The HDR unit must be housed in an adequately shielded room. The shielding and safety requirements are mandated by the NRC (or the state).
  - ➤ The shielding calculations are based on the dose limits specified by the NRC for individual members of the public and for occupational personnel.
  - ➤ The NRC annual effective dose-equivalent limits follow the National Council on Radiation Protection and Measurements guidelines (see Chapter 16).
  - ➤ For HDR, the exposure limit for individual members of the public is 5 mSV (0.5 rem) in 1 year (i.e., the limit for infrequent exposure).
  - ➤ The limit for occupational personnel is 50 mSV (5 rems) in 1 year.
  - ➤ In addition to the annual limits, the NRC requires that the dose in any unrestricted area must not exceed 0.02 mSv (2 mrem) *in any 1 hour*.

  The general principles of calculating primary and secondary barriers are the same as discussed in Chapter 16. The factors relevant to ^{192}Ir source are the following:
  - ➤ Tenth-value layer (TVL) = 5.8 inches of concrete (density 2.35 g cm^{-3}) or 2 cm lead.
  - ➤ Exposure rate constant = 4.69 Rcm^{2}mCi^{-1} h^{-1}.

- *Safety features*: Safety requirements for a dedicated HDR vault or an existing teletherapy room adopted for HDR are mandated by the NRC or state. These include:
  - ➤ Electrical interlock system that retracts the source when the door is opened and does not allow resumption of the treatment unless the door is closed and the interlock is reset.
  - ➤ Mechanism to ensure that only one device can be placed in operation at a given time if the HDR is installed in an existing teletherapy room.
  - ➤ Inaccessibility of console keys to unauthorized persons.
  - ➤ A permanent radiation monitor capable of continuous monitoring of the source status.
  - ➤ Continuous viewing and intercom systems to allow for patient observation during treatment.
  - ➤ Restricted area controls such as signs, locks, visible/audible alarms, and door warning lights indicating "Radiation On."

LICENSING REQUIREMENTS

Purchasers of HDR units must apply for a license or license amendment with the appropriate regulatory agency. In the United States, it is the NRC or the state if it is an Agreement State. Essential items are listed in the application forms. For example:

- Applicant's qualifications: education, training, experience, and a description of personnel training program (initial as well as periodic).
- Administrative requirements: ALARA program, radiation safety officer, radiation safety committee, and a written quality management program.
- Technical requirements: calibration and survey instruments, leak testing and inventory of sources, conditions for patient release, posttreatment survey of patients, and posting of radiation signs.
- Written policies and procedures: general as well as specific tests to assure safe application of the HDR procedure.
- Operating procedures: written procedures to guide the operator step by step in the safe operation of the equipment and treatment delivery.
- Emergency procedures: description of emergency procedures, postings, and locations. These procedures include response to, for example, improper source retraction, electrical power loss, applicator dislodging, timer failure, and other possible emergencies that may occur during the HDR procedure.

HDR SOURCE CALIBRATION

The HDR source must be calibrated at each installation. This calibration must be traceable to the National Institute of Standards and Technology (NIST). Secondary calibration laboratories such as the Accredited Dosimetry Calibration Laboratories (ADCLs) provide chamber calibrations that are "directly traceable" to NIST because ADCLs possess reference class chambers or standard sources that are calibrated by the NIST.

- Calibration of an ^{192}Ir HDR source may be performed with a thimble chamber using open-air geometry but it is a time-consuming procedure and is not suitable for routine calibrations.

- The nuclear medicine well-type chamber ("dose calibrator"), which is commonly used for routine calibration of LDR sources, is not suitable for calibrating HDR sources, because of its overly large sensitive volume and, consequently, too high a sensitivity.

- A well-type reentrant chamber of suitably smaller volume, designed specifically for ^{192}Ir HDR sources, may be used provided it bears a calibration factor provided by the ADCL.

- In the current mode of measurement, the air-kerma strength is calculated as below:

$$S_k = I \times C_{T,P} \times N_{el} \times N_C \times A_{ion} \times P_{ion}$$

where S_k is the air kerma strength of the source, I the current reading, $C_{T,P}$ is the correction for temperature and pressure, N_{el} the electrometer calibration factor, N_C the chamber calibration factor for ^{192}Ir, A_{ion} the ion recombination correction factor at the time of chamber calibration, and P_{ion} the ion recombination correction at the time of source calibration.

- For a routine calibration of the HDR source, it is preferable to use the current mode of measurement because it is free of the source transit effect.

TREATMENT PLANNING

HDR treatment planning involves simulation, 3D computer planning, and plan verification.

- *Simulation*: The simulation process starts with the patient preparation and placement of applicators, catheters, or needles, depending on the procedure. Marker wires are inserted into the applicators all the way to the closed ends. The patient is then simulated using a conventional radiographic simulator (or an isocentric C-arm x-ray unit) and/or a computed tomographic (CT) simulator.

  ➤ In the radiographic simulation procedure, orthogonal radiographs are obtained to localize the applicators and the marker wires. These radiographs allow the radiation oncologist to plan the treatment segment and dwell locations in relation to the distal end of the applicator.

  ➤ In the CT simulation, the applicators are localized three dimensionally in relation to the surrounding organs. The films are reviewed by the physician to make final adjustments to the implant if necessary.

- *3D computer planning*: The computer planning session starts with the input of simulation data.

  ➤ In the case of radiographic simulation, orthogonal radiographs are scanned into the computer and the target volumes as well as organs at risk are outlined on the images. Selected dose specification points are also marked and can be used to optimize dose distributions according to constraints.

  ➤ In the case of CT simulation, the images are directly input into the computer whereby the implant and the surrounding anatomy can be reconstructed three dimensionally. The software allows slice-by-slice delineation of targets, applicators, and organs at risk. The plan is developed and can be viewed in any plane with the overlaid isodose curves. Special CT-compatible applicators are sometimes required to avoid significant artifacts in the simulator images.

- *Dose computation*: Dose distribution around a linear brachytherapy source can be calculated using a number of methods such as Sievert integral, TG-43 formalism (American Association of Physicists in Medicine [AAPM] Task Group No. 43) or Monte Carlo calculations. Of these, the TG-43 formalism and Monte Carlo are most commonly used for calculating dose distribution around the HDR ^{192}Ir source.

➤ Basic data for a number of commercial HDR sources have been measured or calculated using TG-43 and Monte Carlo.

➤ Along and away tables, dose rate constant, radial dose function, and anisotropy function for these sources have been published, which can be used as the basis of a dose computation algorithm.

• *Plan verification*: Independent verification of a computer plan is an essential part of HDR quality assurance (QA). Some of these checks consist of:

➤ Verifying the accuracy of input data such as dose prescription, catheter lengths, dwell times, and current source strength.

➤ Independent spot check of dose calculation, manually or by a second computer program. Verification of the dose at the prescription point (or another suitable point) within ±5% is considered reasonable, considering the severe dose gradients around the source.

CLINICAL APPLICATIONS

HDR brachytherapy can be used essentially for any cancer that is suitable for LDR brachytherapy. The most common uses of HDR are in the treatment of:

- Endobronchial obstruction by lung cancer
- Cancer of the esophagus
- Cervical cancer
- Postoperative treatment of endometrial carcinoma (vaginal cuff irradiation)
- Localized prostate cancer
- Post-lumpectomy breast cancer

QUALITY ASSURANCE

A policy and guidance directive for the HDR brachytherapy license has been published by the NRC, which provides a template for designing a quality management program acceptable to the NRC (or Agreement State). In addition, the relevant AAPM reports (TG-40, TG-56, and TG-59) should be consulted.

• The AAPM recommends QA tests at three frequencies: daily, quarterly, and annually.

• Unless HDR treatments are given every day, it is sufficient to perform "daily QA" tests only on days when patients are treated. These tests are described in Chapter 22 of the Textbook (Section 22.3).

• Quarterly QA essentially consists of source calibration and a more thorough review of equipment function. The quarterly interval coincides with the frequency with which HDR sources are replaced.

• The annual QA is a comprehensive review of all equipment, procedures, and patient records, approaching the thoroughness of initial acceptance testing/commissioning of the system.

REVIEW QUESTIONS • Chapter 22

✔ **TEST YOURSELF**

Review questions for this chapter are provided online.

In multiple choice questions, more than one option may be correct.

1. According to the ICRU, high-dose-rate (HDR) brachytherapy is classified as brachytherapy with a prescription dose rate of:
   a) 2 cGy/min or higher
   b) 10 cGy/min or higher
   c) 20 cGy/min or higher
   d) 40 cGy/min or higher

2. An HDR ^{192}Ir source has an apparent activity of 10 Ci. What is its air kerma strength in units of cGycm^2 h^{-1}? [Assume exposure rate constant of ^{192}Ir to be 4.69 Rcm^{2}mCi^{-1} h^{-1}.]
   a) 4.11×10^4
   b) 4.50×10^4
   c) 4.89×10^4
   d) 5.37×10^4

3. Assuming dose rate constant (Λ) for the source in the above problem to be 1.12 cGyh^{-1}U^{-1} (1 U = 1 cGycm^2 h^{-1}), the geometry factor (G) to be 1.023, and the radial dose function (g) to be unity, what is dose rate in tissue in cGy/second at a distance of 1 cm, measured transversely from the center of the source?
   a) 9.5
   b) 11.4
   c) 12.8
   d) 13.1

4. According to the NRC regulations regarding HDR unit, the leakage radiation levels at a distance of 10 cm from accessible surface surrounding the safe, with the source in the shielded position, must not exceed:
   a) 1 mR/hour
   b) 2 mR/hour
   c) 5 mR/hour
   d) 10 mR/hour

5. According to the NRC regulations regarding room shielding for the HDR, the dose in any unrestricted area outside the room must not exceed:
   a) 2 mrem/hour
   b) 2 mrem in any 1 hour
   c) 10 mrem/hour
   d) 10 mrem in any 1 hour

6. A new 10 Ci Ir^{192} HDR source is used in a Gyn-brachytherapy treatment that takes 16 min. If 80% of this time is due to source dwell times, how long would the total treatment 90 days later to deliver the same dose, using the same treatment plan and source?
   a) Same time
   b) 26 minute
   c) 33 minute
   d) 37 minute
   e) 47 minute

7. A single HDR dwell position is planned inside a balloon applicator placed in a lumpectomy cavity for a partial breast brachytherapy procedure. The balloon is filled to a 2.0 cm radius, and the prescription point is taken to be 1.0 cm from the balloon/tissue interface along the perpendicular bisector of the center of the source. If the balloon is asymmetric such that the source is displaced 2 mm toward the prescription point, what is the percent deviation from the prescribed dose?

   a) No change
   b) <0.5
   c) 3.4
   d) 12.9
   e) 14.8

8. For the implant above, the planning protocol requires the skin dose to be limited to 145% of the prescribed dose. If the source is placed in the center of the balloon, what is the minimum distance permitted from the balloon to the skin surface (along the perpendicular bisector of the source center)?

   a) 1 mm
   b) 3 mm
   c) 5 mm
   d) 7 mm
   e) 10 mm

9. What advantage(s) does ^{192}Ir have over both ^{60}Co and ^{137}Cs for HDR brachytherapy source material?

   a) Larger half-life
   b) Higher specific activity
   c) Higher average energy
   d) Higher HVL
   e) All of the above

10. What sites are treated with HDR brachytherapy?

    a) Lung cancer
    b) Esophageal cancer
    c) Pituitary adenoma
    d) Cervical cancer

PROSTATE IMPLANTS

Prostate Implants: Technique, Dosimetry, and Treatment Planning

 TOPIC OUTLINE

The following topics will be discussed in this lecture:
- ➤ Seed implants
  - Volume study
  - Treatment planning
  - Implant procedure
  - Radiation protection
- ➤ Implant dosimetry
- ➤ High-dose-rate implants

SEED IMPLANTS

Permanent implants with ^{125}I or ^{103}Pd are used in the treatment of early stage prostate cancer as the sole modality or in combination with external beam radiation therapy. The target volume for implantation is the prostate gland itself, with minimal margins allowed to account for uncertainty of prostate localization.

The modern technique of implantation consists of a transperineal approach in which ^{125}I or ^{103}Pd seeds are inserted into the prostate gland with the guidance of transrectal ultrasonography and perineal template. The procedure is nonsurgical and performed on an outpatient basis. The implant is done in an approved operating room with the patient requiring a spinal anesthetic.

VOLUME STUDY

Localization of prostate by a series of transverse ultrasound images constitutes a *volume study*.

- Prior to the volume study, evaluation is made from computed tomographic (CT) scans of the prostate gland size and the pubic arch in relation to the prostate. In the case of a large gland and possible pubic arch interference to needle implantation, the patient may need hormonal therapy for a few months to shrink the gland to allow for an adequate implant.

- The patient is placed in the dorsal lithotomy position and the transrectal ultrasound probe (5–6-MHz transducer) is securely anchored to obtain transverse images of the prostate gland from base to apex at 5-mm intervals.

TREATMENT PLANNING

A treatment-planning system specifically designed for prostate implants allows the target outlines from the volume study to be digitized into the computer.

- The implant is typically planned with an interseed spacing of 1 cm (center to center) and a needle spacing of 1 cm.

- The seed strength can be adjusted to deliver a prescribed *minimum peripheral dose*—the dose to the isodose surface just covering the prostate target volume.

- Based on the approved computer plan, a worksheet is prepared specifying the number of needles, seeds in each needle, and the template coordinates for needle positions. Figure 23.1 shows an example of preimplant treatment plan for ^{125}I along with the dose–volume histogram (DVH) and statistics.

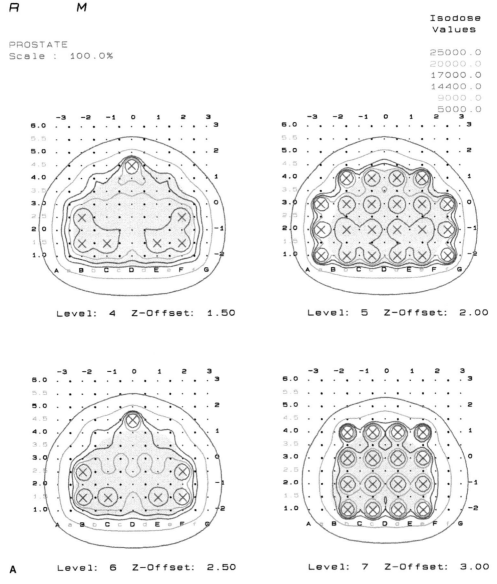

Figure 23.1. A sample of pretreatment plan with ^{125}I seeds showing (**A**) seeds and isodose curves in four ultrasound cross sections of prostate gland and (**B**) dose–volume histogram for target (prostate) and normal tissues (rectum). (*continued*)

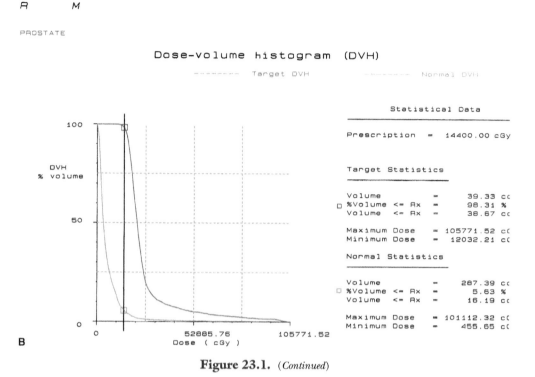

Figure 23.1. (*Continued*)

- Distribution of seeds and isodose curves is reviewed in each ultrasound cross section to assure adequate coverage of the target volume and sparing of normal tissue. DVHs for the target and the critical structures are useful to provide overall statistical evaluation of the treatment plan.

- Critical structures or *organs at risk* in a prostate implant are the urethra, rectum, and bladder. These structures must be outlined in the plan so that they can be viewed in the isodose plans and DVHs. Careful planning is important to avoid high doses to these structures.

- Postimplant dosimetry should be performed using CT scans to assess stability of the implant after swelling of the prostate gland has gone down. Figure 23.2 shows postimplant changes in the isodose plan as result of source movement.

- Treatment plans are calculated using a point source model for the seeds.

- Source anisotropy is a serious problem because of the low photon energy and severe attenuation along the length of the seeds. This problem is somewhat reduced by the randomness of source orientation that naturally develops after implantation and also by using sources that have been designed with reduced anisotropy.

IMPLANT PROCEDURES

The implant procedure is carried out as an outpatient treatment in an operating room with the patient in the dorsal lithotomy position under spinal anesthesia. Figure 23.3 shows the implantation apparatus consisting of a transrectal ultrasound probe and a template to guide specifically designed sterile 18-gauge, 21-cm long needles.

- The needles loaded with seeds are inserted one at a time into the prostate using the ultrasound and template guidance.

- After verifying the needle position, the needle is slowly withdrawn while the plunger is held stationary. This action results in the injection of the seeds and the spacers into the tissues along the track of the withdrawing needle.

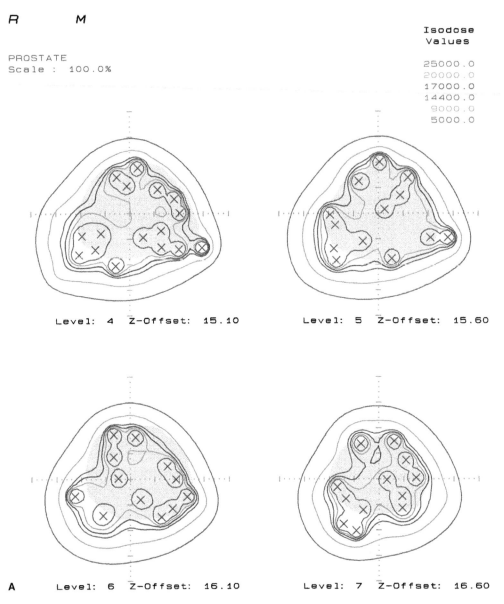

Figure 23.2. A sample of posttreatment plan of the same patient as in Figure 23.1, showing (**A**) seeds and isodose curves in the four ultrasound cross sections of the prostate gland and (**B**) dose–volume histogram for target (prostate) and normal tissues (rectum). (*continued*)

- Final verification of the implant is made with anteroposterior fluoroscopy in the operating room.
- Cystoscopy is performed at the conclusion of the procedure to retrieve any stray seeds in the bladder or the urethra.

RADIATION PROTECTION

The American Association of Physicists in Medicine (AAPM) code of practice for brachytherapy (TG-56) is a comprehensive document on the physics and quality assurance of brachytherapy procedures. The technique and dosimetry of permanent seed implants are discussed in the AAPM TG-64 Report. Before implementing a prostate implant program, one should consult these documents together with the relevant Nuclear Regulatory Commission regulations.

R   M

PROSTATE

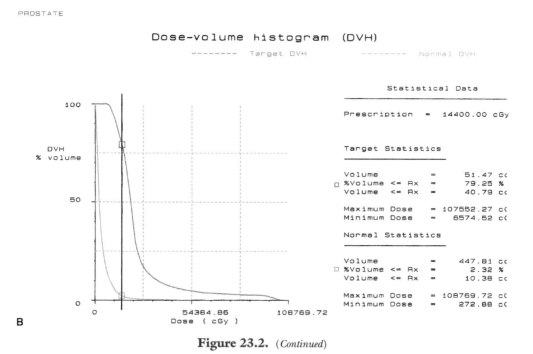

Dose-volume histogram (DVH)

-------- Target DVH   -------- Normal DVH

Statistical Data		
Prescription	=	14400.00 cGy

Target Statistics

Volume	=	51.47 cc
%Volume <= Rx	=	79.25 %
Volume <= Rx	=	40.79 cc
Maximum Dose	=	107552.27 cc
Minimum Dose	=	6574.52 cc

Normal Statistics

Volume	=	447.81 cc
%Volume <= Rx	=	2.32 %
Volume <= Rx	=	10.38 cc
Maximum Dose	=	108769.72 cc
Minimum Dose	=	272.88 cc

DVH % volume

100

50

0

0   54384.86   108769.72
Dose (cGy)

B

Figure 23.2. (*Continued*)

- During the implant procedure, a medical physicist or dosimetrist assisting in the procedure must assure that the total number of seeds is accounted for at all times.
- A thin-window Geiger-Müller tube or a scintillation counter should be available to locate any dropped or misplaced seed.
- Personnel should not be allowed to leave the operating room without being surveyed to prevent accidental transport of any seed outside the room.
- At the conclusion of the procedure, the trash, the room, and the personnel should be surveyed for any misplaced seed.
- The essential requirement for releasing a permanent implant patient from the hospital is that the total exposure to any other individual from the released patient does not exceed 0.5 rem over the life of the implant.

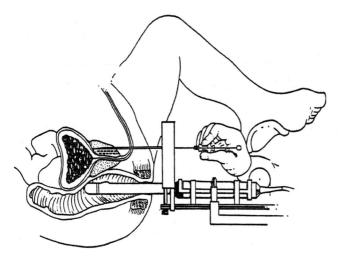

Figure 23.3. Schematic diagram showing ultrasound-guided transperineal template implant procedure. (From Grim PD, Blasko JC, Ragde H. Ultrasound-guided transperineal implantation of iodine-125 and palladium-103 for the treatment of early-stage prostate cancer. *Atlas Urol Clin N Am.* 1994; 2:113–125, with permission.)

- Patients are instructed at the time of discharge to observe certain precautions. For example, they are advised:

  - Not to have prolonged physical contact with pregnant women or young children for a period of 2 months.

  - To abstain from sexual intercourse or use condoms for the first few weeks in case a seed is discharged during intercourse.

IMPLANT DOSIMETRY

- *Source calibration*: Brachytherapy sources are calibrated by the vendor before shipment and bear a calibration certificate with stated limits of uncertainty, usually 10%. Although vendor calibrations are, in most cases, traceable to the National Institute of Standards and Technology, the user is advised to check the calibration values of a sample of sources from the batch as a matter of quality assurance.

  - Agreement within ±5% with the vendor calibration is acceptable, in which case the vendor values may be used for patient dose calculations. In case of a larger disagreement, the user must resolve the difference with the vendor and if unsuccessful, use the in-house calibration, with full documentation of the procedure used.

  - The most suitable method of routine calibration of brachytherapy sources is the well ionization or reentrant chamber.

  - The well-chamber response depends significantly on the energy of radiation, source construction, and source position along the chamber axis.

  - The well chamber calibration for given types of sources may be obtained from the Accredited Dose Calibration Laboratories (ADCLs) that maintain traceability with the National Institute of Standards and Technology. Alternatively, the chamber may be calibrated in-house by using a standard source of the same type, which has been calibrated by an Accredited Dose Calibration Laboratory.

  - The standard source should not only be the same radionuclide but also have the same construction or model.

  - In addition, the calibration geometry (source position along the chamber axis) should be the same for the standard source as for the source to be calibrated. If different source positions are used, appropriate corrections should be determined as a function of source position.

- *Dose computation algorithm*: Dose distribution around ^{125}I, ^{103}Pd, or ^{192}Ir is not isotropic. Analytical methods of dose calculations such as Sievert integral are not suitable for these sources because of complexity in source construction, filtration, and low energy of the emitted radiation. The AAPM Task Group 43 formalism and Monte Carlo are better suited for these sources. The general TG-43 equation (Equation 15.16 in the Textbook) for the calibration of dose at a point $P(r,\theta)$, which includes anisotropy effects, is as follows:

$$\dot{D}(r,\theta) = \Lambda S_k \frac{G(r,\theta)}{G(1,\pi/2)} g(r) F(r,\theta)$$

where $\dot{D}(r,\theta)$ is the dose rate at point P in a medium (e.g., water), Λ the dose rate constant, S_k the air kerma strength of the source, G the geometry factor, g the radial dose function, and F the anisotropy function.

  - For a point source, the above equation reduces to:

$$\dot{D}(r) = \Lambda S_k \frac{g(r)}{r^2} \bar{\phi}_{an}(r)$$

where $\bar{\phi}_{an}(r)$ is the average anisotropy factor. Current values of Λ, $g(r)$ and $\bar{\phi}_{an}(r)$ for prostate implant sources are provided in Tables 15.4–15.7 of the Textbook.

- *Total dose*: As the sources decay with a half-life $T_{1/2}$, the dose rate decreases exponentially with time t as:

$$\dot{D} = \dot{D}_0 e^{-0.693\,t/T_{1/2}}$$

where $\dot{D}$ is the dose rate at any time t and $\dot{D}_0$ the initial dose rate. The cumulated dose D_c in time t is given by:

$$D_c = \dot{D}_0(1.44\,T_{1/2})\,(1 - e^{0.693\,t/T_{1/2}})$$

For a permanent implant, the total dose D_{total} is delivered after complete decay of the sources and is given by:

$$D_{total} = 1.44\,\dot{D}_0 T_{1/2}$$

➤ For respective total doses prescribed, the dose rate for a ^{103}Pd implant is typically about three times that for an ^{125}I implant.

➤ In the case of ^{103}Pd, because of its shorter half-life, the bulk of the prescribed dose (approximately 70%) is delivered in the first month.

HIGH-DOSE-RATE IMPLANTS

The high-dose-rate (HDR) ^{192}Ir brachytherapy for prostate cancer is an alternative technique to the low-dose-rate brachytherapy using seeds.

- *Volume study*: The patient is placed in a lithotomy position and receives epidural anesthesia. The volume study involves the following steps:

  ➤ A transrectal ultrasound probe is used to evaluate the prostate gland. Coronal and sagittal images allow the determination of prostate volume.

  ➤ A prostate gland template is sutured transperineally and HDR guide needles are implanted into the prostate gland with ultrasound guidance (Figure 23.4A). Ten to fifteen needles are usually required to cover the prostate gland.

    - The bladder is filled with Hypaque and dummy source wires are loaded into the guide needles to obtain intraoperative x-ray localization radiographs. The patient is sent to the recovery room and subsequently simulated to obtain orthogonal films for HDR treatment planning.

- *Treatment planning*: Treatment-planning algorithms for HDR have been discussed in Chapter 22. These programs are based on either orthogonal films or CT data. Dwell times of the source in each needle are calculated to provide optimized dose distribution.

  ➤ CT-based treatment planning provides full 3D dose distributions including slice-by-slice isodose curves, isodose surfaces, and DVH.

- *HDR procedure*: After the treatment plan has been optimized and approved, the guide needles are connected to the HDR afterloader through adapters and transfer catheters (Figure 23.4B,C) and the treatment is delivered as planned.

  ➤ At the conclusion of the treatment, the transfer catheters are disconnected from the adapters and the patient is sent to his or her room.

  ➤ The total dose typically ranges from 10 to 25 Gy (minimum isodose surface) given in three to four fractions. This dose is given in addition to the 45 Gy of external beam radiation therapy.

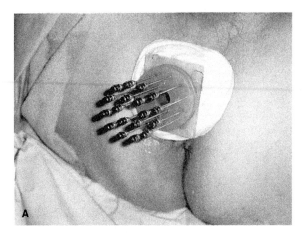

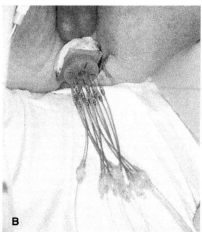

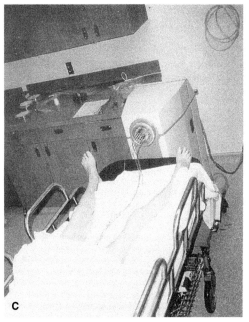

Figure 23.4. Prostate implant procedure using ultrasound-guided high-dose-rate (HDR) procedure showing (**A**) implant needles in place, (**B**) flexible adapters screwed into guide needles, and (**C**) flexible adapters connected to the HDR remote afterloaders. (From Syed AMN, Puthawala AA, Barth N, et al. High dose rate brachytherapy treatment of the prostate: preliminary results. *J Brachytherapy Int.* 1997; 13:315–331, with permission.)

REVIEW QUESTIONS • Chapter 23

✔ **TEST YOURSELF**

Review questions for this chapter are provided online.

In multiple choice questions, more than one option may be correct.

1. The air kerma strength (μGym^2 h^{-1}) of a brachytherapy source depends on:

   a) Photon energies emitted
   b) Exposure rate constant of the source
   c) Active length of the source
   d) Tissue attenuation and scattering

2. The dose rate constant, Λ, of a brachytherapy source depends on:

   a) Photon energies emitted
   b) Exposure rate constant of the source
   c) Source construction
   d) Source encapsulation

3. The geometry factor, G, for a brachytherapy source:

   a) Depends on source construction
   b) Depends on active length
   c) Depends on photon attenuation and scattering in the medium
   d) Follows inverse square law with distance from the source

4. The radial dose function, g, for a brachytherapy source depends on:

   a) Photon energies emitted
   b) Active length
   c) Photon attenuation in source encapsulation
   d) Photon attenuation and scattering in the medium along the transverse axis

5. The anisotropy factor, F, for a brachytherapy source:

   a) Depends on photon energies emitted
   b) Accounts for angular dependence of photon attenuation and scattering in the encapsulation
   c) Accounts for angular dependence of photon attenuation and scattering in the medium
   d) Is normalized to the dose at the transverse axis of the source

6. A ^{125}I brachytherapy seed has an apparent activity of 0.3 mCi. Given the exposure rate constant of ^{125}I source to be 1.46 Rcm^{2}mCi^{-1} h^{-1}, what is the air kerma strength of the seed in units of μGym^2 h^{-1}?

   a) 0.38
   b) 0.42
   c) 0.44
   d) 0.50

7. If the seed in the above problem is implanted in tissue, what is the dose rate in tissue in cGy/hour at a distance of 0.5 cm along the transverse axis of the seed? (Given the dose rate constant for the seed to be 0.965 cGyh^{-1}U^{-1} [where U is air kerma strength in units of μGym^2 h^{-1}], the geometry factor G to be 0.97, and the radial dose function g to be 1.04.)

   a) 0.37
   b) 0.67
   c) 0.97
   d) 1.41

8. What fraction of the dose from an ^{125}I permanent implant is delivered in the first month (30 days)?

   a) <5%
   b) 11.3%
   c) 29.5%
   d) 39.7%
   e) 70%

9. Why are ^{125}I and ^{103}Pd typically used for prostate implants?

   a) The cost/source is small compared to alternatives.
   b) Large dose anisotropy protects structures superior and inferior to implant.
   c) The smaller source size for each allows more flexibility in the implant.
   d) Reduced radiation safety issues.
   e) Lower energies reduce the dose to surrounding critical structures.

10. Which critical structure(s) is/are of most concern for permanent prostate implants?

    a) Bladder
    b) Rectum
    c) Femoral heads
    d) Urethra
    e) Small bowel

11. A prostate implant with ^{103}Pd seeds delivers a total prescription dose (after complete decay) of 125 Gy. What is the prescription dose delivered in the first month? [Given half-life of ^{103}Pd to be 17 days.]

    a) 37.0 Gy
    b) 69.9 Gy
    c) 88.2 Gy
    d) 114.0 Gy

12. In the above problem, in how many days about 70% of the total dose is delivered?

    a) 25
    b) 30
    c) 53
    d) 58

INTRAVASCULAR BRACHYTHERAPY

REFERENCE

Khan FM. *The Physics of Radiation Therapy,* 4th edition, 2009. Chapter 24 "Intravascular Brachytherapy"

Intravascular Brachytherapy: Techniques and Dosimetry

 TOPIC OUTLINE

The following topics will be discussed in this lecture:

➤ Clinical application
➤ Treatment volume
➤ Irradiation techniques
➤ Dosimetry
➤ Measurement of dose distribution

Note: Since the development of drug-eluting stents (DES), intravascular brachytherapy (IVBT) is being phased out as a primary treatment for restenosis. I debated whether this topic should be included in the Lectures. However, there have been reports in the recent literature that the use of IVBT after DES can further decrease the likelihood of restenosis. In view of this and the possibility that IVBT may be used in future studies, I have kept the topic in.

CLINICAL APPLICATION

Intravascular brachytherapy (IVBT) is used to reduce the incidence of *restenosis* (re-narrowing of artery) following the removal or reduction of artery blockage with angioplasty (a procedure to widen the narrowed blood vessel using a balloon catheter).

• Most restenosis after angioplasty or stenting is caused by thrombosis or blood clotting at the percutaneous transluminal coronary angioplasty site (PTCA), which can be prevented partially by using anticlotting drugs. However, another process, which begins within days after angioplasty, is the neointimal growth of tissues prompted by the wound-healing process following tissue injury by angioplasty. This component of restenosis cannot be prevented by anticoagulants or stents.

• Incidence of restenosis because of neointimal hyperplasia may be reduced by one of the following procedures:

➤ Use of IVBT following angioplasty and coronary stent implantation.

➤ Implantation of DES following angioplasty.

➤ Use of IVBT following angioplasty and DES implantation.

TREATMENT VOLUME

Target volume for IVBT is confined to the region of angioplasty. Typically, it is 2 to 5 cm in length of artery and 0.5 to 2 mm in thickness of arterial wall. Occasionally, these dimensions may be exceeded depending on the location and extent of the disease. With 3 to 5 mm of luminal diameter, the radial range of treatment may extend as far as to approximately 5 mm from the center of the artery.

- The depth of dose prescription for intracoronary irradiation is recommended by the American Association of Physicists in Medicine (AAPM TG-60) to be 2 mm from the center of the source and for the peripheral arteries 2 mm beyond the average lumen radius.

IRRADIATION TECHNIQUES

Intravascular brachytherapy techniques may be classified into two categories: temporary implants (sealed sources or liquid-filled balloons) and permanent implants (radioactive stents). Each method has its advantages and limitations, but the catheter-based sealed source is the most commonly used method of treatment.

- *Radiation sources*: A variety of β- and γ-ray sources are available for IVBT. Typical dosimetric requirements of a temporary intravascular implant are the following:

   a. Deliver a target dose of 15 to 20 Gy to a 2- to 3-cm length of the involved arterial wall at a radial distance of approximately 2 mm from the source center;

   b. Minimize the dose to tissues outside the region of angioplasty (target volume);

   c. Provide target dose rates on the order of 5 Gy/minute or greater to minimize the time of completion of the procedure.

   ➤ Above requirements suggest the suitability of high-energy β-ray sources (e.g., strontium-90, yttrium-90, and phosphorus-32) or high activity γ-ray sources (e.g., iridium-192).

   ➤ γ-Ray source could be a high-dose-rate unit with the source dimensions small enough to allow IVBT.

   ➤ β-Ray sources have several advantages over γ-ray sources: higher specific activity, higher dose rate, longer half-life, and greater radiation safety for the patient as well as personnel.

   ➤ A major disadvantage of β-ray sources is the extremely rapid radial dose fall-off within the target region.

   ➤ γ-Ray sources provide relatively more uniform target dose but require high activity to yield reasonably high dose rate (≥5 Gy/minute). Consequently, radiation protection problems with such sources become more significant.

   ➤ High-dose-rate afterloaders using γ-ray sources could provide sufficiently high dose rate but they would require expensive shielding of the catheterization laboratories.

- *Radiation delivery systems*: Several techniques have been developed for IVBT including catheter-based endovascular devices, β-ray emitting liquid-filled balloons, and radioactive stents. Of these, only the following three catheter-based systems are approved for clinical use by Food and Drug Administration.

   ➤ *Cordis Checkmate*: The Cordis Checkmate System consists of three components: a) a nylon ribbon containing an array of ^{192}Ir seeds, b) a delivery catheter, and c) a ribbon delivery device. The iridium seeds are 3 mm in length and 0.5 mm diameter. The seeds are strung in a nylon ribbon with an interseed spacing of 1 mm. The number of seeds in a ribbon can be altered to provide source lengths of 19 to 80 mm. Each ^{192}Ir seed has an activity of approximately 33 mCi, thus making it possible to keep the treatment time within 15 to 25 minutes.

     - The ribbon delivery device is mounted on a cart and uses a hand-crank mechanism to advance the ribbon into a closed-end delivery catheter (Figure 24.1).

   ➤ *Guidant Galileo*: The Guidant Galileo System (Figure 24.2) uses a β-ray source, ^{32}P.

     - The ^{32}P source is hermetically sealed in the distal 27-mm tip of a flexible 0.018-inch nitinol wire. A spiral centering balloon catheter, which centers the source wire, is flexible to

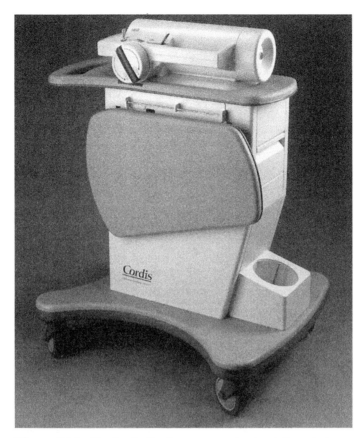

Figure 24.1. The Cordis Checkmate system showing delivery device on a cart. (From Ali NM, Kaluza GL, Raizner AE. Catheter-based endovascular radiation therapy devices. *Vasc Radiother Monitor.* 2000;2:72–81, with permission.)

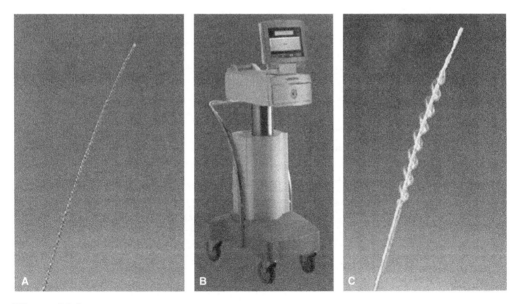

Figure 24.2. Guidant Galileo system: (**A**) source wire, (**B**) source delivery unit, and (**C**) spiral centering catheter. (From Ali NM, Kaluza GL, Raizner AE. Catheter-based endovascular radiation therapy devices. *Vasc Radiother Monitor.* 2000;2:72–81, with permission.)

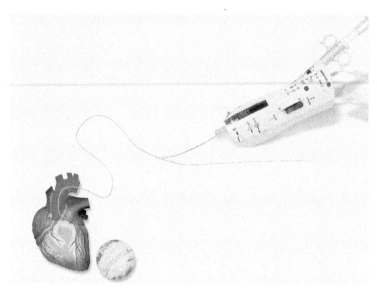

Figure 24.3. Novoste Beta-Cath System with source train and transfer device. (Courtesy of Novoste: www.novoste.com.)

navigate through the arteries and also has perfusion capabilities to limit myocardial ischemia during the procedure.

➤ *Novoste Beta-Cath:* The Novoste Beta-Cath System uses β-ray sources of ^{90}Sr/^{90}Y isotope. The system consists of two main components: a) a transfer device for housing and hydraulic delivery of a radiation source train, and b) a delivery catheter to transport the source train (Figure 24.3).

- The major advantages of the Novoste system include:
  - Use of the ^{90}Sr/^{90}Y source, which is one of the highest energy β-ray emitters with a long half-life (28 years).
  - High dose rate. Consequently, the treatment time is short (approximately 5 minutes).

- The major disadvantage is the lack of a catheter-centering device, which could result in extreme dosimetric hot and cold spots within the target volume.

DOSIMETRY

- *Dose-calculation formalisms:* The AAPM TG-43 formalism is generally applicable to the problem of dose calculation for catheter-based IVBT systems.

➤ *Catheter-based γ-ray emitters:* The following equation is modified from the general TG-43 equation to incorporate the reference point for the IVBT source calibration and its dose rate constant. For a linear γ-ray source:

$$D(r, \theta) = S_k \Lambda_{r_0} [G(r, \theta)/G(r_0, \theta_0)] g_{r_0}(r) F(r, \theta)$$

where D is the dose at a point (r, θ), S_k the air kerma strength, Λ the dose rate constant, G the geometry factor, g the radial dose function, F the anistropy factor, and (r_0, θ_0) are the coordinates of the reference point.

- As discussed in Chapter 15, the reference distance r_0 in conventional brachytherapy is 1 cm. But for IVBT, the AAPM TG-60 recommends $r_0 = 2$ mm. The reference angle in each case is $\theta_0 = \pi/2$ (along the transverse direction).

- In the dose calculation formalism for IVBT, it should be noted that the dose rate constant Λ_{r_0} is specified at 2 mm, and that the dosimetric function, $g(r_0)$, is normalized to $r = 2$ mm.

➤ *Catheter-based β-ray emitters*: Because the quantity air kerma strength does not apply to β-ray emitting sources, the AAPM TG-60 Report recommends the following equation for the calculation of dose at a point (r, θ) for a linear β-ray source:

$$D(r, \theta) = D(r_0, \theta_0) [G(r, \theta) / G(r_0, \theta_0)] g(r) F(r, \theta)$$

where $D(r_0, \theta_0)$ is the dose rate in water at the reference point (r_0, θ_0). The quantity, $D(r_0, \theta_0)$ is determined by calibration of the β-ray source at the reference point of $r_0 = 2$ mm and $\theta_0 = \pi/2$ (along the transverse direction).

- *Calibration*

  ➤ *Catheter-based γ-ray sources*: The calibration procedure of γ-emitting seeds for conventional brachytherapy is discussed in Chapters 15 and 23. The same procedure may be used for the IVBT γ-ray sources, provided the dose rate is specified in water at the reference point of (2 mm, $\pi/2$) as recommended by TG-60.

    - A well-type reentrant chamber may be used for calibrating IVBT sources. The Accredited Dose Calibration Laboratories (ADCLs) provide the chamber calibration for a specific IVBT source in terms of absorbed dose to water at a depth of 2 mm per unit current reading.

  ➤ *Catheter-based β-ray sources*: The strength of β-ray sources for IVBT is specified in terms of dose rate in water at the reference point (r_0, θ_0), where $r_0 = 2$ mm and $\theta_0 = \pi/2$.

    - A well-type reentrant chamber with a source holder for a specific IVBT β-ray source may be used for calibration in terms of absorbed dose to water at the reference point (2 mm, $\pi/2$). The chamber must bear a calibration factor from the standards laboratory (ADCL) in terms of absorbed dose to water at the reference point (2 mm, $\pi/2$) for the particular IVBT source.

MEASUREMENT OF DOSE DISTRIBUTION

Dose distribution around IVBT sources is best measured by film dosimetry. Because of the high dose rate and steep dose gradients near the source, the film must have very thin emulsion, slow speed, and high resolution. Radiochromic films (discussed in Chapter 8) meet these requirements and are the detectors of choice for measuring dose distribution around brachytherapy sources in contact geometry.

REVIEW QUESTIONS • Chapter 24

✔ **TEST YOURSELF**

Review questions for this chapter are provided online.

In multiple choice questions, more than one option may be correct.

1. The AAPM recommends the point of target dose specification for intracoronary arteries irradiated with catheter-based intravascular brachytherapy to be:

   a) On the surface of the arterial wall
   b) 2 mm into the arterial wall
   c) 5 mm into the arterial wall
   d) 2 mm from the center of the source
   e) 5 mm from the center of the source

2. The AAPM recommends the point of target dose specification for peripheral arteries irradiated with catheter-based intravascular brachytherapy to be:

   a) On the surface of the arterial wall
   b) 2 mm beyond the average lumen radius
   c) 5 mm beyond the average lumen radius
   d) 5 mm from the center of the source

3. From the following groups of sources, select the one that delivers an increasing order of target dose rate per unit activity for intraluminal brachytherapy:

   a) ^{192}Ir, ^{32}P, ^{90}Sr/^{90}Y, ^{48}V
   b) ^{192}Ir, ^{48}V, ^{90}Sr/^{90}Y, ^{32}P
   c) ^{90}Sr/^{90}Y, ^{32}P, ^{192}Ir, ^{48}V
   d) ^{48}V, ^{90}Sr/^{90}Y, ^{192}Ir, ^{32}P

4. For the same target dose specified at a radial distance of 2 mm from the source in a catheter-based intravascular brachytherapy, which of the following sources would deliver the least dose at a radial distance of 5 mm?

   a) ^{192}Ir
   b) ^{90}Sr
   c) ^{32}P
   d) ^{103}Pd

5. According to the AAPM TG-60, an intravascular brachytherapy source should be calibrated in terms of:

   a) Apparent activity
   b) Air kerma strength at a radial distance of 1 cm
   c) Dose rate in free space at a radial distance of 2 mm
   d) Dose rate in water at a radial distance of 2 mm

6. Select the most appropriate detector for measuring dose distribution around an intravascular brachytherapy source:

   a) Farmer-type ion chamber
   b) Extrapolation chamber
   c) TLD chips
   d) Radiochromic film

IMAGE-GUIDED RADIATION THERAPY

REFERENCE
Khan FM. *The Physics of Radiation Therapy*, 4th edition, 2009. Chapter 25 "Image-Guided Radiation Therapy"

IGRT: On-Board Imagers, Online Tumor Tracking, and Imaging Dose

 TOPIC OUTLINE

The following topics will be discussed in this lecture:

➤ Image-guidance technologies
  • Portal and radiographic imagers
  • In-room CT scanner
  • Kilovoltage cone-beam CT
  • Megavoltage cone-beam CT
  • Helical tomotherapy
  • Ultrasound imaging
➤ Management of respiratory motion
  • Four-dimensional CT
  • Real-time tumor tracking
➤ Management of imaging dose
  • Imaging dose specification
  • Imaging dose risk evaluation

IMAGE-GUIDANCE TECHNOLOGIES

Broadly, image-guided radiation therapy (IGRT) may be defined as a radiation therapy procedure that uses image guidance at various stages of its process: patient data acquisition, treatment planning, treatment simulation, patient setup, and target localization before and during treatment. Some of these IGRT-enabling technologies that are used for identifying and correcting problems arising from inter- and intrafractional variation in patient anatomy and target location are discussed below.

PORTAL AND RADIOGRAPHIC IMAGERS

The accelerator-mounted imaging systems are called *on-board imagers*. Modern accelerators (e.g., Varian's Trilogy, Elekta's Synergy, and Siemens ONCOR) are equipped with two kinds of imaging systems: 1) kilovotage x-ray imager in which a conventional x-ray tube is mounted on the gantry with an opposing flat-panel image detector, and 2) megavoltage (MV) electronic portal imaging device with its own flat-panel image detector (Figure 25.1).

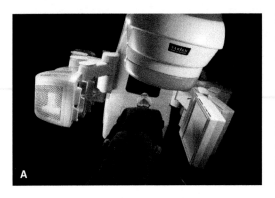
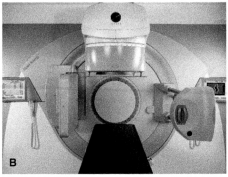

Figure 25.1. **A:** Varian's Trilogy accelerator. (Courtesy of Varian Oncology Systems, Palo Alto, CA, USA.) **B:** Elekta's Synergy unit. (Courtesy of Elekta Inc., Sweden.) Both accelerators are equipped with kilovoltage imaging systems capable of two-dimensional radiography, fluoroscopy, and cone-beam computed tomography modes.

- On-board kV imager provides a choice of imaging modalities including 2D radiographic, fluoroscopic, and 3D cone-beam CT imaging.
- On-board MV imager can provide electronic portal verification before each treatment, online monitoring of target position during treatment delivery, and 3D cone-beam CT imaging.

IN-ROOM CT SCANNER

An in-room CT scanner is a conventional CT scanner on rails that is housed in the treatment room and shares the couch with the accelerator (Figure 25.2).

To acquire a pretreatment CT, the treatment couch is rotated into alignment with the on-rail CT scanner and the scanner is moved in the axial direction relative to the patient for CT scanning. After acquiring CT data, the couch is rotated back into alignment with the accelerator gantry for treatment. Thus, neither the couch nor the patient is moved relative to the treatment isocenter in this process.

- Advantage of the in-room CT scanner is that it allows acquisition of high-resolution 3D volumetric data of patient anatomy in the *treatment coordinates*.

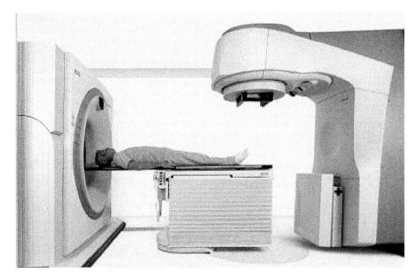

Figure 25.2. Siemens CT Vision consisting of a Primus linear accelerator and a modified SOMOTOM diagnostic computed tomograph scanner that travels on two parallel rails in the treatment room. (Photograph from www.siemens.com/medical.)

- CT data acquired in treatment coordinates are useful not only in target localization prior to treatment but also in reconstructing dose distribution, thus allowing comparison with the reference treatment plan before each treatment or periodically, as needed.

- Frequent verification of isodose plans enables one to make setup corrections or modify treatment parameters to minimize variation between the planned and the actual treatment. This procedure falls into the category of what is called the *image-guided adaptive radiation therapy*.

KILOVOLTAGE CONE-BEAM CT

The kilovoltage cone-beam CT (kVCBCT) involves acquiring planar projection images from multiple directions as the gantry is rotated through 180° or more. 3D volumetric images are reconstructed from the multiple planar radiographs by using a filtered back-projection algorithm.

- Advantages of a kVCBCT system are its ability to:
  - Acquire images in treatment coordinates;
  - Produce volumetric CT images with good contrast, submillimeter spatial resolution, and soft tissue visibility at low imaging doses;
  - Reconstruct dose distribution compatible with the reference treatment plan; and
  - Use 2D radiographic and fluoroscopic modes to verify portal accuracy, track patient motion online, and allow positional and dosimetric adjustments before and during treatment.

MEGAVOLTAGE CONE-BEAM CT

Megavoltage cone-beam CT (MVCBCT) uses the MV x-ray beam of the linear accelerator and its electronic portal imaging device to reconstruct 3D volumetric images from multidirectional planar images.

- MVCBCT is useful for online or pretreatment verification of patient positioning, anatomical matching of planning CT and pretreatment CT, avoidance of critical structures such as spinal cord, and identification of implanted metal markers if used for patient setup.

- Although kVCBCT has better image quality (resolution and contrast), MVCBCT has the following potential advantages over kVCBCT:
  - Less susceptibility to artifacts caused by high Z (atomic number) objects such as metallic markers in the target, metallic hip implants, and dental fillings;
  - No need for extrapolating attenuation coefficients from kV to MV photon energies for dosimetric corrections.

HELICAL TOMOTHERAPY

Helical tomotherapy is an intensity-modulated radiation therapy (IMRT) delivery technique that combines features of a linear accelerator and a helical CT scanner (Chapter 20). The linear accelerator (e.g., 6-MV x-ray beam) is mounted on a CT-like gantry and rotates through a full circle (Figure 25.3).

With the simultaneous rotation of the gantry, the treatment couch is translated slowly through the doughnut aperture, thus creating a helical motion of the beam with respect to the patient. A computer-controlled multileaf collimator (a long narrow slit with multileaves) provides the required intensity modulation of the beam.

- Continuous helical motion of the beam around the longitudinal axis of the patient minimizes the problem of interslice match lines.

- Helical tomotherapy is a unique device capable of delivering both the IMRT and the IGRT in the same treatment geometry.

- Because tomotherapy images are reconstructed from the same MV x-ray beam as used for actual treatment, they are called *MVCT images*.

- Compared to the diagnostic CT images, the noise level in MVCT images is higher and the low-contrast resolution is poor.

- The scan dose for MVCT images is in the range of 1 to 2 cGy.

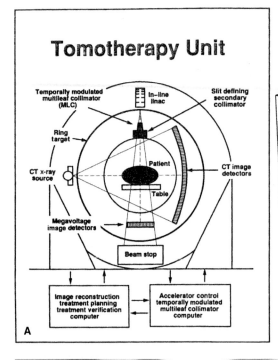

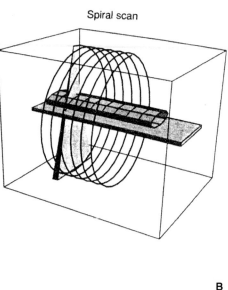

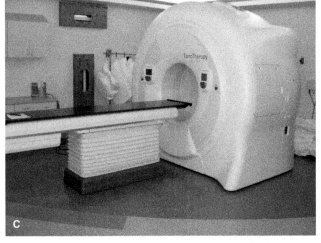

Figure 25.3. A, B: Schematic diagram of the tomotherapy unit. (From Mackie TR, Holmes T, Swerdloff S, et al. Tomotherapy: a new concept for the delivery of conformal radiotherapy using dynamic collimation. *Med Phys.* 1993; 20:1709–1719, with permission.) **C:** Photograph of tomotherapy unit (Tomotherapy Inc., Madison, WI, USA) at the University of Minnesota.

- In spite of the poor image quality, these relatively low-dose MVCT images provide sufficient contrast for verifying the patient's position at the time of treatment.
- MVCT images are less susceptible to imaging artifacts caused by high atomic number objects such as surgical clips, hip implants, or dental fillings.
- Because of the predominance of Compton interactions in the MV range of x-ray energies, the MVCT numbers are linear with respect to the electron density of the imaged material.
- The MVCT numbers have been shown to be reliable for accurately calculating dose distributions from the MVCT images.

ULTRASOUND IMAGING

Ultrasound is a noninvasive, nonradiographic real-time imaging technique for localizing soft tissue structures and tumors, primarily in the abdomen, pelvis, and breast. EXAMPLES: BAT System by Nomos and the SonArray 3D Ultrasound Target Localization System by ZMed Inc.

- Basic problems with an ultrasound imaging system are the following:
  - Image quality is poor.
  - Ultrasound images have unfamiliar appearance for most observers and are often difficult to interpret.
  - Ultrasound transducer pressure on the body surface can cause anatomic distortions.
- A 3D ultrasound system is definitely an improvement over the traditional 2D ultrasound systems. However, the basic limitations of the ultrasonic imaging, namely, the image quality and the anatomic distortions caused by the transducer pressure remain.

MANAGEMENT OF RESPIRATORY MOTION

Respiratory motion affects all tumor sites in the thorax, abdomen, and pelvis. Tumors in the lung, liver, pancreas, esophagus, breast, kidneys, prostate, and other neighboring sites are known to move due to respiration.

- Although tumor displacement varies depending on the site and organ location, it is most prevalent and prominent in lung cancers.
- Management of respiratory motion is addressed by the American Association of Physicists in Medicine (AAPM) TG-76 report. The task group recommends the following:
  1. Respiratory management techniques should be considered if a) the range of motion is greater than 5 mm in any direction; and b) significant normal tissue sparing can be gained through the use of a respiratory management technique.
  2. Assessment of tumor mobility should be assessed in three dimensions.
  3. If the magnitude of motion is not significant (<5 mm in any direction), the extra effort of using respiratory management is unwarranted.
  4. If a patient-specific tumor-motion measurement is made, this information should be used in designing planning target volume margins in treatment planning.
  5. Before deciding on respiratory management, assessment should be made if an individual patient can tolerate the respiratory management technique.
  6. For proper management of the respiratory motion problem, it is essential that the relevant personnel (radiation oncologist, physicist, dosimetrist, and therapist) be all well trained in the procedure and be available for participation, assistance, and/or consultation, as needed.
  7. Quality assurance has a crucial role in all aspects of radiation therapy including the techniques used in the management of respiratory motion.

FOUR-DIMENSIONAL CT

Four-dimensional computed tomography (4D CT) is the process of acquiring CT scans synchronously with the patient's respiratory phases. The 4D images (the fourth dimension being time) are reconstructed from scans acquired at each respiratory phase of the breathing cycle.

- One commonly used method of acquiring 4D CT images is to use a reference signal from up and down motion of the surface where the motion could be correlated with the target motion.
- Gating thresholds may be set when the target is in the desired position of the respiratory cycle. Treatment beam is turned on and off in accordance with the programmed gating thresholds.

REAL-TIME TUMOR TRACKING

The main objective of real-time tumor-tracking is to detect the respiratory motion and dynamically reposition the radiation beam to follow the tumor's changing position.

- Because of the difficulty of detecting the tumor itself, surrogate markers (external fiducials on the skin surface or internal fiducials implanted directly into the tumor) are used in most cases.
- For the method to work, the time delay between the detection of motion and the corrective action should be short (on the order of 100 ms).

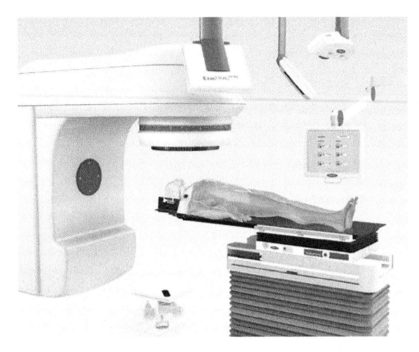

Figure 25.4. Novalis Body System (BrainLab AG, Heimstetten, Germany).

EXAMPLES:

- **ExacTrac/Novalis Body System:** This commercially available system was developed by BrainLab AG, Heimstetten, Germany (Figure 25.4).

It is a room-mounted system that provides IGRT capabilities for the delivery of stereotactic radiosurgery or stereotactic radiotherapy. Essential features include two real-time tracking systems: optical tracking and fluoroscopy-based tracking.

- **CyberKnife:** The CyberKnife (Accuray Inc., Sunnyvale, CA, USA) is an image-guided frameless stereotactic radiosurgery system for treating cranial or extracranial lesions (Figure 25.5).

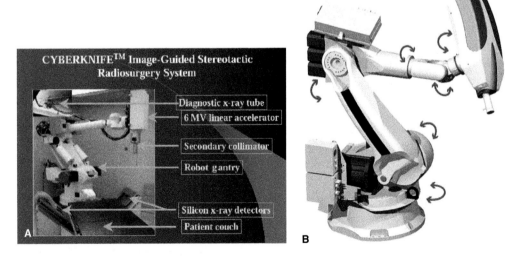

Figure 25.5. The CyberKnife radiosurgery system (Accuray Inc., Sunnyvale, CA, USA). (Picture from http://en.wikipedia.org/wiki/Image:CyberKnifeSchematic2.gif.) **B:** The CyberKnife showing linear accelerator mounted on a six-axis robotic manipulator. (From Gerszten PC, Burton SA, Ozhassoglu C. CyberKnife radiosurgery for spinal neoplasms. *Prog Neurol Surg.* 2007;20:340–358.)

The system consists of an orthogonal pair of x-ray cameras coupled to a small X-band linear accelerator (6-MV x-rays) mounted on a robotic arm.

➤ The imaging system in CyberKnife consists of two diagnostic x-ray tubes mounted orthogonally (90° offset) in the ceiling and two opposing amorphous silicon (aSi) flat panel detectors. The system is capable of acquiring and processing multiple images for patient setup as well as for tracking target motion during treatment.

➤ The robotic arm has six degrees of freedom and is capable of maneuvering and pointing the linac beam almost anywhere in space.

➤ Treatment beams in CyberKnife are not restricted to isocentric geometry. They can be directed independently, without a fixed isocenter.

• **Electromagnetic field tracking**: A tumor-tracking system has been devised that does not involve the use of ionizing radiation. It is based on real-time localization of electromagnetic transponders (beacons) implanted into the tumor (Figure 25.6).

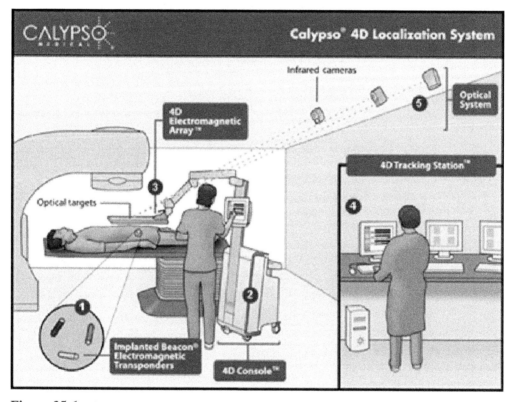

Figure 25.6. Electromagnetic field tracking system, Calypso 4D Localization System (Calypso Medical Technologies Inc., Seattle, WA, USA).

➤ Electromagnetic transponders are tiny (1.8 mm × 8.6 mm) oscillating circuits. When excited by an electromagnetic field, they emit a unique resonant frequency signal that can be detected by a magnetic array positioned close to the patient.

➤ Magnetic array contains both the source coils to generate signals to excite the transponders and the sensor coils to receive the unique frequency signals returned by the responders.

➤ Position of the magnetic array relative to the linear accelerator is measured dynamically by the infrared cameras. The system is fast enough to track tumor motion during the breathing cycle.

➤ Phantom studies have demonstrated submillimeter accuracy of the system in tracking moving objects.

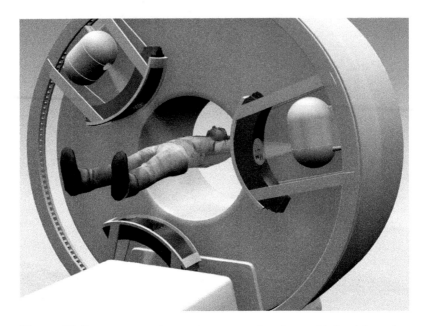

Figure 25.7. A schematic of magnetic resonance imaging—guided real-time volumetric tracking system (Renaissance System; ViewRay Inc., Gainesville, FL, USA).

- **MRI-guided IGRT**: A system that integrates magnetic resonance imaging (MRI)–based real-time volumetric tracking with a treatment delivery system has been devised (Renaissance™ System; ViewRay Inc., Gainesville, FL, USA) (Figure 25.7).

The system is specifically designed for MRI-guided IMRT, using a low-field open MRI unit for real-time imaging and three ^{60}Co sources, each equipped with computer-controlled multileaf collimators, for delivering γ-ray IMRT.

- ➤ MRI-guided IGRT allows image acquisition dynamically to track patient's anatomy in 3D while the treatment beam is on.

- ➤ Because of the MRI providing superior soft tissue contrast and involving no ionizing radiation for imaging, this technology is ideally suited for real-time volumetric tracking of soft tissue targets.

MANAGEMENT OF IMAGING DOSE

One problem with IGRT is the potential for excessive dose to the patient as a result of various radiographic imaging procedures used for patient positioning, target localization, and real-time tumor tracking. The AAPM Task Group (TG-75) has addressed the issue of imaging dose for IGRT procedures.

IMAGING DOSE SPECIFICATION

Imaging dose involving kilovoltage x-rays is dependent on a number of variables, for example, type of imaging modality, beam quality, technique, and duration and frequency of the procedures used. The following dosimetric quantities, recommended by the AAPM TG-75, are consistent with those for diagnostic imaging procedures.

- *Planar kilovoltage imaging*: entrance skin dose or air kerma, in units of mGy.

- For kV beams, air kerma and absorbed dose are essentially the same. Entrance dose refers to dose in free air, that is, without scatter.

- *Kilovoltage CT*: air kerma on the axis of rotation in mGy, with or without scatter. A special quantity, called computed tomography dose index (CTDI), has been defined for specifying CT doses. It represents the total dose (with or without scatter) deposited at a point within a single slice during a complete scan. Mathematically:

$$CTDI = (1/h) \int_{-\infty}^{\infty} D(z)\,dz$$

where $D(z)$ is the dose at a position z along the axis of rotation and h the nominal slice thickness. A more practical equation involves integration of air kerma over a length of 100 mm. Thus a measured quantity, $CTDI_{100}$, is given by:

$$CTDI_{100} = (1/h) \int_{-50}^{50} K_{air}(z)\,dz$$

where K_{air} is the air kerma. $CTDI_{100}$ may be obtained with an ion chamber that integrates the dose in a single slice during an axial scan over a length of 100 mm.

> ➤ If the measured values of $CTDI_{100}$ in the above equation include scatter contributions from the phantom, we obtain $CTDI_w$.

> ➤ If $CTDI_{100}$ is measured at the center in free air (without the phantom), then we get the axial dose in air or $CTDI_{air}$. The $CTDI_{air}$ thus defined is comparable to entrance air kerma.

- *Dose area product*: the dose area product is defined as the product of dose and area exposed in planar imaging.
- *Dose length product*: for axial imaging (e.g., CT), the integral dose is expressed as the dose length product—the product of dose and the axial length imaged.
- *Effective dose*: it is recommended that doses to patients received from different modalities should be compared and summed only in units of "effective dose."

  Effective dose is mathematically defined as:

$$E = \sum_T w_T H_T$$

where H_T is the average organ dose to tissue T for a given imaging procedure and w_T the weighting factor representing relative sensitivities of the organs. The unit of effective dose is millisievert (mSv).

> ➤ A practical form of the above equation is:

$$E = D \cdot F$$

where D is the imaging dose in mGy and F the conversion factor in units of mSv/mGy.

> ➤ Summing of effective doses from imaging and therapy remains problematic. Computation of effective dose in patients undergoing radiation therapy has rarely been attempted. The AAPM TG-75 considers this to be an important issue in IGRT. It states: *"Because this comparison appears to be of great interest to the radiation therapy community, we consider that theoretical and/or empirical estimates of effective dose from the therapy beam during treatment should be made."*

IMAGING DOSE RISK EVALUATION

As discussed in Chapter 16, harmful effects of ionizing radiation are classified into two general categories: *stochastic* effects and *nonstochastic* or *deterministic* effects. Whereas no threshold dose can be predicted for stochastic effects, it is possible to set threshold limits for nonstochastic effects. The National Cancer Institute has published an advisory on the risks associated with interventional fluoroscopy that may be relevant to some of the IGRT procedures.

REVIEW QUESTIONS • Chapter 25

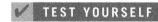

In multiple choice questions, more than one option may be correct.

1. Potential advantages of kilovoltage cone-beam CT (kVCBCT) over megavoltage cone-beam CT (MVCBCT) include:

   a) Better contrast and spatial resolution
   b) Better soft-tissue visibility at much lower doses
   c) Better correlation between CT numbers and electron density of tissues
   d) Less susceptibility to artifacts due to metallic objects in tissues

2. Potential advantages of megavoltage CT (MVCT) images acquired from a helical tomotherapy unit over diagnostic CT (kVCT) images include:

   a) Better contrast and spatial resolution
   b) Lower noise level in images
   c) Better localization of target position in relation to implanted fiducial markers
   d) Better correlation between CT numbers and electron density of tissues
   e) Less susceptibility to artifacts caused by metallic objects in tissues

3. For image guidance before a pelvis treatment which of the following is true?

   a) MVCBCT can visualize implanted markers.
   b) kVCBCT can visualize implanted markers.
   c) kVCBCT delivers higher doses to the femoral heads than MVCBCT.
   d) kVCBCT delivers higher skin doses than MVCBCT.

4. A linear accelerator in CyberKnife generates a 6-MV x-ray beam. The microwave frequency it uses for accelerating electrons is in the range of:

   a) 500 to 1,000 MHz
   b) 2 to 4 GHz
   c) 8 to 12 GHz
   d) 15 to 20 GHz

5. According to the AAPM Task Group TG-76, real-time tumor-tracking or respiratory gating is warranted if the magnitude of target motion in any direction is in excess of:

   a) 1 mm
   b) 2 mm
   c) 3 mm
   d) 5 mm

6. In planar kilovoltage imaging:

   a) Entrance skin dose means incident dose plus scatter.
   b) Entrance air kerma is approximately the same as entrance skin dose.
   c) Dose area product (DAP) is the integral dose received by the irradiated volume.
   d) Skin dose is higher than air kerma.

7. The quantity, computed tomography dose index (CTDI), refers to:

   a) The limit of axial dose that should not be exceeded in a complete CT scan.
   b) Dose in free space required at the axis of rotation to generate a single CT slice.
   c) Surface-to-axial dose ratio in a complete CT scan.
   d) Total dose (with or without scatter) deposited at a point within a single slice during a complete CT scan.

PROTON BEAM THERAPY

Proton Beam Therapy: Dosimetry and Treatment Planning

 TOPIC OUTLINE

The following topics will be discussed in this lecture:

➤ Basic physics
➤ Radiobiology
➤ Proton accelerators
➤ Beam delivery systems
➤ Dosimetry
➤ Treatment planning
➤ Concluding remarks

BASIC PHYSICS

According to the Big Bang theory, hydrogen was the first element to form in the universe (~100 seconds after the creation of the universe at approximately 13.7 billion years ago). Proton is the nucleus of the hydrogen atom. It carries a unit positive charge (1.6×10^{-19} coulombs) and has a mass of 1.6×10^{-27} kg (~1840 times the mass of electron). The existence of proton was first demonstrated by Ernest Rutherford in 1919.

- *Nature of the particle*
  - ➤ According to the current theory of fundamental particles—the *Standard Model*—proton has a substructure (discussed in Chapter 1).
  - ➤ Proton consists of three quarks (two up and one down) held together by gluons.
  - ➤ Proton is the most stable particle (half-life of greater than 10^{32} years) and decays into a neutron, a positron, and a neutrino.
- **Proton interactions**: As protons travel through a medium, they interact with atomic electrons and atomic nuclei of the medium through Coulomb force. Rare collisions with atomic nuclei causing nuclear reactions are also possible.
  - ➤ *Inelastic collisions* with atomic electrons (ionization and excitation)—predominant contributor of absorbed dose
  - ➤ *Inelastic collisions* with nuclei (bremsstrahlung)—negligibly small

➤ *Elastic scattering*—primarily by nuclei

➤ *Nuclear reactions*—possible but rare

• **Stopping power**: The average rate of energy loss of a particle per unit path length in a medium is called the *stopping power*. The linear stopping power $(-dE/dx)$ is measured in units of MeV cm^{-1}.

➤ Related to the stopping power is the *linear energy transfer* (LET) of the particle. LET is the energy transferred to the medium per unit path length (less that carried away by δ-rays) and is usually expressed as keV μm^{-1} in water.

➤ Stopping power in various materials may be calculated by Bethe-Bloch formula (1947), refined subsequently by Berger et al. in International Commission on Radiation Units and Measurements (ICRU) Report 49 (1993).

➤ Mass stopping power (S/ρ) is inversely proportional to the square of the velocity v of the particle:

$$S/\rho = \frac{1}{\rho}[dE/dx] \propto 1/v^2$$

➤ As the particle loses energy, it slows down and the rate of energy loss per unit path length increases. As the particle velocity approaches zero near the end of its range, the rate of energy loss becomes maximum.

• *Particle range*: Range of a charged particle of kinetic energy T can be calculated from inverse of stopping power as a function of energy:

$$R = \int_0^T \left[\frac{1}{dE/dx}\right]^{-1} dx$$

➤ Values of stopping powers and ranges in various materials are given in ICRU Report 49 (1993).

• *Multiple Coulomb scattering*:

➤ Angular distribution of protons through multiple Coulomb scattering is given by Molière's theory (1947).

➤ Distribution of angles may be approximated by a gaussian function characteristic of multiple small-angle scattering (primarily by nuclei).

• *Dependence of stopping power and scattering on atomic number*:

➤ Mass stopping power for protons is greater in low atomic number (Z) materials than in high-Z materials.

➤ High-Z materials scatter protons through larger angles than the low-Z materials.

➤ If we want to scatter a proton beam with minimum loss of energy (principle of scattering foils), we should use high-Z materials.

➤ If we want to decrease proton energy with minimum scattering, we should use low-Z materials.

➤ Scattering and reduction in beam energy can be controlled through a combination of high-Z and low-Z materials.

• *Bragg peak*: The depth dose distribution follows the rate of energy loss in a medium. For a monoenergetic proton beam, there is a slow increase in dose with depth initially, followed by a sharp increase near the end of range. This sharp increase or peak in dose deposition at the end of particle range is called the *Bragg peak* (Figure 26.1).

➤ To provide wider depth coverage, the Bragg peak can be spread out by superposition of several beams of different energies (Figure 26.2). These beams are called the *spread-out Bragg peak* (SOBP) beams.

➤ The SOBP beams are generated by using a monoenergetic beam of sufficiently high energy and range to cover the distal end of the target volume and adding to it beams of decreasing energy and intensity to cover the proximal portion.

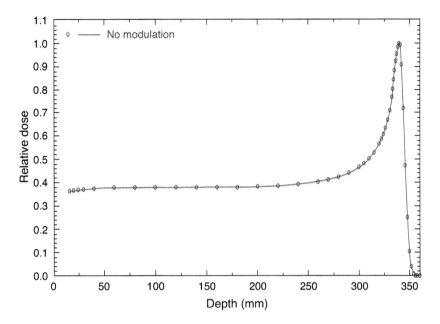

Figure 26.1. Central axis depth dose distribution for an unmodulated 250-MeV proton beam, showing a narrow Bragg peak. (Data from synchrotron at Loma Linda University, CA, USA. From Miller DW. A review of proton beam radiation therapy. *Med Phys.* 1995;22:1943–1954.)

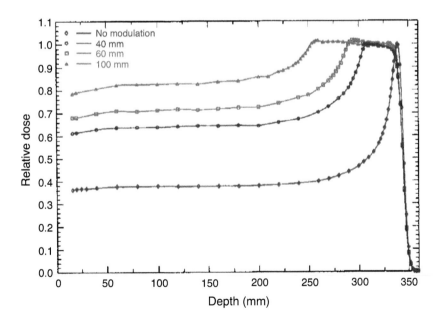

Figure 26.2. Central axis depth dose distribution for a combination of unmodulated 250-MeV and 4-, 6-, and 10-cm range-modulated proton beams. (Data from synchrotron at Loma Linda University, CA, USA. From Miller DW. A review of proton beam radiation therapy. *Med Phys.* 1995;22:1943–1954.)

➤ Beyond the Bragg peak or SOBP, the depth dose curve drops off sharply to zero dose value.

➤ A slight decrease in slope of the depth dose curve occurs near the end of SOBP because of energy-loss straggling of the particles near the end of the range.

RADIOBIOLOGY

Relative biological effectiveness (RBE) of any radiation is traditionally defined as the ratio of the dose of 250 kVp x-rays to produce a specified biologic effect to the dose of the given radiation to produce the same effect. In modern radiotherapy, the reference radiation for RBE comparison is often chosen to be ^{60}Co γ-rays or megavoltage x-rays for which the RBE has been determined to be approximately 0.85 ± 0.05 (relative to 250 kVp x-rays).

• *RBE of protons*: Although the RBE depends on the type and quality of radiation, dose fractionation, and the biologic end point, the factor of critical importance related to RBE is the LET. The higher the LET, the greater is the RBE. Because charged particles, in general, have higher LET than the megavoltage x-rays, the RBE of charged particles is ≥1.0.

➤ Most treatment facilities use an RBE of 1.1 for protons relative to ^{60}Co or megavoltage x-ray beams in their dose prescriptions for all proton energies, dose levels, tissues, and regions covered by SOBP.

➤ This universal RBE factor of 1.1 for proton beams has been adopted for practical reasons—to bring clinical response to proton and photon beams into rough agreement.

PROTON ACCELERATORS

Clinical proton accelerators in the energy range of 160 to 250 MeV include:

– Cyclotrons

– Synchrotrons

– High-gradient electrostatic accelerators (under development)

– Laser plasma particle accelerators (under development)

• *Cyclotron*: The schematic of cyclotron operation is shown in Figure 26.3.

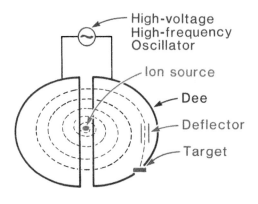

Figure 26.3. Diagram illustrating the principle of operation of a cyclotron.

➤ Principle of cyclotron operation is outlined below:

Positively charged particles (e.g., protons or deuterons) injected at the center of the two dees ➤ Particles accelerated in the gap between dees by the electric field ➤ Particles travel in a circular orbit by the action of the magnetic field ➤ Polarity of the electric field switched at the exact time the beam enters the gap from the opposite direction ➤ Magnetic field confines beam in orbits of ever-increasing radii ➤ Beam extracted when the desired maximum energy is achieved.

➤ Cyclotron used in radiotherapy is a fixed-energy machine, designed to generate proton beams of a maximum energy of approximately 250 MeV (range ~38 cm in water).

➤ This energy is sufficient to treat tumors at any depth by modulating the range and intensity of the beam with *energy degraders.*

➤ Energy degraders consist of plastic materials of variable thickness and width to appropriately reduce the range of protons as well as achieve differential weighting of the shifted Bragg peaks to create SOBP beams suitable for treating tumors at any depth.

➤ The cyclotron is *isochronous*—all the particles in the accelerator revolve at the same frequency regardless of their energy or orbit radius. This means that the accelerator runs continuously during treatment and can deliver high dose rates as needed.

➤ Cyclotron operates at a fixed maximum energy and requires energy degraders to treat more superficial tumors and to create SOBP beams at any depth.

• *Synchrotron*: As a particle reaches very high velocity (in the relativistic range) in a cyclotron, further acceleration causes the particle to gain in mass. This increases the transit time between the dees. As a result, the relativistic particles get out of step with the frequency of the alternating potential applied to the dees. This problem is solved in the synchrotron. In the synchrotron, the frequency of the accelerating potential is adjusted to compensate for the decrease in particle velocity.

➤ In the synchrotron, a proton beam of 3 to 7 MeV, typically from a linear accelerator, is injected and circulated in a narrow vacuum tube ring by the action of magnets located along the circular path of the beam (Figure 26.4A).

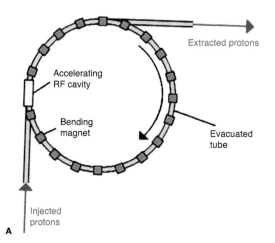

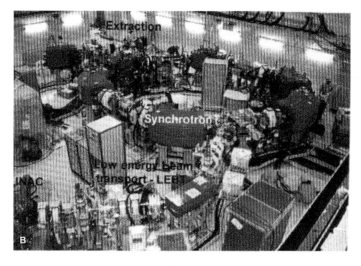

Figure 26.4. **A:** Schematic diagram illustrating the principle of proton acceleration in a synchrotron. Protons are accelerated in the radio frequency cavity powered by a sinusoidal voltage. **B:** Synchrotron manufactured by Hitachi Ltd., Japan. (From Flanz J. Particle accelerators. In: Delaney TF, Kooy HM, eds. *Proton and Charged Particle Radiotherapy.* Philadelphia, PA: Lippincott Williams & Wilkins; 2008:27–32.)

➤ The proton beam is accelerated repeatedly through the radiofrequency (RF) cavity (or cavities), powered by a sinusoidal voltage with a frequency that matches the frequency of the circulating protons.

➤ Protons are kept within the tube ring by the bending action of the magnets. The strength of the magnetic field and the RF frequency are increased in synchrony with the increase in beam energy; hence the name synchrotron.

➤ When the beam reaches the desired energy, it is extracted. A commercial unit, manufactured by Hitachi Corporation is shown in Figure 26.4B.

➤ Synchrotrons have a distinct advantage over cyclotrons in that they accelerate the charged particles to precise energies needed for therapy. In other words, the synchrotron is operated to produce the SOBP beams at any desired depth without the use of energy degraders.

BEAM DELIVERY SYSTEMS

A single proton accelerator can provide proton beam in several treatment rooms (Figure 26.5).

• Beam transport to a particular room is controlled by bending magnets that can be selectively energized to switch the beam to the desired room.

• There is very little loss of beam intensity in the transport system—usually less than 5%.

• The particle beam diameter is kept as small as possible during transport. Just before the patient enters the treatment room, the narrow beam is spread out to its required field cross section in the treatment head—the *nozzle*.

• Beam spreading is done in two ways: passive scattering or scanning.

➤ *Passive scattering*: The beam is scattered using thin sheets of high atomic number materials (e.g., lead—to provide maximum scattering and minimum energy loss).

• Dual scattering foils are required to obtain large fields of acceptable cross-beam uniformity.

• Custom blocking (e.g., Cerrobend) is used to shape the fields.

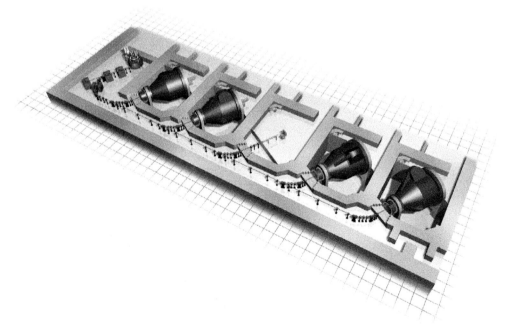

Figure 26.5. Schematic of proton beams from cyclotron transported to various rooms. (Courtesy of Varian Medical Systems, Palo Alto, CA, USA.)

- Range modulators (low Z) are used to spread the Bragg peak.
- Range shifters (low Z) are used to adjust the depth of the Bragg peak.

➤ *Scanning*: In this technique, magnets are used to scan the beam over the volume to be treated.

- Uniform fields are produced without loss of range by magnetically scanning a narrow beam of protons. EXAMPLES:
  - *Spot scanning*, in which a pencil beam is moved by sweeping magnets to specific static positions to deliver the dose.
  - *Raster scanning*, in which a pencil beam scans the field in a raster.

DOSIMETRY

- *Absorbed dose calibration*: General formalism for the determination of absorbed dose to water for proton beams is the same as for the photon and electron beams (discussed in Chapter 8). Current protocol for the calibration of proton beam is included in the International Atomic Energy Agency (IAEA) Report 398 (2000).

➤ Calibration is performed with an ionization chamber (plane-parallel or cylindrical) in a water phantom.

➤ Chamber is calibrated by the reference calibration laboratory (National Institute of Standards and Technology or Accredited Dosimetry Calibration Laboratory) in terms of absorbed dose to water in a ^{60}Co γ-ray beam.

➤ Reference calibration is based on absolute dosimetry of a ^{60}Co beam using a calorimeter.

➤ Absorbed dose to water $D_{w,Q}$ at the reference depth z_{ref} in water irradiated by a proton beam of quality Q and in the absence of the chamber is given by

$$D_{w,Q} = M_Q N_{D,w,Q_0} k_{Q,Q_0}$$

where M_Q is the reading of the ion chamber at the depth z_{ref} (at midpoint of SOBP) under reference conditions given in Table 26.1 of the Textbook, corrected for temperature and pressure, electrometer calibration factor, polarity effect, and ion recombination; N_{D,w,Q_0} the ion chamber calibration factor (absorbed dose to water/dosimeter reading) for the reference beam of quality Q_0 (^{60}Co), and k_{Q,Q_0} the chamber specific quality factor that corrects chamber response for differences between the reference beam quality Q_0 and the quality Q of the given beam.

- *Beam quality index*: The IAEA protocol specifies proton beam quality by the effective energy, defined as the energy of a monoenergetic proton beam that has the same *residual range, R_{es},* as that of the given clinical proton beam. The effective energy thus determined is close to the maximum energy in the proton energy spectrum at the reference depth.

➤ The residual range R_{es} is obtained from the measured depth dose curve. Figure 26.6 shows a typical depth dose distribution of a clinical proton beam with an SOBP.

➤ The reference depth z_{ref} is located at the midpoint of the SOBP.

➤ The practical range R_p is defined as the depth at which the dose beyond the Bragg peak or SOBP falls to 10% of its maximum value.

➤ The residual range R_{es} is determined from the measurement of R_p and z_{ref}:

$$R_{es} = R_p - z_{ref}$$

- *Quality correction factor, k_{Q,Q_0}:*
Beam quality factor k_{Q,Q_0} is defined as the ratio of calibration factors for the given ion chamber in terms of absorbed dose to water irradiated by beams of quality Q and Q_0:

$$k_{Q,Q_0} = \frac{N_{D,w,Q}}{N_{D,w,Q_0}} = \frac{D_{w,Q}/M_Q}{D_{w,Q_0}/M_{Q_0}}$$

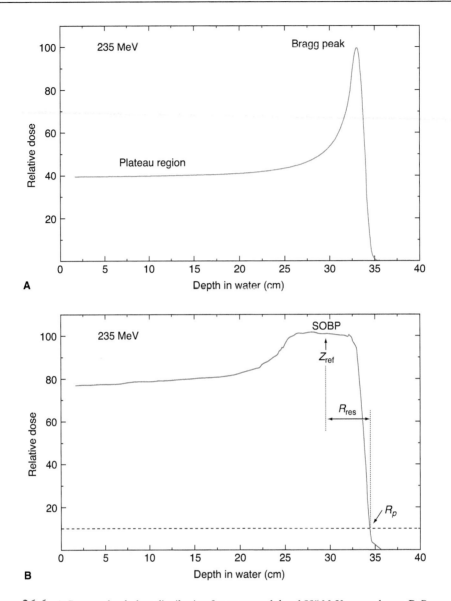

Figure 26.6. A: Percent depth dose distribution for an unmodulated 235-MeV proton beam. **B:** Percent depth dose distribution for a modulated proton beam, illustrating reference depth z_{ref}, residual range R_{es}, and the practical range R_p. (From International Atomic Energy Agency. *Absorbed Dose Determination in External Beam Radiotherapy.* Technical Report Series No. 398. Vienna: International Atomic Energy Agency; 2000.)

k_{Q,Q_0} values have been calculated using the following equation with ^{60}Co γ-ray radiation as the reference quality for Q_0:

$$k_{Q,Q_0} = \frac{(s_{w,air})_Q (\overline{W}_{air})_Q P_Q}{(s_{w,air})_{Q_0} (\overline{W}_{air})_{Q_0} P_{Q_0}}$$

Where $s_{w,air}$ is the Spencer-Attix water/air stopping power ratio, $\overline{W}_{air}$ the mean energy required to create an electron–ion pair in air, and P the chamber perturbation factor (accounting for air cavity, displacement factor, chamber wall, and central electrode). The currently accepted values of $\overline{W}_{air}/e$ for protons and photons (or electrons) are 34.23 and 33.97 J/C, respectively.

➤ When the reference beam quality Q_0 is the ^{60}Co γ-ray radiation, the factor k_{Q,Q_0} is referred to simply as k_Q. Calculated values of k_Q as a function of R_{es} for various cylindrical and plane-parallel ionization chambers are given in Table 31 of the IAEA protocol.

- *Depth dose distributions*: Typically, these include central axis depth dose distributions, transverse beam profiles, isodose curves, and output factors.
  - ➤ A variety of instruments are available for measuring relative dose distributions in proton fields: ion chambers, thermoluminescent dosimeters (TLDs), silicon diodes, radiographic films, radiochromic films, and diamond detectors.
  - ➤ Not all the detectors have the same accuracy or precision and, in general, require appropriate corrections and care in their use to provide dosimetry with acceptable accuracy.
  - ➤ The use of a particular detector is dictated by the irradiation conditions and the dosimetry objectives.

TREATMENT PLANNING

Basic principles of radiotherapy treatment planning for protons are essentially the same as for photons and electrons. These include acquisition of 3D imaging data set, delineation of target volumes and organs at risk, setting up of one or more beams, selection of beam angles and energies, design of field apertures, optimization of treatment parameters through iterative or inverse planning, display of isodose distributions and dose–volume histograms, and so on, depending on the complexity of a given case.

Because of the very sharp dose drop-off at the end of the beam range and laterally at the field edges and uncertainties in the CT-based water-equivalent depths, calculated beam ranges, patient setup, target localization, and target motion assume greater importance for protons than for photons.

- *Dose calculation algorithms*: Several dose calculation algorithms for proton beam treatment planning have been developed. On the basis of formalisms used, they fall into three major categories:
  - ➤ Pencil beam
  - ➤ Convolution/superposition
  - ➤ Monte Carlo
- *Clinical applications*: Proton beam therapy has been used to treat almost all tumors that are traditionally treated with x-rays and electrons, for example, tumors of the brain, spine, head and neck, breast, lung, gastrointestinal malignancies, prostate, and gynecological cancers.
  - ➤ Because of the ability to obtain a high degree of conformity of dose distribution to the target volume with practically no exit dose to the normal tissues, the proton radiotherapy is an excellent option for tumors in proximity of critical structures such as tumors of the brain, eye, and spine.
  - ➤ Protons give significantly less integral dose than photons and, therefore, should be a preferred modality in the treatment of pediatric tumors where there is always a concern for a possible development of secondary malignancies during the lifetime of the patient.
  - ➤ Proton dose distributions can be optimized by the use of intensity-modulated proton therapy, achieving dose conformity comparable to intensity-modulated radiation therapy but with much less integral dose.
  - ➤ A three-field intensity-modulated proton therapy plan used in the treatment of a patient with a head and neck tumor is shown in Figure 26.7 as an example.

CONCLUDING REMARKS

- Proton therapy provides an excellent option for tumors in proximity of critical structures such as tumors in the brain, eye, and spine.
- Protons give less integral dose than photons by a factor of about 3. Accordingly, it is a preferred modality for the treatment of pediatric tumors.
- Sharper dose drop-off beyond the Bragg peak is a double-edged sword—better dose conformity but greater chances of geometric miss in depth.

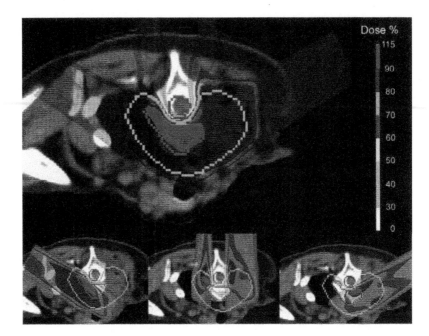

Figure 26.7. An example of an intensity-modulated proton therapy (IMPT) treatment plan for a tumor in the head and neck region. Three fields with nonhomogeneous fluences are delivered to obtain a conformal dose distribution for the planning target volume located between two critical structures, the esophagus and the spinal cord. (From Pedroni E. Pencil beam scanning. In: Delaney TF, Kooy HM, eds. *Proton and Charged Particle Radiotherapy*. Philadelphia, PA: Lippincott Williams & Wilkins; 2008:40–49.)

- Cost of proton treatments is a factor of about 2.5 times higher than photon treatments.
- After approximately 10^{22} years from now, all matter outside the black holes will come apart. Even the most stable particle, the proton, will disintegrate into electron, positron, and neutrino. It will take approximately 10^{90} years for all black holes to evaporate away and disappear completely.

> *This is the way the world ends*
> *Not with a bang but a whimper*
>
> TS Eliot, *The Hollow Men*

REVIEW QUESTIONS • Chapter 26

✔ **TEST YOURSELF**

Review questions for this chapter are provided online.

In multiple choice questions, more than one option may be correct.

1. Interactions of protons with atoms include:

   a) Ionization and excitation
   b) Bremsstrahlung
   c) Compton scattering
   d) Elastic scattering without loss of energy
   e) Pair production

2. Compared to electrons, protons:

   a) Carry greater charge, numerically
   b) Scatter through larger angles
   c) Produce less bremsstrahlung
   d) Have a sharper lateral distribution

3. Mass stopping power for protons:

   a) Is greater in low-atomic number (Z) materials than in high-Z materials
   b) Is directly proportional to their kinetic energy
   c) Is inversely proportional to the square of their velocity
   d) Drops-off sharply near the end of their range

4. Radiobiologic effectiveness of protons is:

   a) Related to their linear energy transfer (LET)
   b) Constant with depth
   c) About the same as that of electrons in the clinical range of energies
   d) Greater than that of ^{60}Co γ-rays

5. For a therapeutic proton beam:

   a) The RBE of 1.1 is larger than a neutron beam RBE due to higher LET at the Bragg peak.
   b) Range compensators are made of low-Z materials for a passive scattering system.
   c) Organ motion is one of the disadvantages of an active scanning beam system.
   d) Synchrotron system cannot produce SOBP at any depth without the use of energy degraders.

6. According to the IAEA protocol (TRS-398), the beam quality index for proton beam calibration should be based on:

   a) Ionization ratio at 10-cm depth
   b) Percent depth dose, ($\%$dd $(10)_P$), for a 10×10 cm^2 field at 100 cm SSD
   c) TPR$_{20,10}$ for a 10×10 cm^2 field
   d) Residual range parameter, R_{es}, determined from depth dose curve

7. The mean energy required to produce a unit charge of ionization in dry air is denoted by W/e. The currently accepted value of W/e in units of J/C is:

   a) 34.23 for proton beams
   b) 33.97 for photon beams
   c) 34.23 for electron beams
   d) 33.97 for all beams
   e) 34.23 for all beams

ANSWERS

Chapter 1

1. a); c); e)
2. b); d)
3. a); b); c)
4. a); b); c)
5. b); c)
6. a)
7. d)
8. d)
9. c)
10. a)
11. b)
12. a); b); c); e)
13. b); c)
14. c)
15. b)
16. c)

Chapter 2

1. d)
2. c); d)
3. c)
4. a); b); c)
5. c)
6. d)
7. c)
8. b)
9. a)
10. b)
11. d)
12. b); d)
13. c)

Chapter 3

1. b)
2. c)
3. a)
4. c)
5. b); c); d)
6. b); e)
7. c)

8. c)
9. b); d)
10. a); b); d)
11. b)
12. e)

Chapter 4

1. a); b); c)
2. c); d)
3. a); c)
4. d)
5. c)
6. a); b)
7. a); c); d)
8. d)
9. c)
10. c); e)
11. e)
12. c)
13. c)
14. c)
15. b); c)

Chapter 5

1. a); c)
2. b)
3. b)
4. c); d)
5. a)
6. a); c); d)
7. c)
8. a)
9. b); c); d)
10. d)
11. c)
12. b)
13. a); b); c); e)
14. a); b); d)
15. d)
16. a)

Chapter 6

1. c)
2. e)
3. d)
4. e)
5. b)
6. a)
7. d)
8. d)
9. b)
10. b)
11. d)
12. b); c); d)
13. b)
14. b); c)
15. a); c); d)

Chapter 7

1. c)
2. a)
3. b)
4. c)
5. b)
6. a); c)
7. a)
8. b); c)
9. a); c); d)
10. b); d)

Chapter 8

1. c)
2. a); c)
3. a); b); c)
4. b)
5. b)
6. c); e); f)
7. b)
8. a); c)
9. d)
10. e)
11. d)
12. c)
13. d)
14. a); b); d)
15. a); d); e)

Chapter 9

1. b)
2. a); b); c)
3. c)
4. c)
5. c)
6. d)
7. b)

8. d)
9. b)
10. d)
11. a); d); e)
12. d)
13. a); b); d)
14. c)

Chapter 10

1. a); c)
2. a); c)
3. b)
4. b)
5. b)
6. b)
7. a)
8. a)
9. e)
10. c)
11. b)
12. a)

Chapter 11

1. b); c); d)
2. d)
3. b); c)
4. b); d)
5. c)
6. b)
7. d)
8. a); c); d); e)
9. e)
10. d)
11. d)
12. b); d)
13. d)
14. d)
15. a); c); d)
16. a); c); d)
17. b)
18. a); b); c); d)
19. a); c); d)
20. b)
21. a); d)
22. c)

Chapter 12

1. d)
2. d)
3. b)
4. b)
5. c); d)
6. a); d); e)
7. b)
8. c)

9. b); c)
10. b); c); d)
11. d)

Chapter 13

1. d)
2. b)
3. c)
4. a); b); d)
5. a); c); d)
6. b)
7. a); d); e)
8. a)
9. a)
10. b)

Chapter 14

1. b)
2. c)
3. c)
4. c)
5. b)
6. a)
7. b)
8. a); b)
9. c)
10. d)
11. a); b); c); d)
12. a)
13. b)
14. a); c)

Chapter 15

1. d)
2. b)
3. a); b); c)
4. a)
5. a)
6. c)
7. b)
8. c)
9. a)
10. c); d)

Chapter 16

1. a); c); d)
2. e)
3. a)
4. a)
5. c)
6. c)
7. b)
8. c)
9. b)

10. b)
11. c)
12. a); b); d)
13. b)
14. b); c); e); f)
15. a); c); d)
16. c); e)

Chapter 17

1. a)
2. b)
3. b)
4. a); b)
5. b)
6. c)
7. a); c)
8. c); d)
9. c)
10. a); b); d)

Chapter 18

1. b); c)
2. b)
3. c)
4. c)
5. b)
6. c)
7. c)
8. a)
9. c)
10. a)

Chapter 19

1. c)
2. d)
3. d)
4. a)
5. c)
6. d)
7. a); d)
8. b); c)
9. c)

Chapter 20

1. b); c); d)
2. b)
3. c)
4. c)
5. b); c); d)
6. c); d)
7. a); c); d)
8. e)
9. d)
10. d)

11. e)
12. e)

Chapter 21

1. d)
2. c); d)
3. b)
4. d)
5. d)
6. b); d); e)
7. a); d)
8. d)
9. b); c)
10. a); c); d)
11. a); e)

Chapter 22

1. c)
2. a)
3. d)
4. a)
5. b)
6. c)
7. e)
8. c)
9. b)
10. a); b); d)

Chapter 23

1. a); b)
2. a); b); c); d)
3. a); b)
4. a); d)
5. a); b); c); d)

6. a)
7. a)
8. c)
9. e)
10. a);b); d)
11. c)
12. b)

Chapter 24

1. d)
2. b)
3. a)
4. c)
5. d)
6. d)

Chapter 25

1. a); b)
2. c); d); e)
3. a); b); c); d)
4. c)
5. d)
6. b); d)
7. d)

Chapter 26

1. a); b); d)
2. c); d)
3. a); c)
4. a); d)
5. b); c)
6. d)
7. a); b)

INDEX